# MERCHANTS OF MEDICINE

## NOSTRUM PEDDLERS - YESTERDAY & TODAY

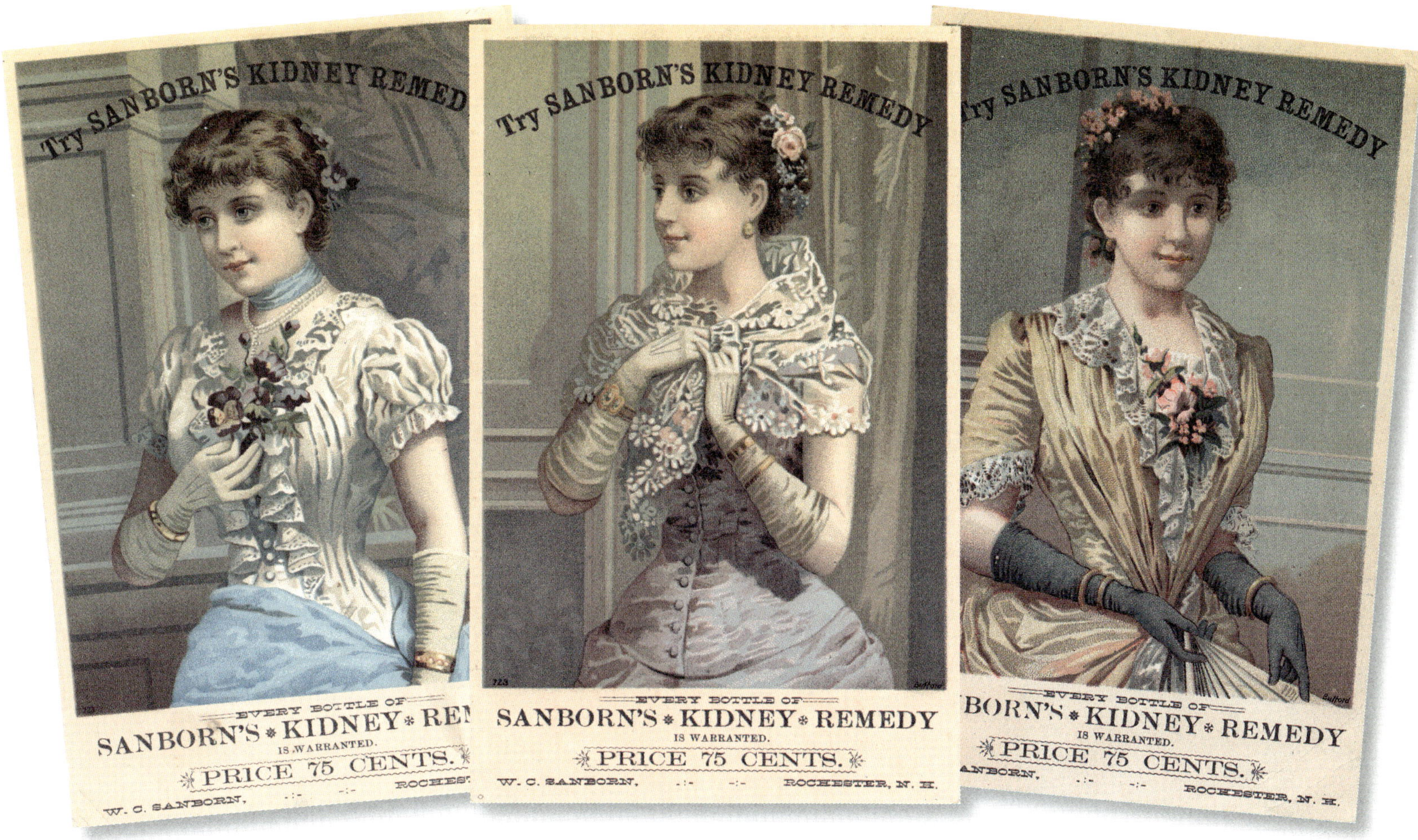


By Dewey R. Heetderks, MD, FACS

Library of Congress Number 2002095378
ISBN 0-9726650-0-5


Dewey R. Heetderks, MD
4907 N. Quail Crest, Grand Rapids, MI 49546
Ph. 616-949-0713 email: Dheetderks@aol.com

Published by
Drukker Press, 4907 N. Quail Crest, Grand Rapids, MI 49546

Printed in the United States of America

# Contents

# Acknowledgements

My wife, Marilyn Heetderks, without whose wonderful encouragement, I could not have produced this book.

Ed and Ervina Boevé whose gracious gift of a patent medicine bottle started this great adventure.

Lee Pool for camera artistry and technical skills that combined to produce excellent photography.

Dennis Kucharczyk for skillful display and creative graphic design excellence.

Peter DeBoer and Lorraine Warlick for editing proficiency.

Jim Doezema for help in negotiating the world of business.

Nick Wolterstorff and Richard Watson for advice and support regarding book publishing.

Bill Agee, John Wolf and Dann Louis who have been antique bottle and ephemera friends from the beginning.

# Foreword

It all started in 1972 when a grateful patient gave me my first urology bottle, "Dr. Kilmer's Swamp Root, Kidney, Liver and Bladder Cure." Little did he know when he pushed my button that I would become an "archeophialist," or antique bottle collector. I thought I had seen all the old urological medicine bottles when I next discovered, in Northport, Michigan, "Foley's Kidney and Liver Cure." However, after accumulating over five hundred medicine bottles, boxes, and tins, I realized that there were many more. My collection now goes from the common to the rare and even to one-of-a-kind specimens. These include medicines labeled as cures, bitters, tonics, alteratives, elixirs, soda waters, and more. Of each type of medicine container, I have acquired most of the known variants. The items shown in this book are a portion of my own collection. Since no one else has sought just urological antique medicines and other artifacts, I can say with a smile that I have the world's largest collection.

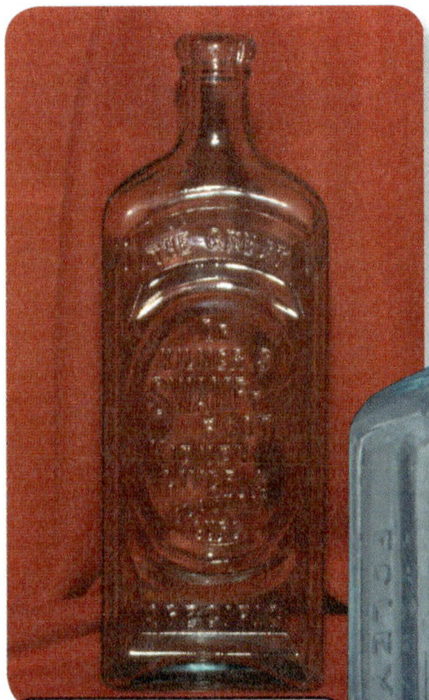

My first urology bottle.

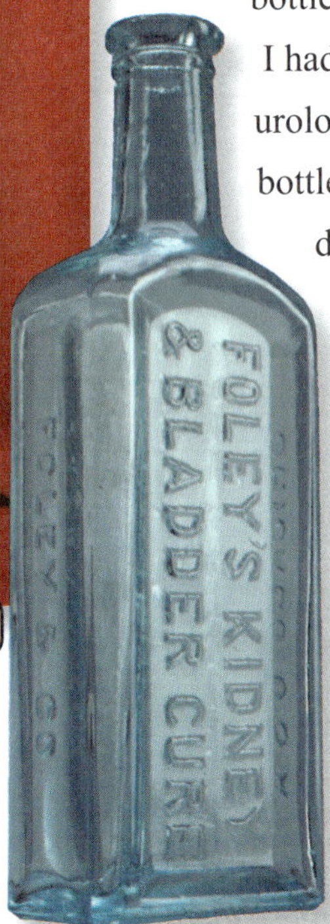


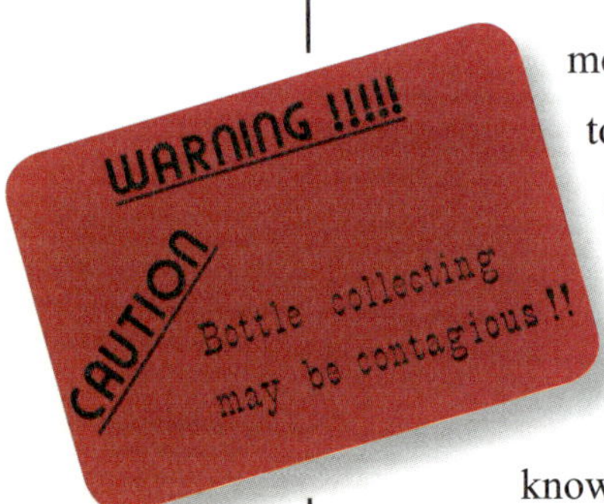


Antique bottle collecting is a national phenomenon. There are bottle shows and auctions each week somewhere around the country. Bottles come from attics, basements, old drug stores, and privies. Several antique bottle magazines provide a means for extensive advertising and resale of medicine bottles, trade cards, almanacs, signs, and books.

The William P. Didusch Urological Museum in Baltimore, Maryland, houses the surgical specialty's old instruments and artifacts. In 1990, Dr. William W. Scott, curator of the museum, invited me to display a portion of my collection of antique urological medicines, showing what people took to care for their supposed urological ills in a doctorless countryside.

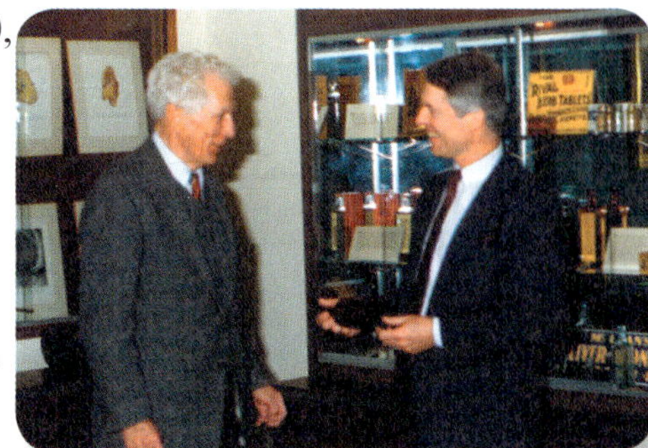

The saga of antique bottle collecting has many twists and turns. For me the enjoyable benefits of the adventure include making new friends and acquaintances, an appreciation of beautiful glass, the fascination with our medical heritage, and the inspiration to write this book.

# Preface

In what follows I would like to do two things. First, I describe the patent medicine era – a colorful and romantic time. Glass manufacturing, America's first industry resulted in the production of beautiful medicine bottles. But, the patent medicine era was also a deceitful era. Itinerant purveyors with robber baron ethics created the "snake oil syndrome" by peddling medicines with the promised magic of exotic substances. To appreciate fully how America was sold its nostrums, the story must be told how human hopes and fears were exploited by marketing ploys such as trade cards, almanacs, and the Indian road show. The rise and fall of the patent medicine era were both interesting and dramatic. In 1906 the Food and Drug Administration and later the Federal Trade Commission outlawed certain substances and required proper labeling of contents.

Second, I'd like to alert the reader to an ever-growing industry that needs more policing than it is presently getting. With deliberate deceit medical quackery exists today as a multi-billion dollar business. Because of budget limitations and departmental differences the Food and Drug Administration and the Federal Trade Commission have an overwhelming task to safeguard the public from quackery. So, today in the 21st century the old warning of "caveat emptor"--let the buyer beware--is still relevant.

We now live in an era involving alternative medicine. It is true that such therapy may have beneficial effects for some patients. However, this is medicine that has not been scientifically tested and proven, resulting unfortunately in two separate health delivery systems-a conventional form and an alternative form. Unusual and unconventional types of alternative medicine afford potions and practices rich in opportunities for quackery. Today, people need to be reminded that "he who forgets the past is doomed to repeat it."

PART ONE

# HUCKSTERING

## A 19th CENTURY

# DECEPTION

"There is a class of minds much more ready to believe that which is at first sight incredible, because it is incredible, than what is generally thought reasonable."

- Oliver Wendell Holmes 1842

"The desire to take medicine is perhaps the greatest feature which distinguishes man from animals."

- Sir William Osler

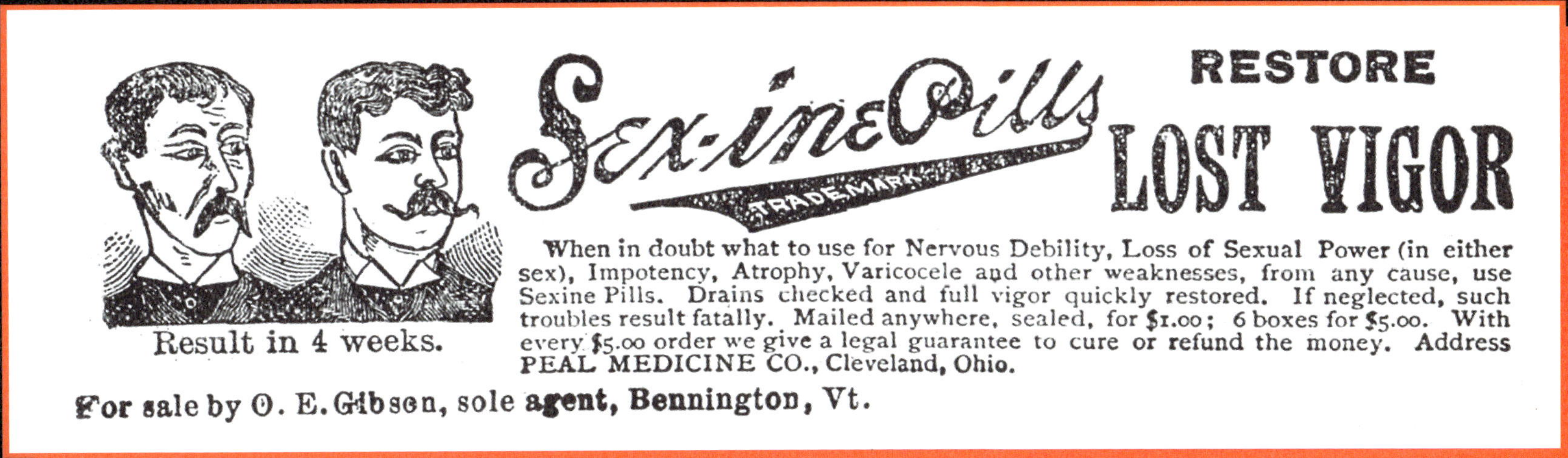


## It is a Nap You Need.

*Hall's Journal of Health* explains the necessity of a couch in the following manner: A room without a couch of some sort is only half furnished. Life is full of ups and downs, and all that saves the sanity of the mentally jaded and physically exhausted fortune fighter is the periodical good cry and momentary loss of consciousness on the upstairs lounge or the old sofa in the sitting-room. There are times when so many of the things that distract us could be straightened out and the way made clear if only one had a long, comfortable couch on whose bosom he could throw himself, boots and brains, stretch his weary frame, unmindful of tidies and tapestry, close his tired eyes, relax the tension of his muscles and give his harrassed mind a chance. Ten minutes of this narcotic when the head throbs, the soul yearns for endless, dreamless, eternal rest, would make the vision clear, nerves steady, the heart light and the star of hope shine again.

# THE PATENT MEDICINE ERA

"There is something wrong with my testicles and I don't know what to make of it. I noticed for some time that they don't hang even and the left one hangs lower. I ain't got the nerve to ask a doctor about it. Please use plain envelope."

Test letter from the Postal Inspector to the Interstate Remedy Company - 1913

Chapter 1

# Patent Medicine What Is It?

The history of patenting began in the sixteenth century when the English first granted patents. Patents were monopolies permitted by the sovereign and in return the proprietor applicant was required to make his secret "open,"or "patent." Patent rights were refined and restricted as English law developed.[2,3]

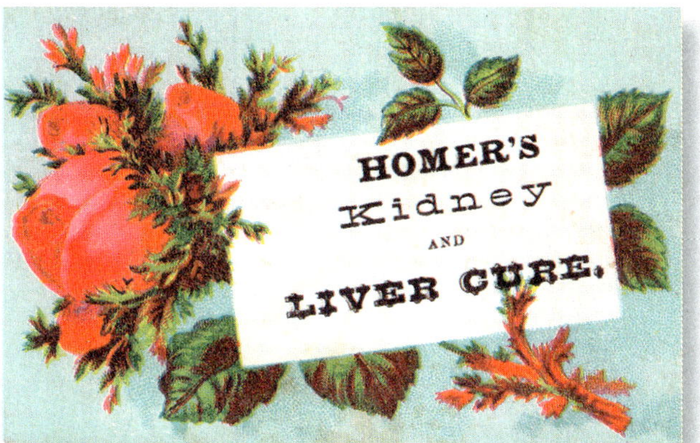


The first patent medicines that were sold in America were imported from England, where "patents of royal favor" were issued to the makers of such concoctions as early as 1710. No nostrum developed in America during the colonial period was granted a King's Patent. The United States Patent Office was established in 1790. Yet, in spite of the ease of obtaining a patent on a medicine, few of the nostrum makers did it. When a patent was obtained, the ingredients of the medicine became a matter of public record. Secrecy was important for protection from imitators anxious to share in the rewards. Also, secrecy offered concealment of toxic ingredients or, in other cases, the significant simplicity of the remedy. After all, one might not want the public to know that a medicine, like "Dr. Townsend's Sarsaparilla," was composed of nothing more than sassafras bark, molasses, and cheap rye whiskey.[2,3]

The first patent for a medicine in the United States was issued in 1796 to Samuel Lee, Jr. of Windham, Connecticut. That was only three years after the young Republic had passed a law offering patents to inventors under the constitutional provision to advance the "Progress of Science and Useful Arts." Lee's patent protected what he labeled simply "Bilious Pills," later said to contain a potent mixture of aloes, soap, nitrate of potassium and gamboge. Other pill makers followed with patents for similar bilious medications. As with Lee's product, they were marketed as a sure cure for anything from yellow fever and dropsy to worms and female complaints.[1] Although relatively few purveyors of the early nostrums bothered to seek patent protection, the medicinal boom was on, and gradually spread over the expanding nation. Today we refer to any dubious remedy from that era as a patent medicine.

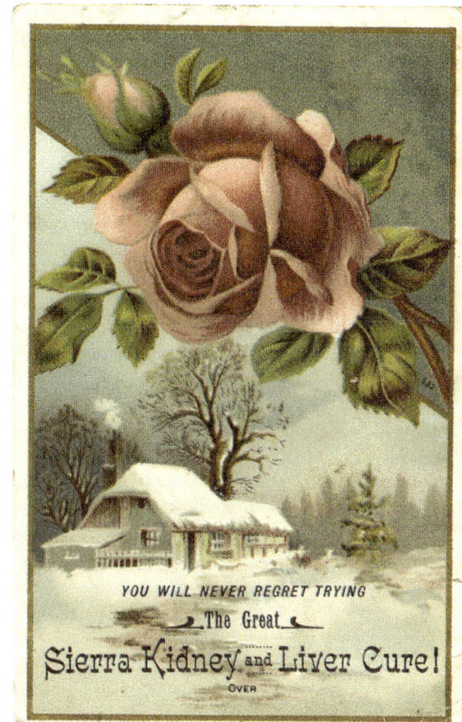
YOU WILL NEVER REGRET TRYING
The Great
Sierra Kidney and Liver Cure!
OVER

A non-patent medicine was distinguished as being a medicine for which a prescription was written by a doctor for an individual patient. The ingredients were known, as the medicine was individually prepared or compounded by a pharmacist. In contrast a patent medicine was simply a ready mixed nostrum whose ingredients were not revealed. Also, the medication was usually self-prescribed.

While the term "patent medicine" has been used in this

"Federal chemists reported that it consisted essentially of sulfuretted linseed oil and turpentine."
*Nostrums and Quackery. Vol.III, p.70, 1936.*

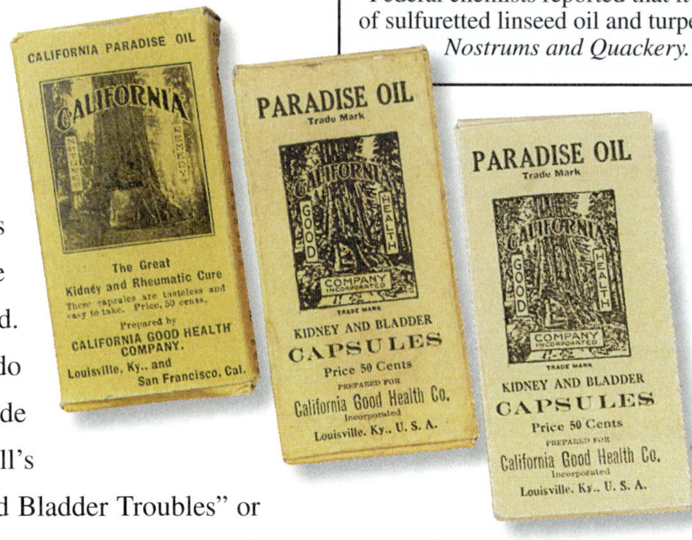


country since colonial times, it is not an accurate designation, since few medications were patented. What the proprietor chose to do instead was to coin a catchy trade name—"Texas Wonder - Hall's Great Discovery For Kidney and Bladder Troubles" or "Black Gin for the Kidneys"—and register the name with the Patent Office. The registered name was a trademark, which gave exclusive ownership of the name to the proprietor. All medicines using the trademark are more correctly called "proprietary medicines" demonstrating exclusive ownership of the name. The composition of the medicine could change, the effects claimed could change, but ownership of the name remained unchanged. With judicious advertising and marketing the name would become the product and could easily be protected under the trademark regulations.[2]

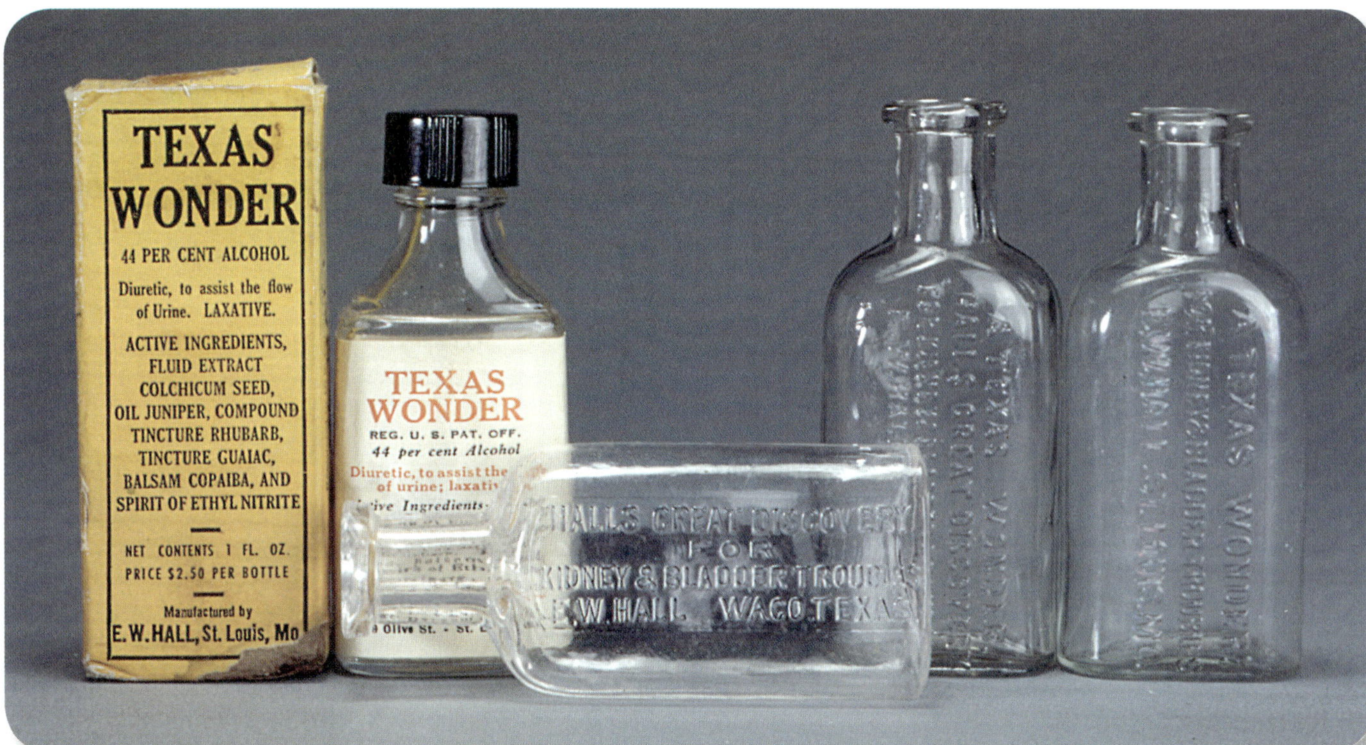


Analyzed by federal chemists revealed an alcohol content of 41.6%. Note the rare Texas Wonder bottle from Waco.

Chapter 2

# Nostrum Container- The Glass Bottle

Even though glass is familiar in so many diverse forms, it is still very difficult to capture an appreciation of its wondrous nature. Glass is a fused mixture of silica and alkaline bases. The physical charms and values of glass arise from its peculiar properties that are so eloquently described, often in poetic style, by George and Helen McKearin. "Glass, . . . in its liquid viscous state, like molasses in January, is extremely ductile and elastic. In this state it can be spun into fibers for the weaving of fabrics; a skilled craftsman can give it any chosen shape and degree of thickness; it can be pressed into a myriad of patterns and even cast in statues. It can be crystal clear or by the addition of metallic oxides be made to take on any hue of the rainbow. It can be highly polished and cut. Because of its refractive powers, precious gems can be so skillfully simulated that only the eye of the expert can detect the imitation. It can be unaffected by any acid except hydrofluoric acid. It is one of the most fragile substances and yet it can be made bullet proof and heat resistant. Even in the 20th century the possible transmutation of solid opaque granules of sand and alkali into a liquid state and back again into a brittle transparent solid, having all these properties, seems a miracle of alchemy."[5]

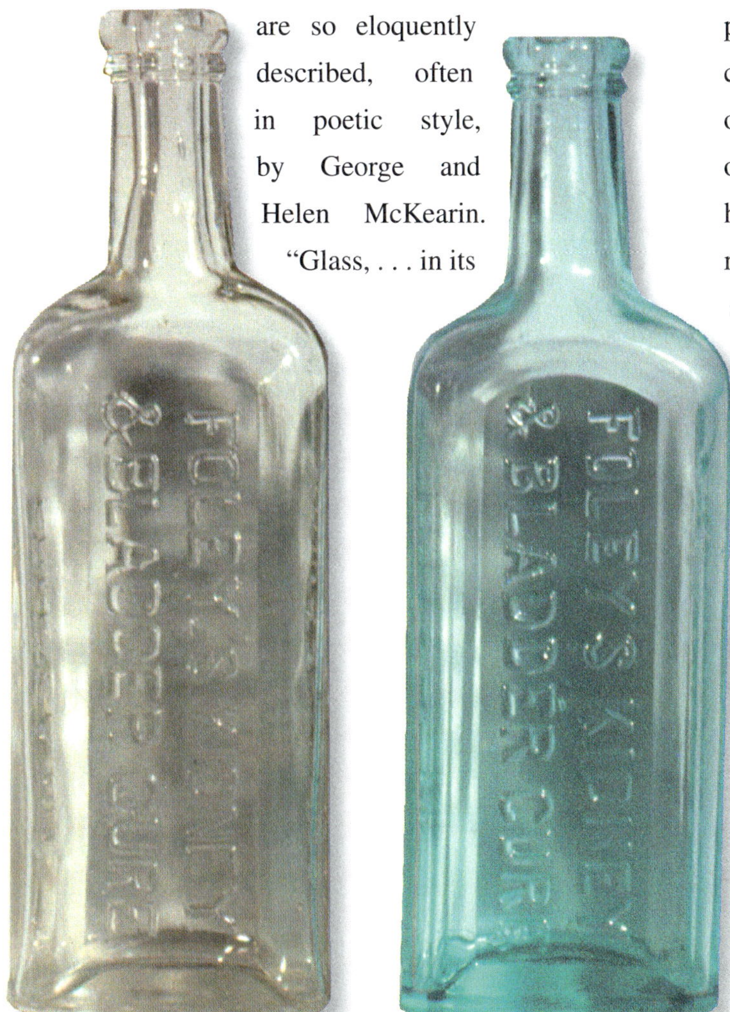


The production of the nostrum container, the common blown medicine bottle, involved the use of a basic type of glass. Its pale green color was due to various metallic impurities found in the raw materials and not due to artificial coloration. The color ranged from pale blue-green to amber, depending on the presence of iron or alumina. It was the cheapest form of glass and it is commonly used today. Manganese was often used to decolorize glass, making colorless clear glass as was used in the bottle on the left.(3,4,5)

**GLASS**

- sand
- soda
- lime

These are the basic ingredients of glass.

When and where this miracle called "glass" was discovered is in part shrouded in mystery and tradition. It is understood, though, that at least 3500 years ago and probably earlier, men knew how to make glass.

**COLOR**

| | |
|---|---|
| Red | copper, selenium, gold |
| Blue | cobalt, copper |
| Yellow | selenium |
| Green | iron |
| Purple | manganese, nickel |
| Black | iron slag |
| Brown | carbon, nickel |

When these elements and compounds are added to glass, they result in a variety of colors.

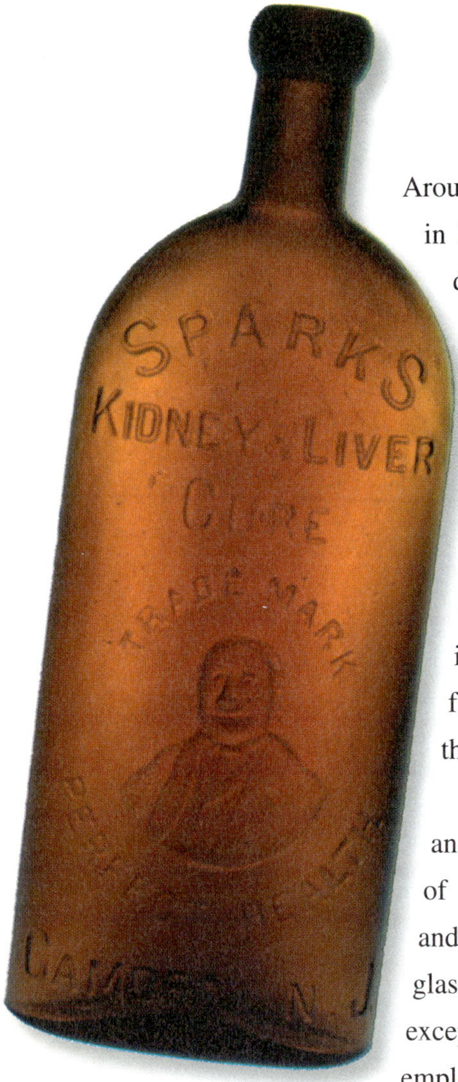


Around 1500 B.C. workshops were set up in Egypt, where glass making flourished during the remainder of the New Kingdom to the eleventh century B.C. Although glass blowing had not yet been discovered, the vessels produced, even initially were by no means primitive. The glass vessels were manufactured by dipping or rolling a solid core of sand-clay or animal dung in glass threads while it was inside a furnace. A shell of glass or a vessel was thus formed.[2,5]

The industry became well established and all the normal pre-Roman techniques of core-forming, casting, cold-cutting and grinding—in fact, every fundamental glass making process except glass blowing was employed almost from the start. So, too, were many varieties of decorations—trailing, relief and intaglio cutting, and casting mosaic designs in patterns fashioned from thin sections of circular glass rods. Yet this industry, although technically proficient, suffered from the fatal defect that its processes were laborious and slow. Thus, what it made was rare and costly, making no impact on the common people, but achieving much favor in royal and aristocratic circles.[2,5]

The Syrians are credited with the invention about 300 B.C. of the blowpipe and blown glass vessels. However, the Romans, as in many areas of the arts, were the major creative forces. With this biggest-of-all invention in glass history the whole character of glass vessels changed. Thin walled containers replaced the heavier ones of earlier periods. The new technique made it possible to mass-produce glass items of a utilitarian nature and glass vessels or bottles became a household commodity. Thus, glass production entered a new era, and glass bottles, from being luxuries, known, used and cherished by comparatively few, were, within less than a century, in common use throughout the Roman Empire and beyond.[2,5]

The art of glass blowing was not extinguished by the advent and spread of the barbarians throughout Europe. However, before the 5th century, when the fall of the Roman Empire was complete, there existed only few isolated glass

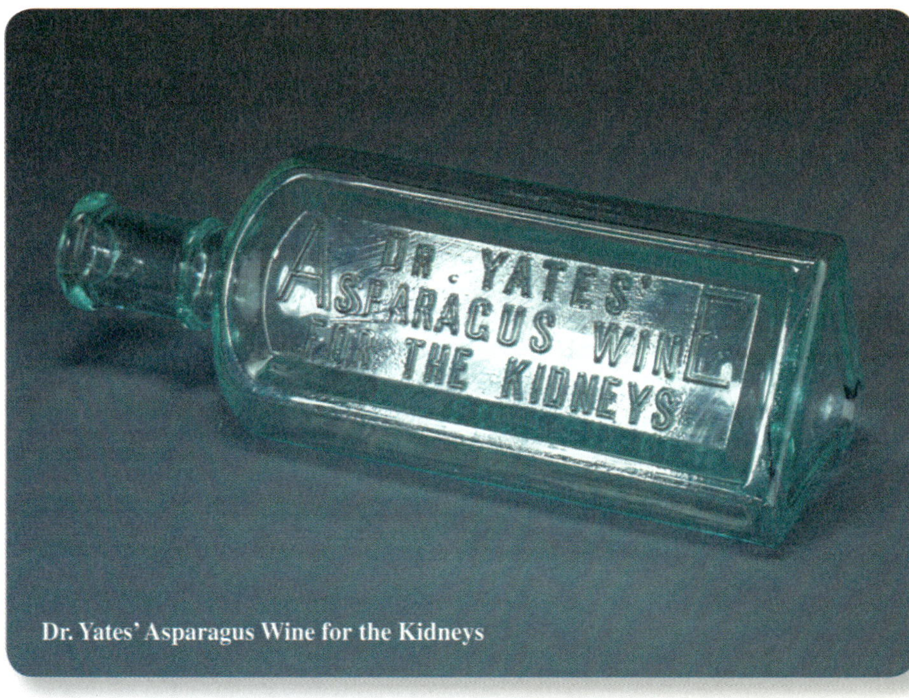


Dr. Yates' Asparagus Wine for the Kidneys

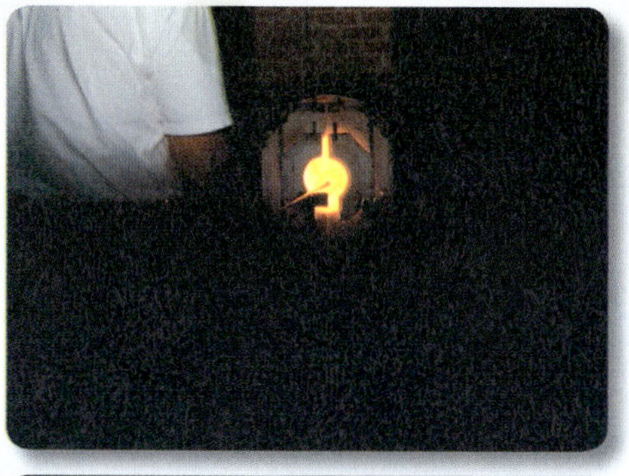

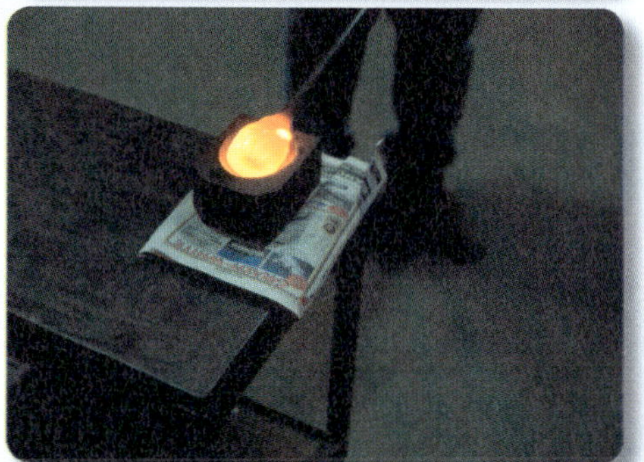

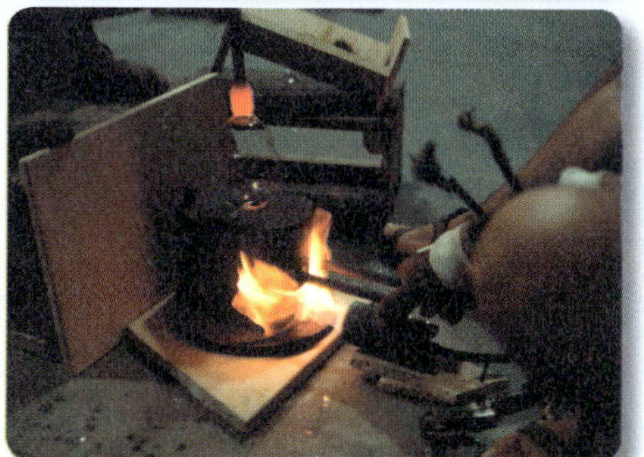

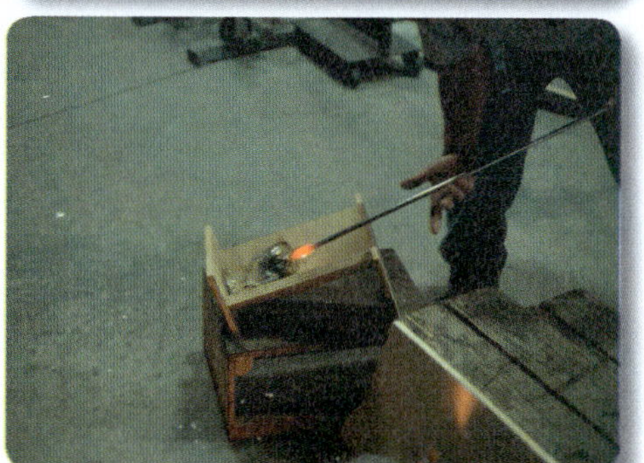

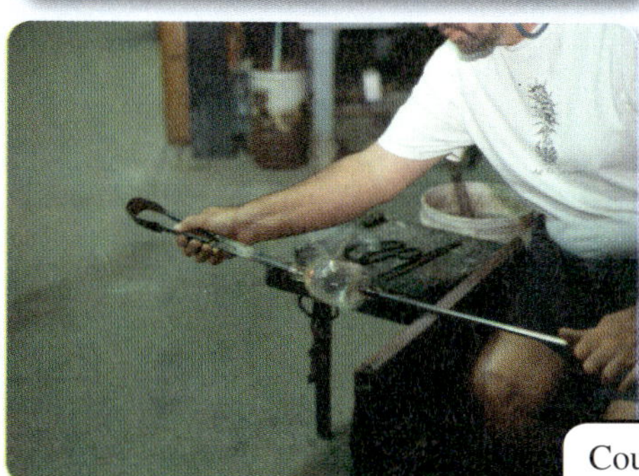

Courtesy of Wheaton Village Museum of American Glass

Essential for glass blowing was the blowpipe. It was generally a 4 to 6 feet long iron tube, narrower at the blowing end. A glob of molten glass was collected on the gathering end. The bottle maker would then expand it by blowing air into it similar to making an air filled bubble with bubble gum. Containers and bottles were thus created taking the desired shape as crafted by the glass blower. The bottle could be free blown or take a more restricted shape-design as provided by a mold. Molds were initially simple forms but later became hinged molds providing embossing for the bottle. The molds were no longer made of wood, but of brass and iron.(3, 4,7)

The hinged mold did not fit together completely and the bottles produced in them showed a mold seam along each side where the glass was forced out of the crack in the process of expansion. Initially, hinged molds were the non-shoulder type. Later, more shoulder and even the bottle neck were formed in the mold. Mold seams reveal this progression in bottle making as the second refired mouth and lip portion of bottle making was always without seams.(3,4)

Bottle making was a two step process the second step, the refiring of the neck and lip of the bottle, required a method of holding the base of the bottle. At first this was done with a second rod (pontil rod) that adhered to the base by means of a small glob of molten glass. When the bottle and the rod were separated, a rough glass pontil scar remained. After 1850 the base of all bottles were held with a "snap case" metal clasper resulting in smooth based bottles.(3,4,7)

Thus, inspection reveals the age of the hand blown bottle. Pontil scarred bottles were made before 1850. Also, the height of the mold seam correlates with the age of the bottle. Smooth based bottles with mold seams up to the shoulder and later up to the neck and lip were made between 1850 and 1903.

making sites. It was nearly a thousand years later that there was a renaissance in the art of glass blowing. Centuries later, in America, glass manufacturing began with workers who came from many countries in which glass making had been highly developed. These workers followed methods and styles of their native lands. Consequently many years elapsed before the influences became blended into something approaching a Native American expression of the medium. Glass making in the colonies had its beginning in Jamestown, Virginia, in 1608 and was America's first industry. English laws governing the colonies included restrictions on glass manufacturing. As Americans struggled for political freedom,

## Age Identification Mold Seams of Bottles

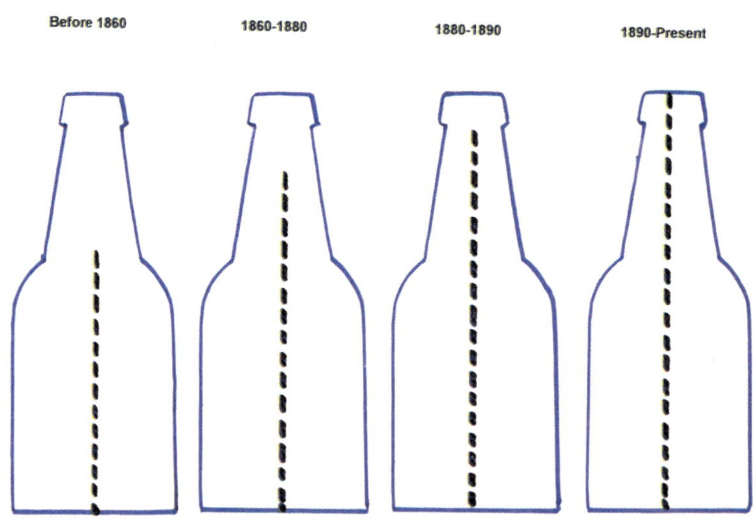


**Before 1860:** Seams extend to just over the shoulders.
**1860-1880:** Seams go most of the way up the neck of the bottle.
**1880-1890:** Seams continue through the top but not through or over the lip.
**1900-present:** Seams extend the full length of the bottle and over the lip.

so also did they pursue economic independence. More than a century was to pass before the colonists ventured their money in glass manufacturing with any degree of success.[4,6,8] The Owens automatic bottle machine was developed in 1903. Bottles were produced with great uniformity having mold seams that extended over the mouth and lip of the bottle. The era of individual hand blown bottles thus came to an end.

Collecting 19th century medicine bottles invariably awakens an interest in the life and times of our ancestors. Some understanding of the reason for the existence of the nostrum trade in the United States helps us appreciate such bottle collecting more fully. Steeped in superstition and fear of disease, people were willing dupes of the illicit medicine man. The bottles used by the purveyors of medicine were hand blown glass containers which varied in size, shape, and color. They were often crudely made with bubbles and imperfections. As such, they are desirable because of their individual beauty and fascinating history.

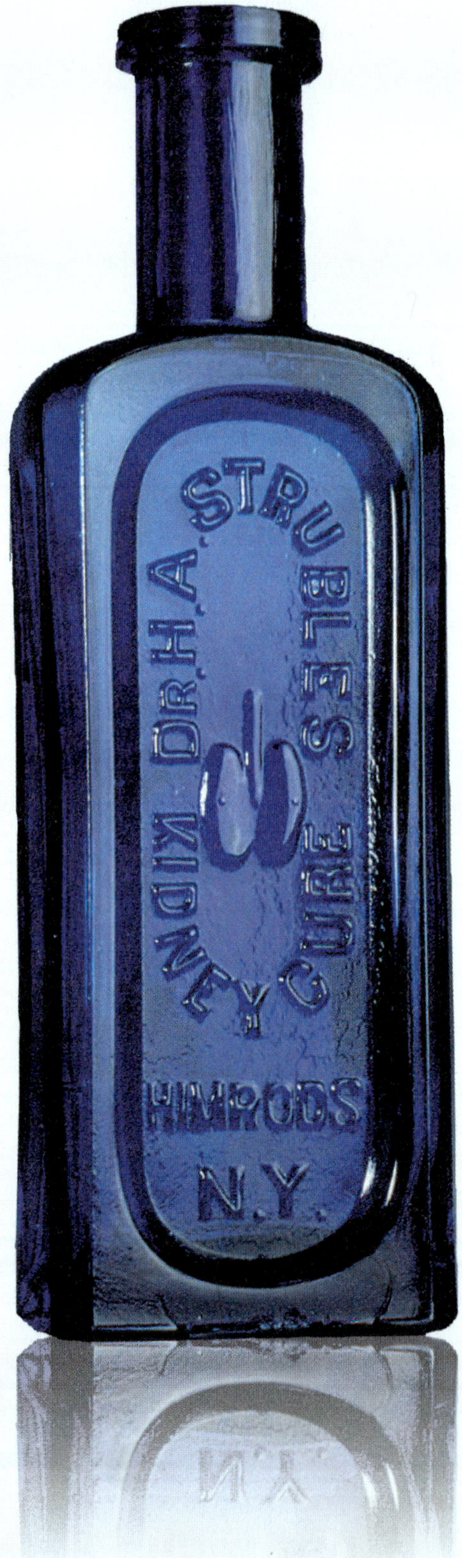


**Dr. Struble's Kidney Cure -** "A fabulous bottle with a great history. Henry Albert Struble, self-appointed doctor of maladies, lived and worked out of the West-Central New York village of Himrod. Dr. Struble was just Al to the locals who knew that jealousy existed between him and the town physician, Dr. Biggers. One summer night Dr. Struble's barn burned and the next day Dr. Biggers proceeded to tell Al that he may have fired his own barn for the insurance. This exchange took place at the post office, Aug. 2, 1917. As Dr. Biggers walked past Struble's house and approached the railroad crossing, Al followed him and murdered him in open daylight. Struble ran back to his house, locked himself in and by the time Doc Willis and the arm of the law broke in, they found the frustrated medicine man had committed suicide in his bedroom. Struble's home still stands today, but the bottle that bears his name will outlive the home in which he dwelled." (1)

Chapter 3

# From Medicine Men To Men of Medicine

As technology thrusts us relentlessly into the future, I find myself, perversely, more interested in the past. We seem to have lost something vital, something of individuality and passion. That may be why we tend to view the patent medicine peddler, rightly or not, as a romantic figure, who, though a deceitful man, enjoyed sanctuary. He had his "Indian medicine," snake oil, pain killer and quick cure for all physical ailments—ailments like torpid liver, gleet, consumption, gravel, dropsy, rheumatism, and even pimples.

There were many reasons why patent medicines and the patent medicine peddler were so well accepted. One was man's continued quest for cheap, quick, painless remedies for good health. It was cheaper to seek a cure in a potion container from a patent peddler than to summon a doctor who might be a one or two day journey away. Ultimately, when the physician had to be called, it was often too late to be helpful. Not infrequently he got the blame for a death which directly or indirectly should have been laid to a patent panacea.

Not all "granny" medicines were harmful. Many were simply harmless—they didn't help or hurt. The problem was the delay of proper treatment. However, some medicines were downright poisonous, being concocted by transient charlatans from whatever ingredients were available. Alcohol and opium were sometimes added which resulted in problems of addiction.[1]

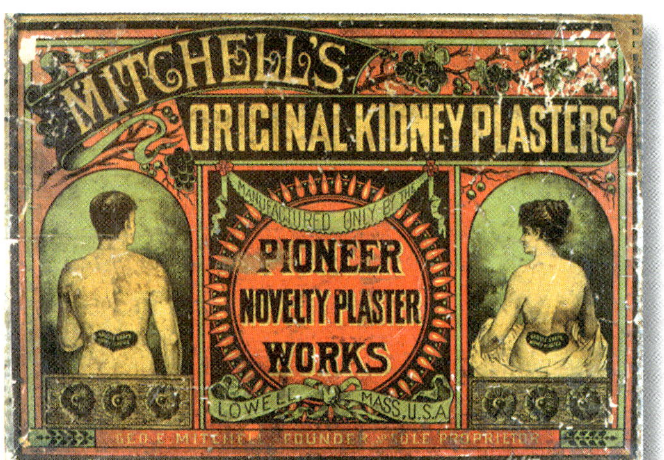


John D. Rockefeller, who around the turn of the 20th century had become the world's richest man and its first billionaire, had an interesting father. William A. Rockefeller, with a flair for showmanship and self-promotion, peddled sham medicines under the names of Doc Rockefeller and Doc Levingston. His deceitful and beguiling ways not only involved his patent peddling, but also his bigamous marriages, each of which lasted over fifty years.[3,8]

The glamour of the long ago and the fascination of the faraway united in the American Indian. Both the belief in botanic medicine and a primitive hostility toward the educated doctor contributed to the conclusion that Indians were "natural" physicians. The Indian suggested strength, independence, and native sagacity. In truth, the concept of Indian pharmacology was greatly exaggerated. The "red man" had many simple applications for wounds, aimed more at placating the supernatural influences than curing

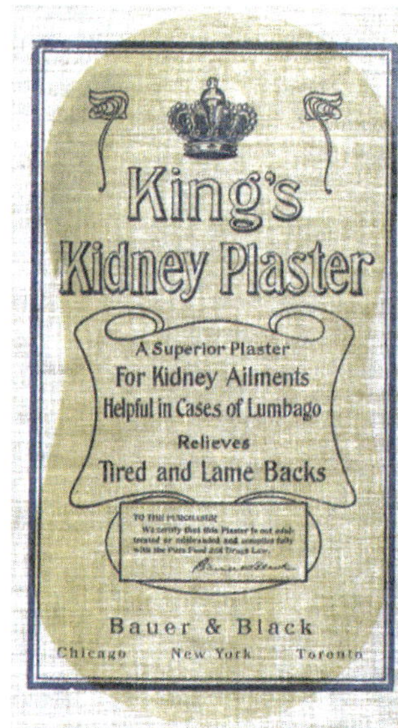


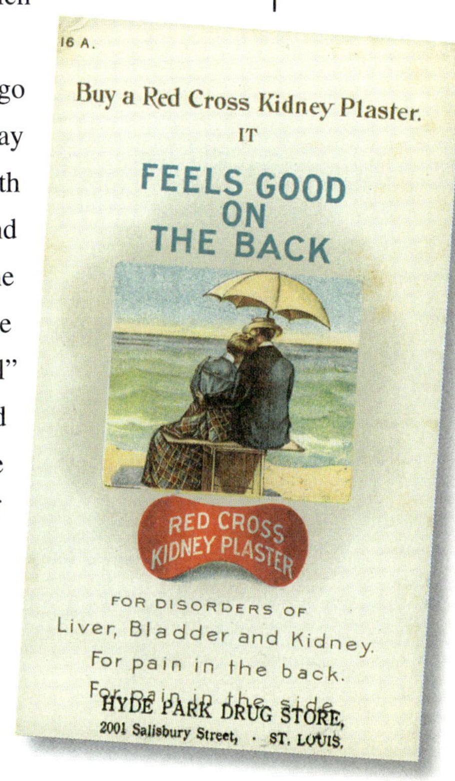

**Alexander's Liver and Kidney Tonic**
This nostrum had two labels which were similar in appearance. The front label was for "Liver and Kidney Tonic" and the reverse label was a "Sure Cure for Malaria."

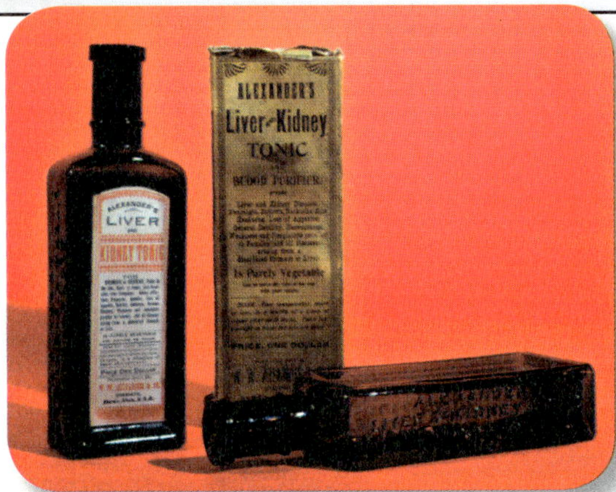


disease. It took the white man's commercial instincts and vivid imagination to create the Indian healer, Indian herbal medicines, and Indian road shows. Probably the most spectacular shows of the patent medicine decades were the Healy and Bigelow Kickapoo Indian galas. They capitalized on curiosity about the West and the life of the Indian.[2,4,7]

The medicine shows had a natural appeal to entertainment-starved pioneers in scattered mountain hamlets and pioneer villages. They gawked at the Indian chiefs and dancing girls, volunteered to have aching teeth pulled free of charge, and fell for the shill who was always there to buy the first bottle of every imaginable kind of salve, syrup, and solution.[1, 5]

After the itinerant pitchman, the other classic source of patent medicine sales was the country store. Nostrum advertising boosted the popular demand for such products that soon appeared on store counters.[1,5] America was predominately rural in the 1800s, its population further dispersed after the Civil War to the vast new lands in the West. Small clusters of farms might not support a pharmacy but any country

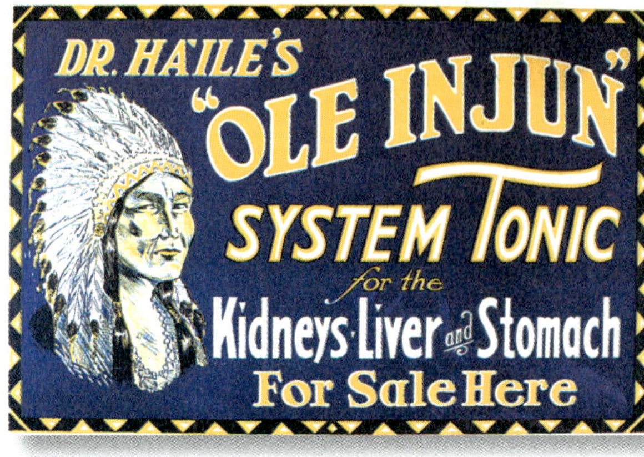


store could carry such medical achievements as "Seminole Indian Liver and Kidney Cure," "Richfield's Asparagus and Buchu Compound Kidney and Bladder Specific," and "The Cherokee Kidney and Liver Cure."

In 1869 America celebrated the completion of the transcontinental railroad. In spite of the controversy over slavery former Confederates and former Yankees stood together to celebrate the uniting of the East and the West. The railroad enabled man to move cross-country at sixty miles per hour and the telegraph that was beside it permitted the dispatch of reports from coast to coast almost instantly. Prior to this event the transport of persons and the movement of information occurred no faster than was possible during the Roman era. The timing of this accomplishment significantly aided the marketing and distribution of patent medicines.

Patent medicine advertising is important because of both its priority and its variety. The nostrum makers demonstrated the power of brand-name merchandising. The power wasn't in the bottle, but in the advertising—American evangelism applied to material things. The nostrum makers were the first to create the public image of a trademark with ideas, pictures, and slogans

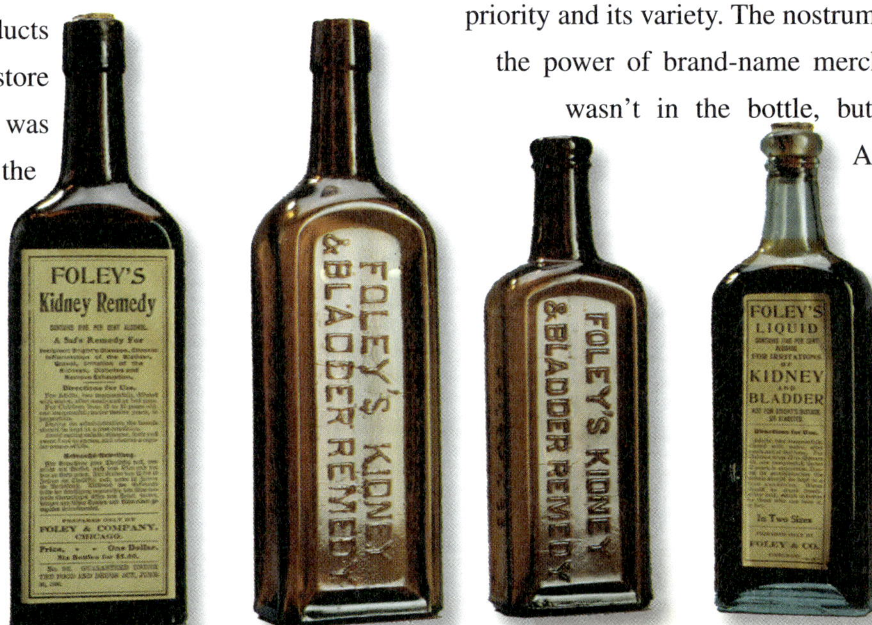

Seminole Indian Liver and Kidney Cure

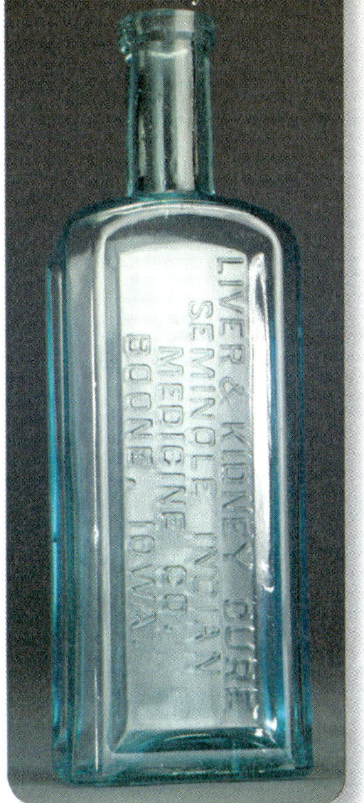


to establish a product personality. The seeds of quackery were rigorously tilled.[6] As one entered this world, it was soon apparent that the adman had been there with board-fence bill posters, rock painters, curbstone artists, and side walk stencilers. Anything that had a smooth surface, that rose above the ground between New York and Philadelphia and could be seen from the train, was decorated with the names of "Dr. J.H. McLean's Liver and Kidney Balm," "Bronson's Crown Kidney Cure," "Dr. Southworth's Celebrated Blood and Bladder Medicine," and "Dr. M.M. Fenner's Kidney and Backache Cure."

The nostrum manufacturers advertised by means of the printed word in all its myriad forms. At their disposal were newspapers, almanacs and pamphlets, trade cards, calendars, posters, and outdoor signs and billboards. Newspaper advertising was a singularly important medium that mutually benefitted both the medicine proprietors and the newspaper industry. Throughout the nineteenth century patent medicines were first in volume of newspaper advertising, ahead of all other products. Soon the newspapers shared an economic bias in favor of the nostrum makers and continued to keep their editorial columns understandably quiet as to the dangers of the nostrum trade.[1]

Both newspapers and almanacs were crammed with testimonials. The message of the testimonial was a personal "before and after pitch" offered by ordinary citizens who endorsed the manufacturers' claims. The vast majority of testimonials were probably genuine and unsolicited, although undoubtedly edited in many cases. There were always enough gullible people available who were pleased to see their names in print. One newspaper editor is said to have advised that "if your brains won't get you into the papers, sign a patent medicine testimonial. Maybe your kidneys will."[9,10]

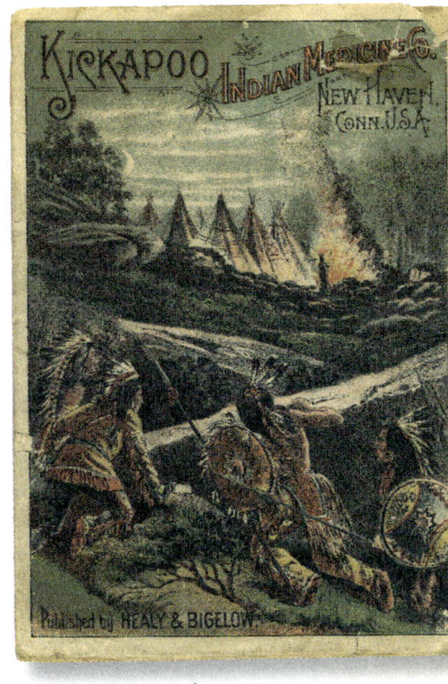


The advertising trade card was used in the last two decades of the nineteenth century and was extraordinarily successful as sales material. The trade card was probably the most artistic and vivid advertising mode used. Wide spread trade card collecting further increased its popularity. Similarly, the ubiquitous almanacs with beautiful covers lithographed in color were widely distributed on the counters of the country stores.[9,10]

Not to be confused with legitimate hospitals and clinics were the "health institutes," laboratories and dispensaries which advertised quick cures for almost everything. A specialty item was the secret deficiencies of "lost manhood." Dr. R.F. Price in his Denver clinic offered to

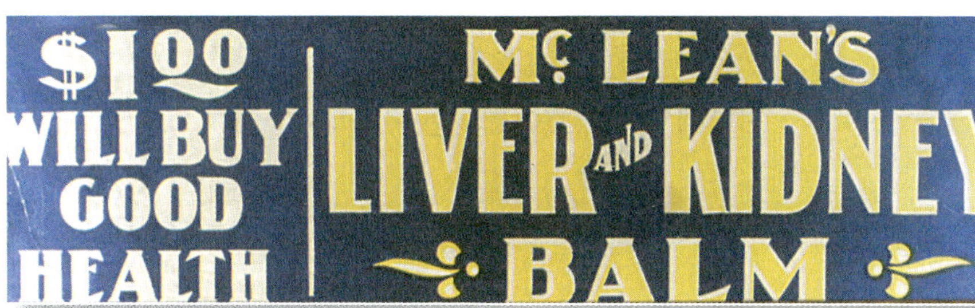

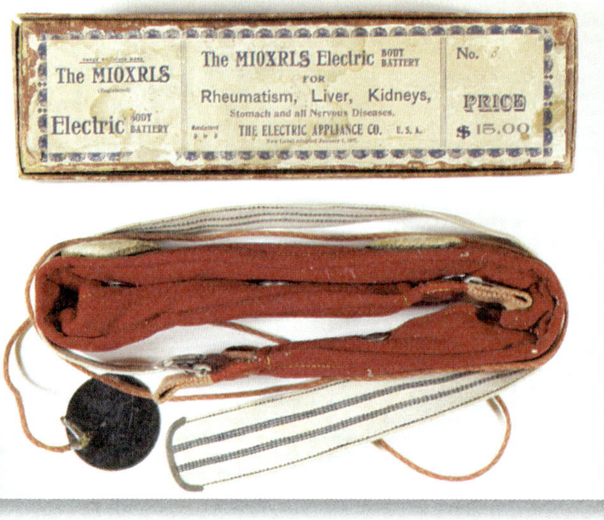


**Mioxrl's Electric Belt**
Positive relief with a written guarantee for a quick and reliable cure.

treat "all diseases arising from indiscretions of early youth" and guaranteed to forfeit $1000.00 for any case of "seminal weakness" he accepted and failed to cure.

After the nostrum peddler came other phases of quackery. The variety was limited only by the imagination of the inventors and the gullibility of the suffering. Displaying their customary ambivalence toward orthodox medicine, the doctors of gadgetry preyed especially upon those who were clutching at medical straws to cure hopeless cases. Whatever special advantage device quackery might have, its fundamental persuasive force came from the combination of admiration and incomprehension. Electrical gadgetry with flashing lights and wiggling dials convinced the anxious patient that a cure was inevitable.[10]

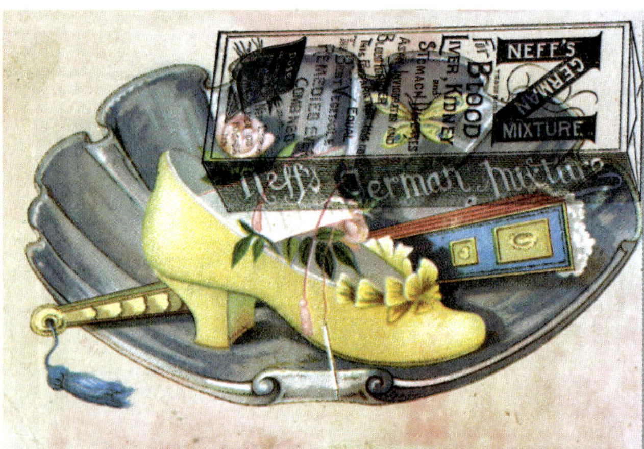


Year after year nostrum advertisers told the public about the failings of orthodox physicians. They pictured regular doctors as heartless brutes, armed with scalpels, leeches and mercurial purges. Both as to science and as to ethics, the early practice of medicine rested on an unsure foundation. The prevailing $18^{th}$ century American methods of therapy, owing much to the influence of the Philadelphia's Dr. Benjamin Rush, stressed extreme bleeding and purging. From the patients' point of view, the arduous impact of disease was aggravated by the arduous impact of therapy. It was medicine's "heroic age." However, not every sick man felt like being a hero. The sick, whether their illness was real or imagined, understandably preferred trying a bottle of the latest blood purifier as opposed to the good doctor's blood letting by knife or leech.

Needless to say, if the old frontier offered a fertile field of endeavor for any profession, medicine was it. As was described by Robert Karolevitz in *Doctors of the Old West*[6], this was a land of vigor and violence, where great physical exertion was commonplace and where the slightest rebuff could erupt into a deadly showdown with knife or gun. It was a vast rugged expanse where drought, malnutrition, and exposure to the harsh elements took a heavy toll. Though

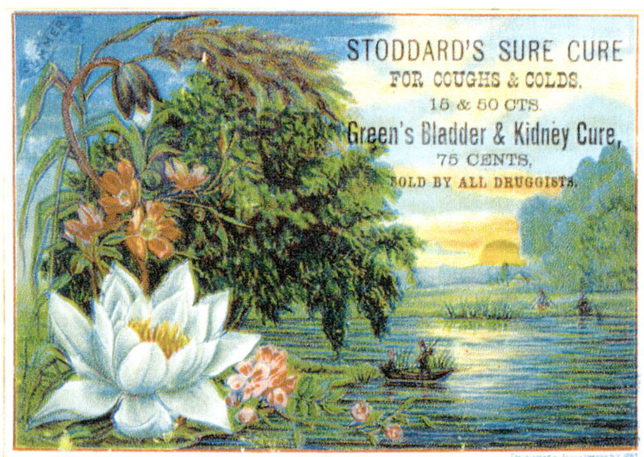


beautiful and rich and productive, it was a land of devastating epidemics, where wasting fevers and refractory diseases were rampant, while such killers as cholera, smallpox and

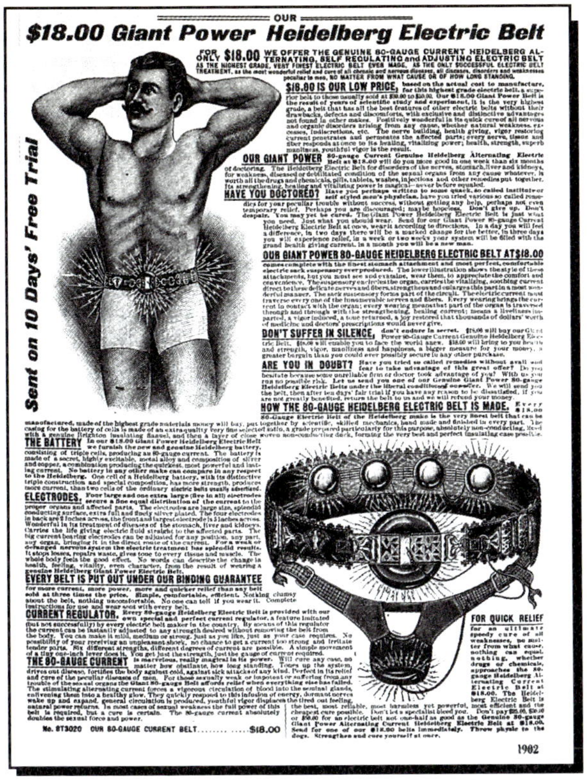


measles struck down young and old alike.

The doctors who volunteered to enter this medical battleground cannot be described in one broad generalization. Mostly, though, they were adventuresome, wealth-seeking young men from "back east" or from Europe. Their medical degree—if they had one—was their passport to a life of excitement in a new land.

There were, of course, the military surgeons who finished tours of duty at frontier outposts and then remained as private practitioners. There were railroad surgeons, medical missionaries, and Indian agency physicians. Included, too, were a few wife deserters and men with tainted backgrounds who hoped for a new start as pioneer doctors where no one questioned a stranger's past.

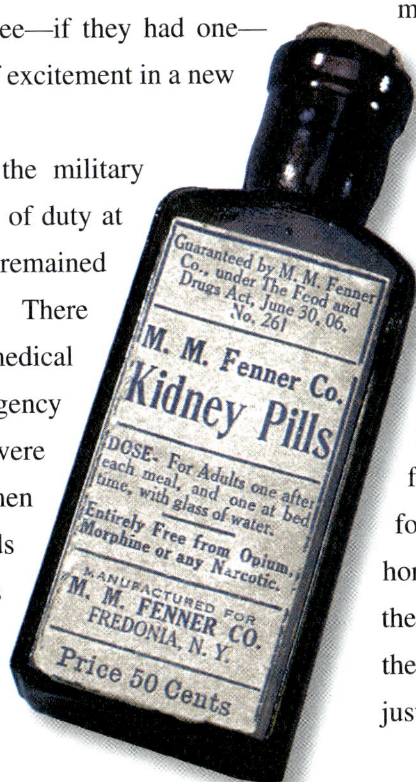


The medicines used by the frontier doctor depended largely upon their training. The followers of homeopathy prescribed many drugs, but not much of any one drug. The allopaths went in for heavy doses of ipecac and mercurous medicines. Botanic physicians were partial to herb and root concoctions. In general, most country doctors carried a small medicine case with a variety of remedies to treat the specific illnesses they knew something about. However, it was a rare medicine kit that didn't contain a liberal supply of whiskey, either for a patient or for the doctor himself.

Generally, all of them came to be known as horse-and-buggy doctors, and a romantic aura of indefatigability, selflessness, and courage grew up around them. But just to keep the record straight, there were also a few who didn't fit the mold. With their medical degree proudly emblazoned on the wall, there were those who foisted upon ignorant patients the most objectionable forms of quackery. All the rest—the vast majority—were honorable, hard working medical servants who overcame the reputations of the black sheep among them and made the title of country doctor one of which they could be justifiably proud.[6]

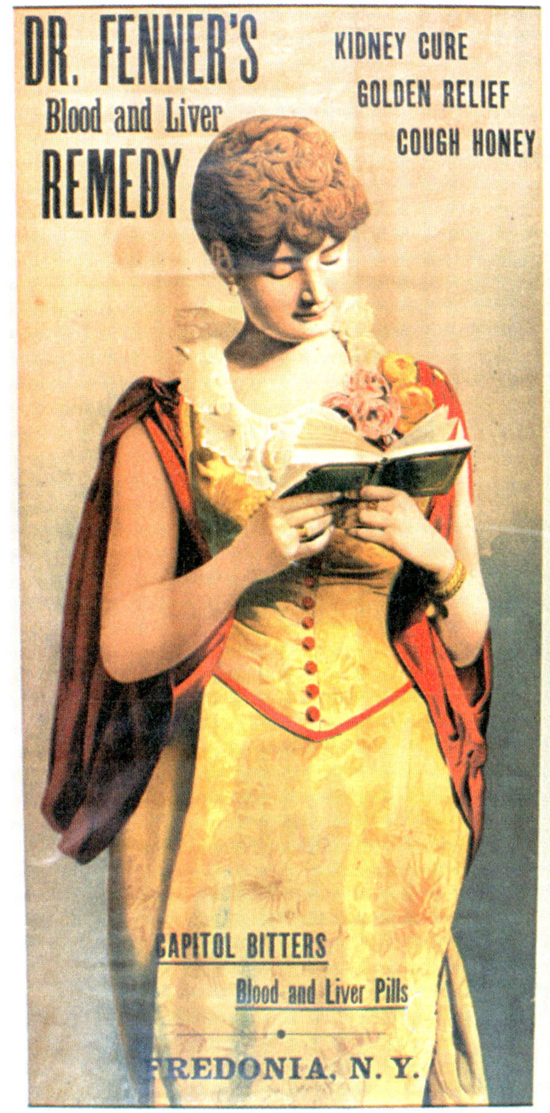

**Dr. M.M. Fenner's Kidney and Backache Cure**
An internationally known product that in 1913 was cited: "falsely and fraudulently represented as a cure for inflammation of the kidneys, catarrh of the bladder, heart disease, leukorrhea." Fine, $25.00. *Nostrums and Quackery. Vol.II, p.216, 1921.*

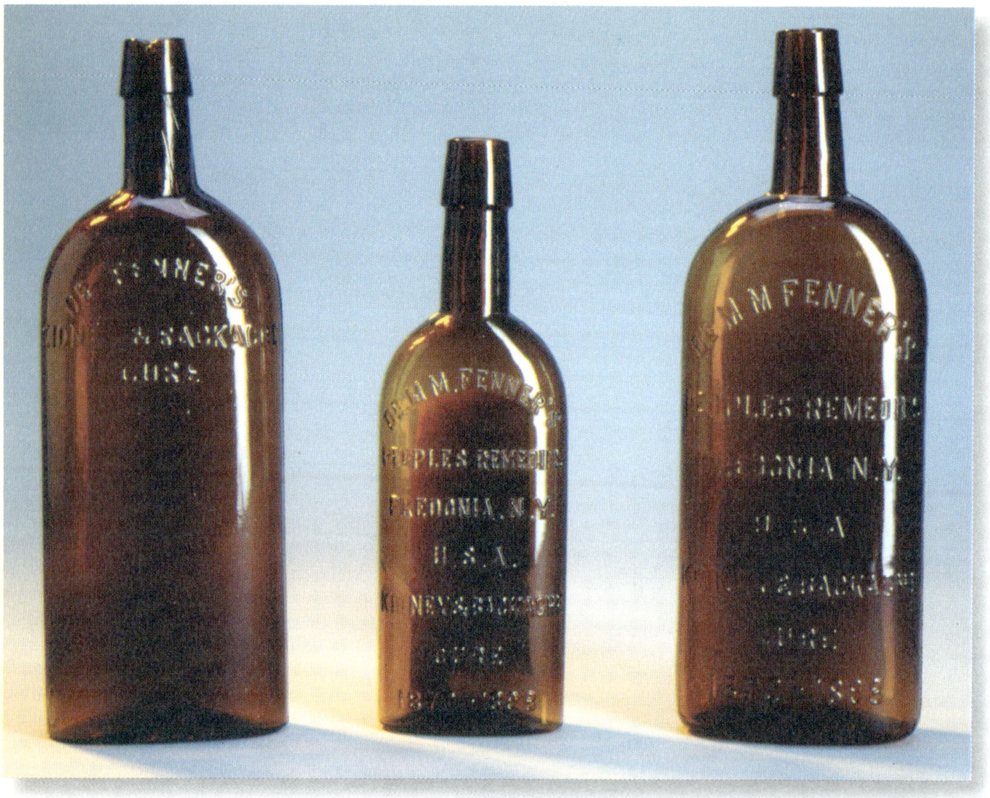

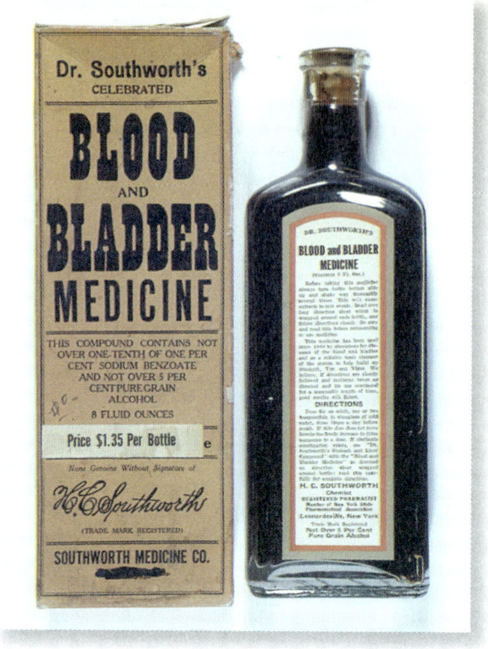


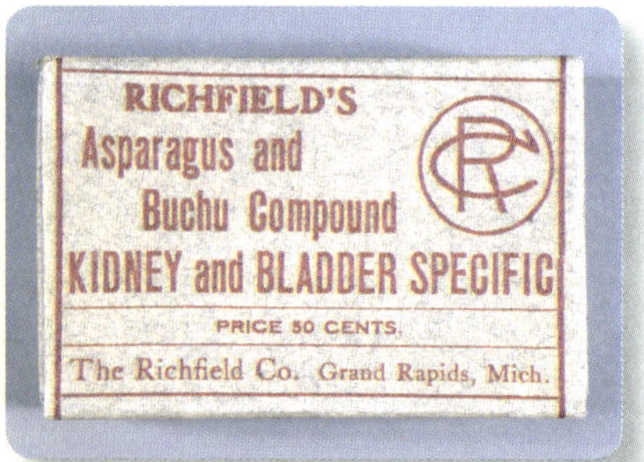


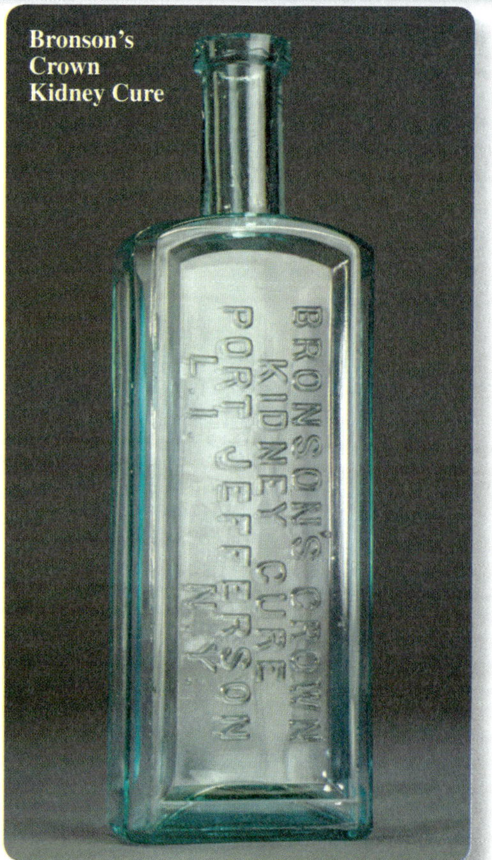


Bronson's Crown Kidney Cure

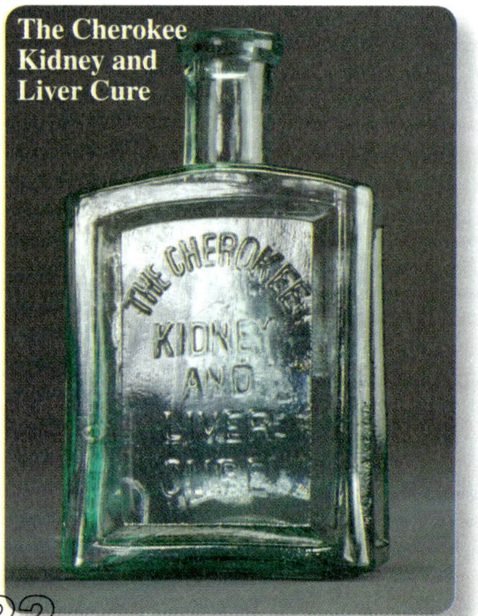


The Cherokee Kidney and Liver Cure

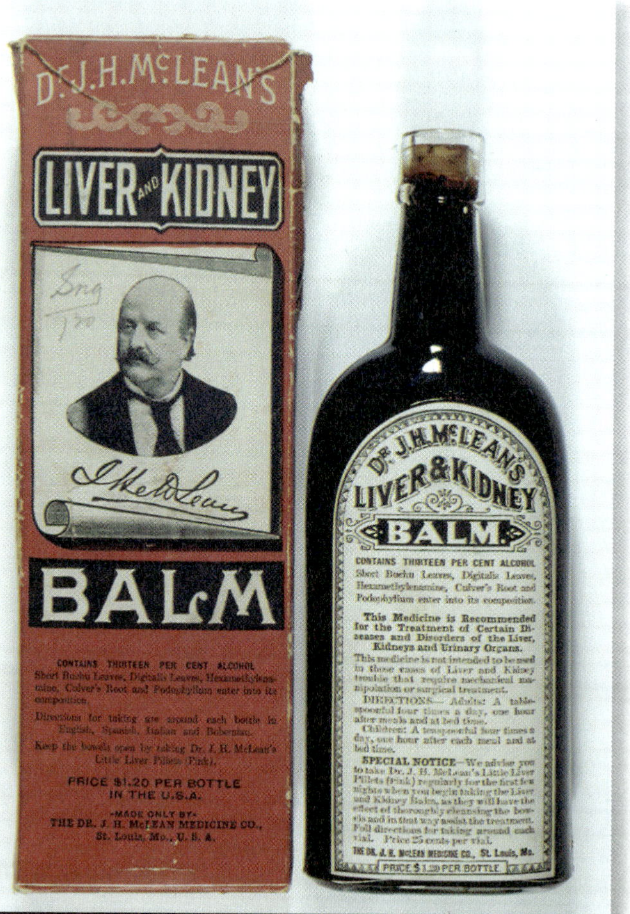


**Dr. J.H. McLean's Liver and Kidney Balm**
In 1916 upon analysis it was found to contain "11.8% alcohol which is the most active constituent contained in the preparation." *Nostrums and Quackery. Vol.II, p.219, 1921.*

Chapter 4

# The Rise and Fall

In the past several centuries America has undergone a great agricultural and scientific revolution. Becoming a farmer and a trader, rather than merely a hunter, man learned the need for rules to insure safety and fair dealing in the food supply.

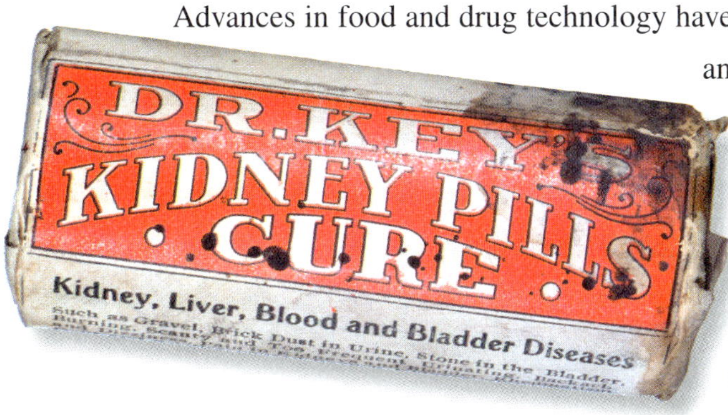


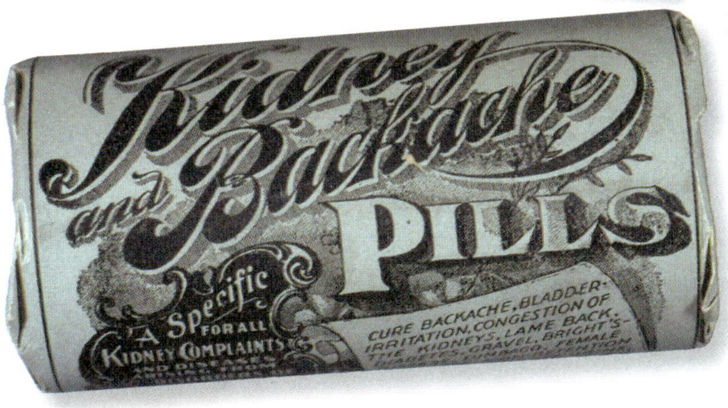


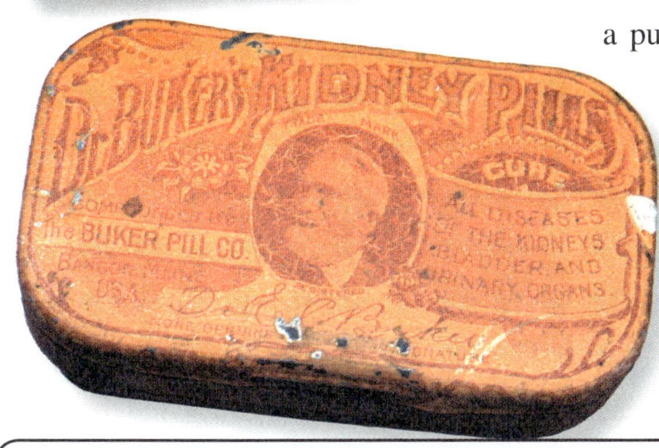


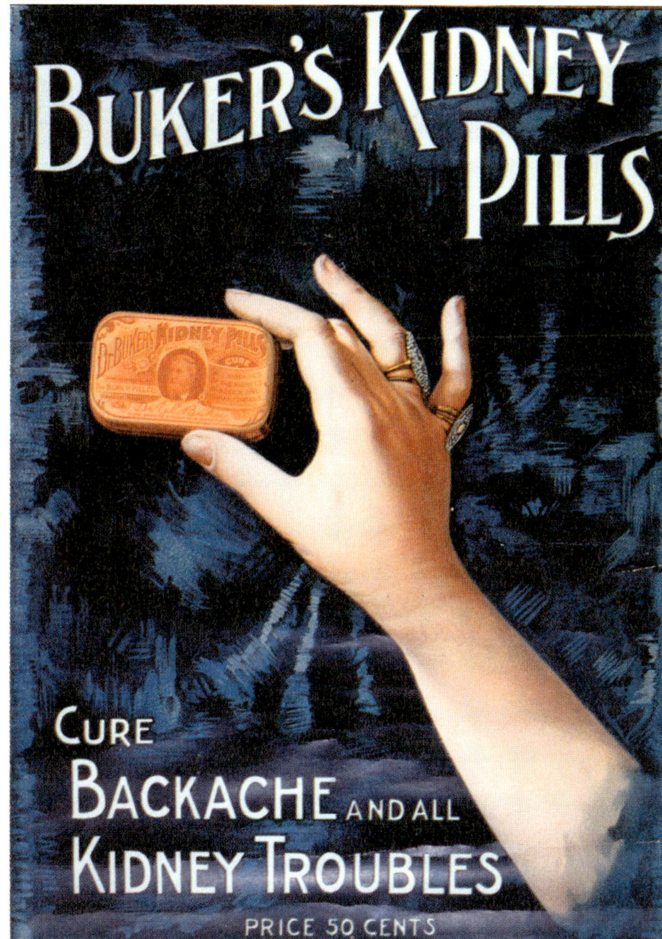


Advances in food and drug technology have provided a variety of foods and medicines our forefathers never knew—but they have also created new problems. When people raised their own food, or bought from a neighbor, they had control over its purity and quality. In modern times, however, no consumer can exercise such control himself. Government must do for all what no individual can do alone.

The birth and battle for a pure food law was long and fierce although food and drug laws are as old as Hebrew and Egyptian laws. More recently records of the Massachusetts Bay Colony tell of Nicholas Knopf, who in 1630 was given his choice of a fine or a flogging for selling "a water of no worth nor value" as a cure for scurvy, an early case of prosecution on the effectiveness of a drug. Massachusetts was also the first state to pass a general law in 1785 against food adulterations. However, it took a flood of diseased meats, poisonous adulterants, quack medicines, and more than 100 bills submitted and rejected by the United States

"The pills and the panaceas of today are colloquially, but incorrectly, called "patent medicines"; incorrectly, because among the thousands of remedies offered to the public for the self-treatment of disease there are probably not half a dozen that are really patented. The reasons are not far to seek. The United States Patent Office is not supposed to grant a patent on a product unless it can be shown that the article on which protection is sought is a new and useful invention. This simple requirement is sufficient in itself to prevent practically all so-called "patent medicines" from being patentable."
*Nostrums and Quackery and Pseudo-Medicine. Vol.III, Introduction p.7, 1936.*

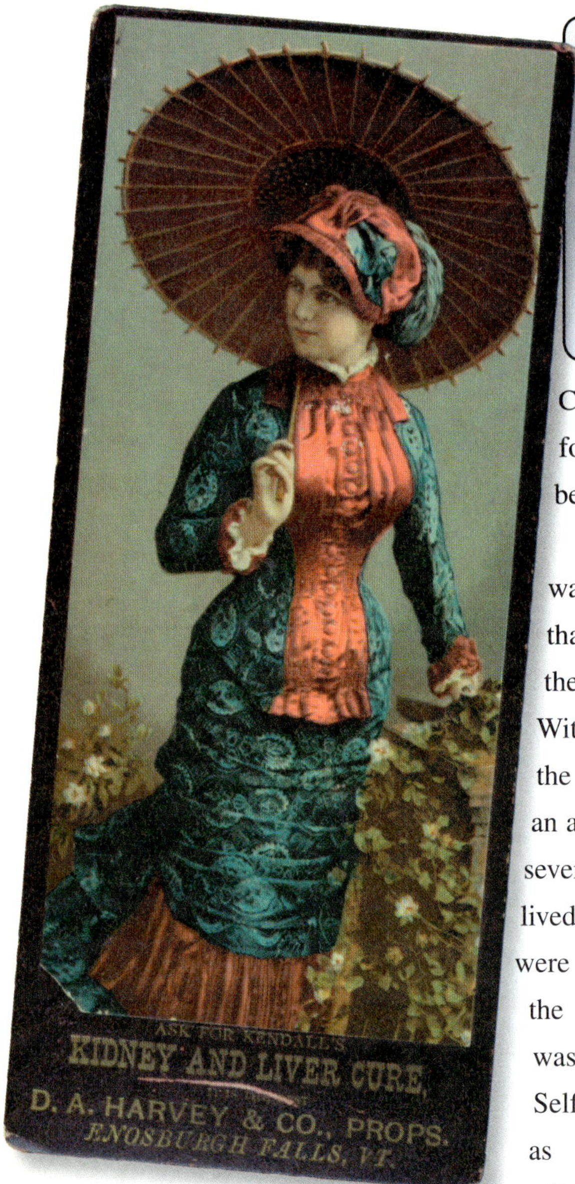


"Take away from the "patent medicine" industry secrecy, and the mystery which goes with it, and you have undermined the foundations on which this monument to human gullibility is raised. For, in applying for a patent on a medicine, one must lay cards on the table, face up! If a patent is granted on a medicine, the names and quantities of the ingredients and the methods of combining these ingredients become a matter of public record, a copy of which any one can obtain from the Commissioner of Patents. But the unknown always inspires awe, and here we have the explanation of the strenuous efforts, so far universally successful, on the part of manufacturers of "patent medicines" to fight every attempt on the part of the public to require a declaration of the ingredients and their quantities on the nostrums."
*Nostrums and Quackery and Pseudo-Medicine. Vol.III, Introduction p.8, 1936.*

Congress, before federal food and drug regulation became law in 1906.[1]

Against this background was an American populace that was rapidly overcoming the effects of the Civil War. With development of the West the settlers soon established an agrarian life style since over seventy percent of Americans lived on farms. Because doctors were few, the country store or the itinerant nostrum peddler was the source of medicine. Self-dosage was practiced as it appealed to the self-reliant. In time, cheap postal rates facilitated self-doctoring by mail-ordering the medicine.

The development of the industrial revolution in America was reflected in the economic forces that produced the booming business of patent and proprietary medicines. It started with the itinerant medicine man who in time evolved into the factory owner. The automatic bottle machine of 1903 greatly improved glass bottle manufacturing. Millions of bottles with a variety of nostrums were produced each year and were then shipped great distances. Transportation of the medicine was facilitated by cheap railroad distribution costs. Promotional

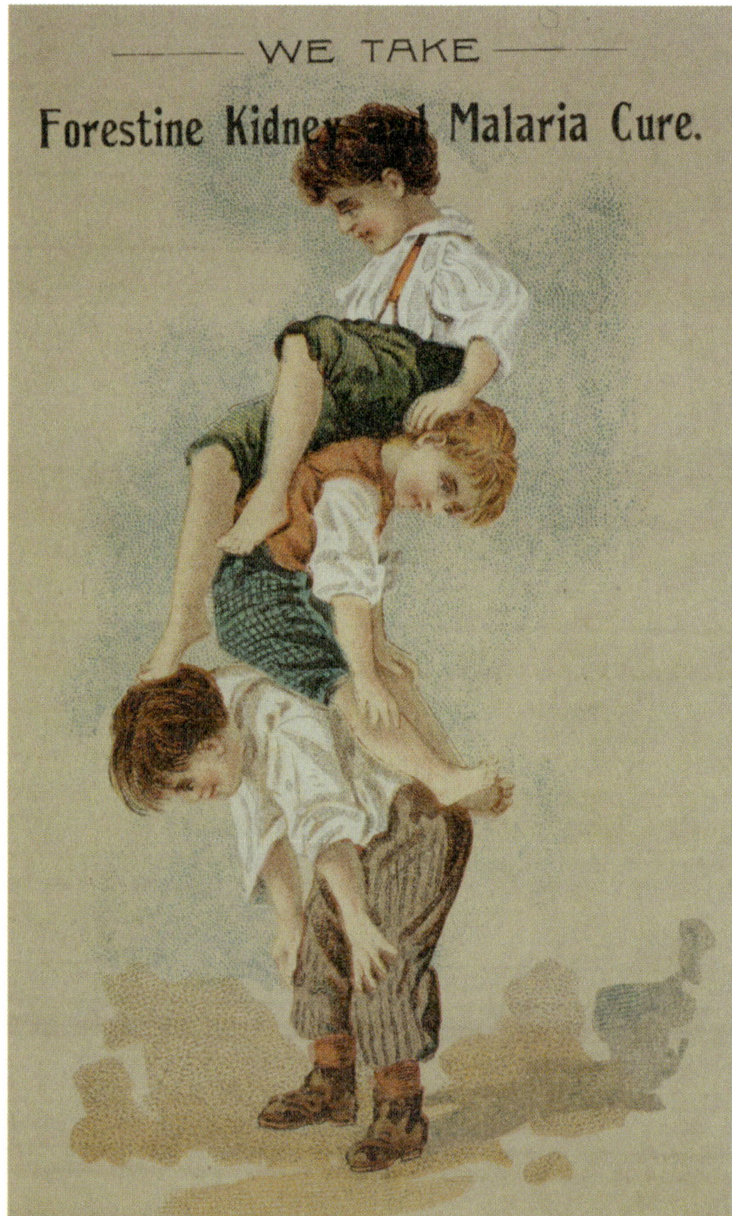


Quoting the patent medicine industry, "While the claims we make for our products may be fraudulent, so long as we keep the composition secret, it will be difficult for the courts to convict us."
*Nostrums and Quackery and Pseudo-Medicine. Vol.III, Introduction p.8, 1936.*

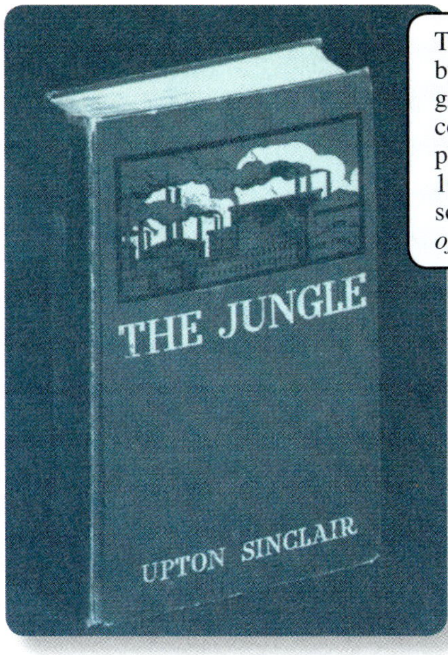

The first edition of *The Jungle* by Upton Sinclair. Described in graphic detail were the horrifying conditions in the meat packing plants of Chicago. More than 100,000 copies of the book were sold by the end of 1906. *Courtesy of The Chicago Historical Society.*

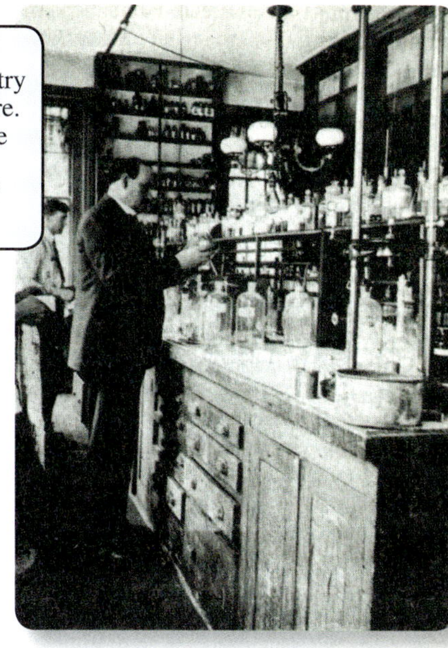

Dr. Harvey Washington Wiley, Chief of the Bureau of Chemistry of the department of Agriculture. He provided leadership to those seeking to regulate the patent medicine industry by means of the Pure Food and Drug Act.

genius permitted medicine proprietors to make patent medicines among the first consumer products to achieve a national market under a single brand name. Bill posting blanketed American cities as aggressive advertising with outrageous claims resulted in rapid product dissemination. In complete harmony with the times of 1905, Sears Roebuck and Company carried twenty full catalogue pages of patent medicines and nostrums. By 1906, at its very pinnacle of success, the traffic in patent and proprietary medicine had reached a volume of over eighty million dollars a year, in a market comprised of over 50,000 different brands.[2]

Eventually there arose a public concern for the safety of patent nostrums. Before 1906 the labels on the bottles themselves were of no help as there was no disclosure of

This article by Samuel Hopkins Adams was the first of the famous series that appeared in *Colliers Weekly*. Entitled the *Great American Fraud*, it discussed the composition and the ill effects of a wide variety of products on the market. The American Medical Association was finally aroused by the article series to join in and actively pursue the patent medicine industry.

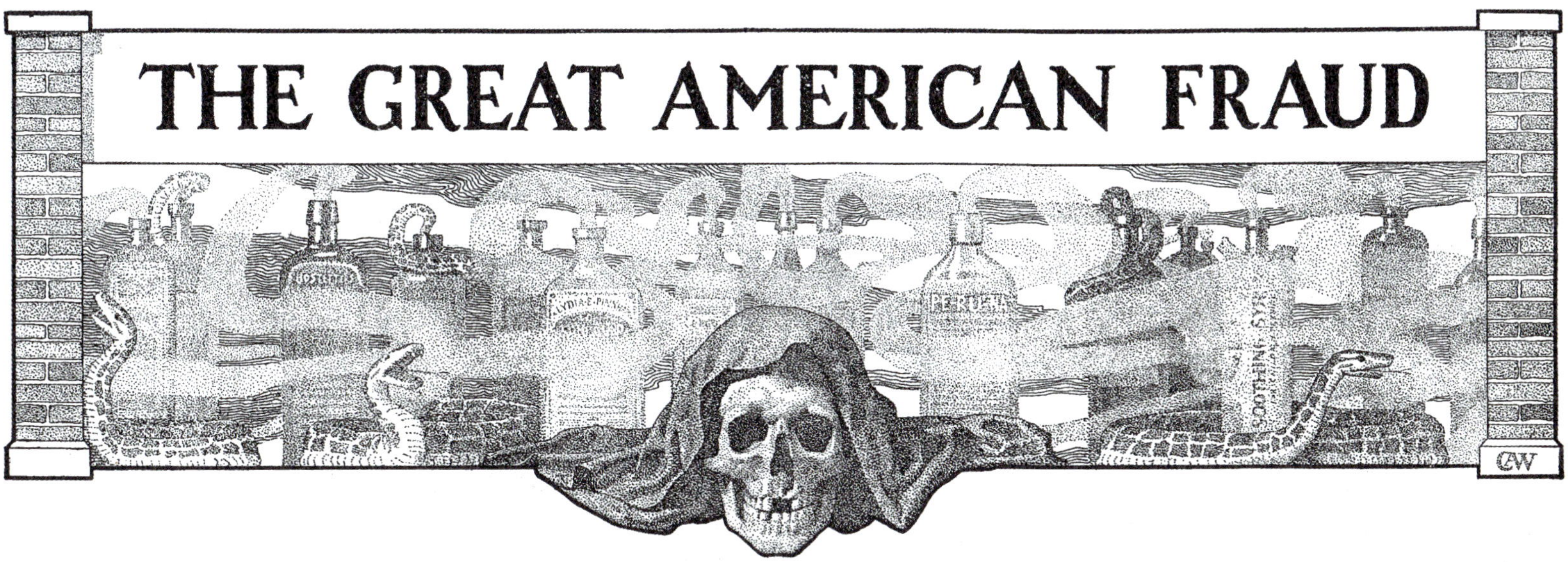

Collier's for October 7 1905

# THE GREAT AMERICAN FRAUD

By SAMUEL HOPKINS ADAMS

*This is the introductory article to a series which will contain a full explanation and exposure of patent medicine methods, and the harm done to the public by this industry, founded mainly on fraud and poison. Results of the publicity given to these methods can already be seen in the steps recently taken by the National Government, some State Governments, and a few of the more reputable newspapers. The object of the series is to make the situation so familiar and thoroughly understood that there will be a speedy end to the worst aspects of the evil. The second article, "Peruna and the 'Bracers,'" will be published in COLLIER'S for October 21*

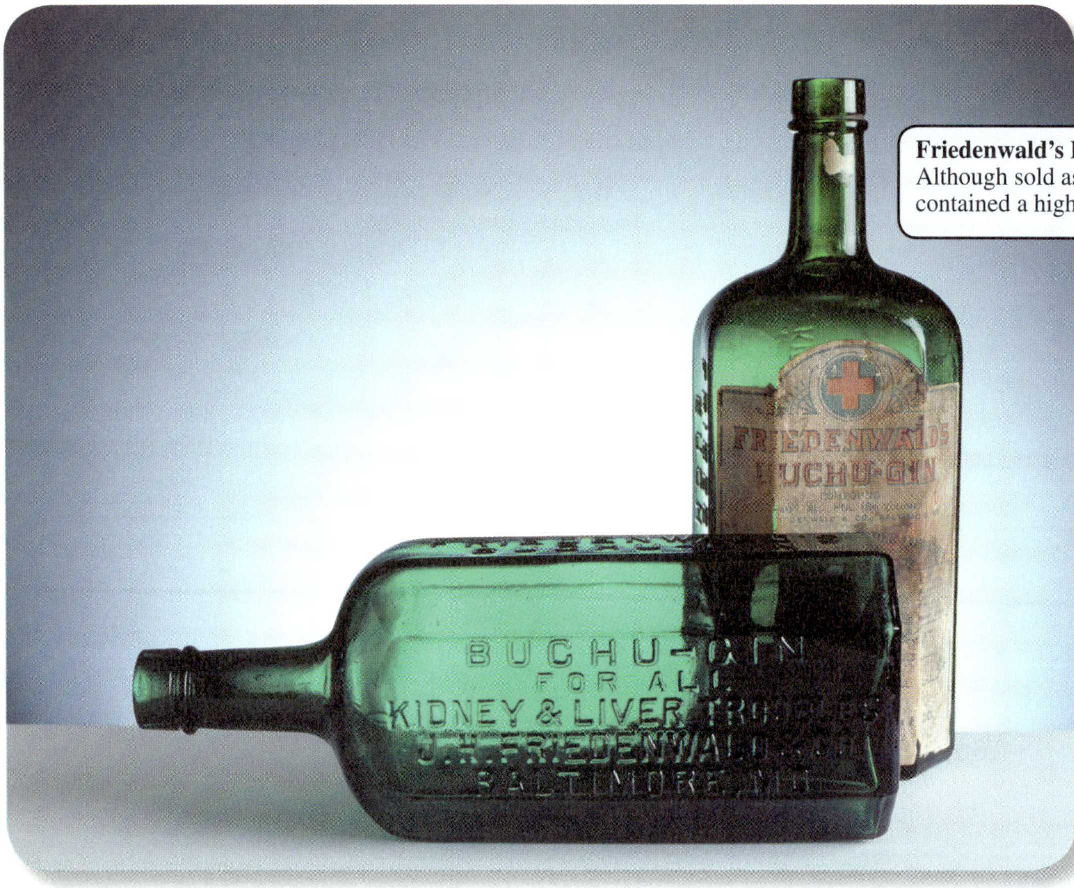


**Friedenwald's Buchu-Gin For All Kidney And Liver Troubles**
Although sold as a medicinal, there was no question that the nostrum contained a high percentage of alcohol.

ingredients. Popular journalists and writers exposed not only the medical dangers present in leading products on the market but also the industry's shoddy advertising practices. A significant series of articles on patent medicines written by Samuel Hopkins Adams appeared in *Colliers Weekly* from October 1905 to February 1906 entitled *"The Great American Fraud."* In addition, *Ladies Home Journal* and *Good Housekeeping* aroused public opinion with their articles, editorials and cartoons. Coincidentally, Upton Sinclair's brutally realistic novel about the meat packing industry appeared when the debate was at its peak. The book, *The Jungle*, dramatized the shockingly soiled and spoiled meat products that were being processed.[3]

The combined efforts of reformers were initially focused on fighting adulterated

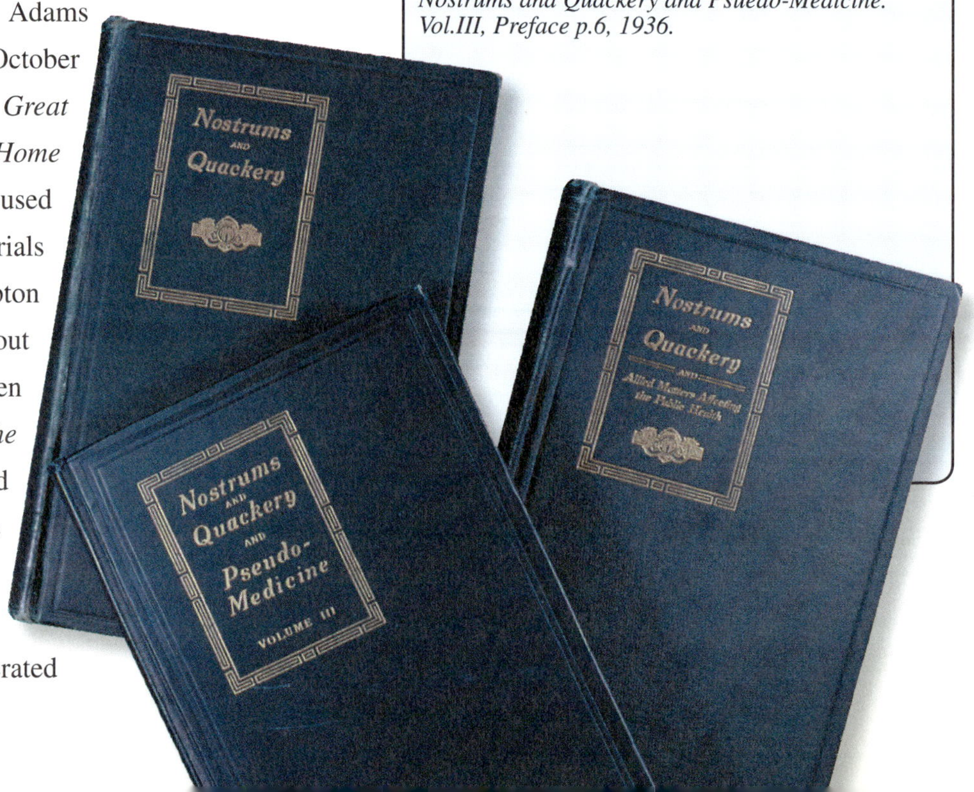


**Nostrums and Quackery Volumes I, II, III published by the American Medical Association**

"It is often charged-wholly without justification-that the medical profession's opposition to quackery and nostrum exploitation is motivated by self-interest. The facts are that if the medical profession looked at the "patent medicine" business from a dollar-and-cents viewpoint it would raise no opposition to it for, next to the "patent medicine" maker himself and the newspapers that take such a large share of the nostrum maker's profit, there is no other social group that is so widely benefited as the medical profession by "patent medicine" advertising. Every piece of advertising devised to convince the public that a pain in the lower part of the back means kidney disease will send, probably, as many people to the family physician as it will send to the drug counter. The medical profession is not opposed to the "patent medicine" industry because it cuts into its income-for it doesn't-but because it is bad for the health of the public."
*Nostrums and Quackery and Psuedo-Medicine. Vol.III, Preface p.6, 1936.*

food and liquor and unsanitary conditions in the food processing industry. Strenuous opposition to a Federal food and drug law came from many food manufacturers, as well as the makers of patent medicines who were the largest advertisers in the country. Enlisted for the government cause was a physician—chemist Dr. Harvey Washington Wiley who became Chief of the Bureau of Chemistry of the Department of Agriculture.[4] A man of great energy, talent, and prestige, Dr. Wiley advanced considerably the movement for an effective national law. With the support of President Theodore Roosevelt, the final vote in Congress was almost unanimous. The Pure Food and Drug Act was signed into law on June 30, 1906.[5]

However, the passage of the Act of 1906 did not result in the demise of the nostrum industry. The law did provide an increased means of surveillance and control of the burgeoning business. It required the manufacturer to state on every label the quantity of alcohol, opium, cocaine, and certain other specific substances, if present. No statement on the label could be false or misleading. If a drug was listed, it must be present in the strength and purity asserted, or the medicine would be considered "adulterated." The Sherley Amendment of 1912 further identified and outlawed unclear and misleading statements on the label. A claim like "sure cure" could no longer be used. A popular medicine like "Warner's Kidney and Liver Cure" was renamed "Warner's Kidney and Liver Remedy". Also, they removed the alcohol entirely and substituted glycerin to

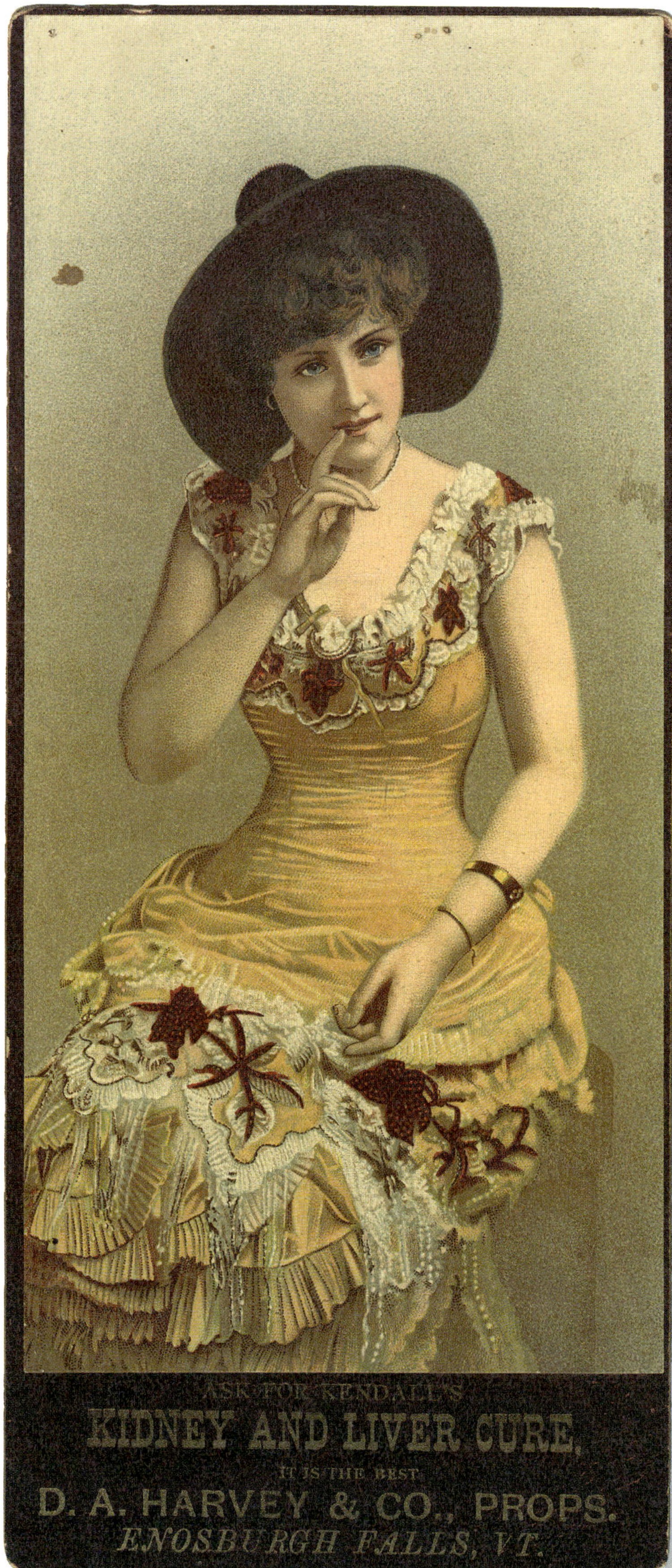

make it more palatable.

The American Medical Association made a significant effort to educate the public concerning the dangers of the nostrum industry by its publication entitled *Nostrums and Quackery.*[6] It appeared in three separate volumes beginning in 1912, followed by 1921, and 1936. The publication contained hundreds of actual cases where the purveyors of quackery continued to deceive the public. The work recorded many nostrums, subjected to chemical analyses, which revealed that they were not only useless but in many cases harmful preparations. These books were written in the language of the layman and received wide distribution. Thus the combined efforts of the Food and Drug Administration as well as an increased public awareness did much to restrain the makers of quack medicines.

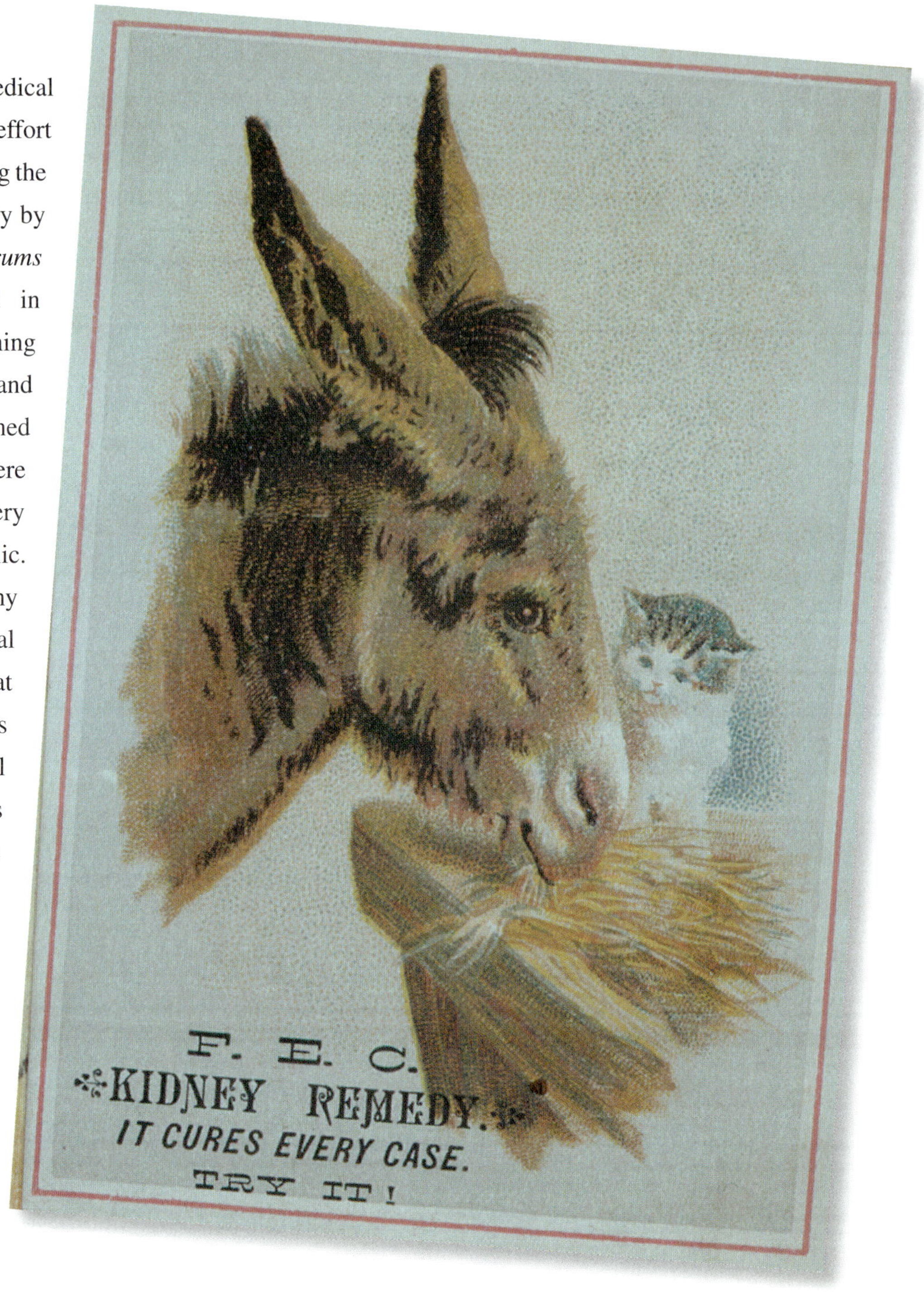

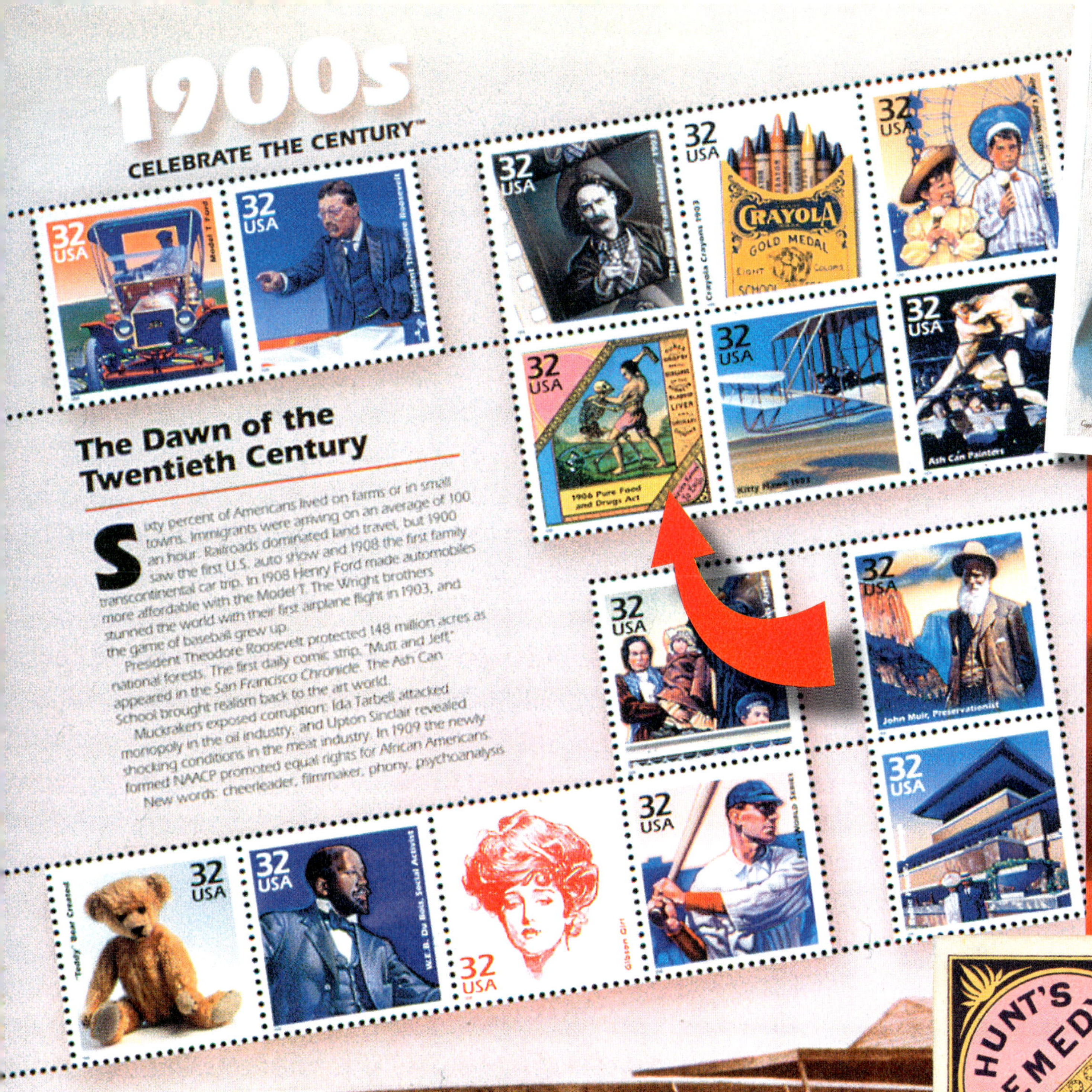
1900s
CELEBRATE THE CENTURY™
The Dawn of the Twentieth Century
Sixty percent of Americans lived on farms or in small towns. Immigrants were arriving on an average of 100 an hour. Railroads dominated land travel, but 1900 saw the first U.S. auto show and 1908 the first family transcontinental car trip. In 1908 Henry Ford made automobiles more affordable with the Model T. The Wright brothers stunned the world with their first airplane flight in 1903, and the game of baseball grew up.
President Theodore Roosevelt protected 148 million acres as national forests. The first daily comic strip, "Mutt and Jeff," appeared in the San Francisco Chronicle. The Ash Can School brought realism back to the art world.
Muckrakers exposed corruption: Ida Tarbell attacked monopoly in the oil industry, and Upton Sinclair revealed shocking conditions in the meat industry. In 1909 the newly formed NAACP promoted equal rights for African Americans.
New words: cheerleader, filmmaker, phony, psychoanalysis
32 USA
Model T Ford
President Theodore Roosevelt
Crayola Crayons 1903
CRAYOLA
GOLD MEDAL
1906 Pure Food and Drugs Act
Kitty Hawk 1903
Ash Can Painters
John Muir, Preservationist
"Teddy" Bear Created
W.E.B. Du Bois, Social Activist
Gibson Girl
First World Series

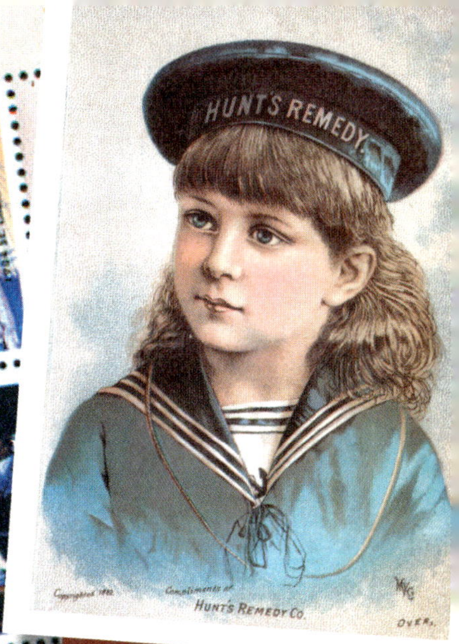
HUNT'S REMEDY
HUNT'S REMEDY CO.

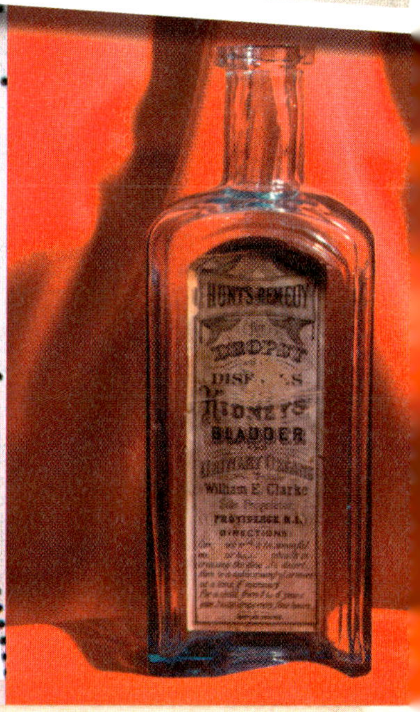

**Hunt's Remedy**

Dr. Simon Hunt of Providence, RI, collaborated with a local pharmacist, William C. Clark, to compound a favorite prescription. They began bottling it for public distribution in 1870 and continued till after the turn of the century.

In 2000 the United States Postal Service published a stamp series that "Celebrated The Century" by decades. The 1900s decade sheet includes a stamp for the Pure Food and Drug Act of 1906. This stamp is represented by a Hunt's Remedy trade card. The man on the card is pictured using a bottle of the nostrum to beat a skeletal representation of death.

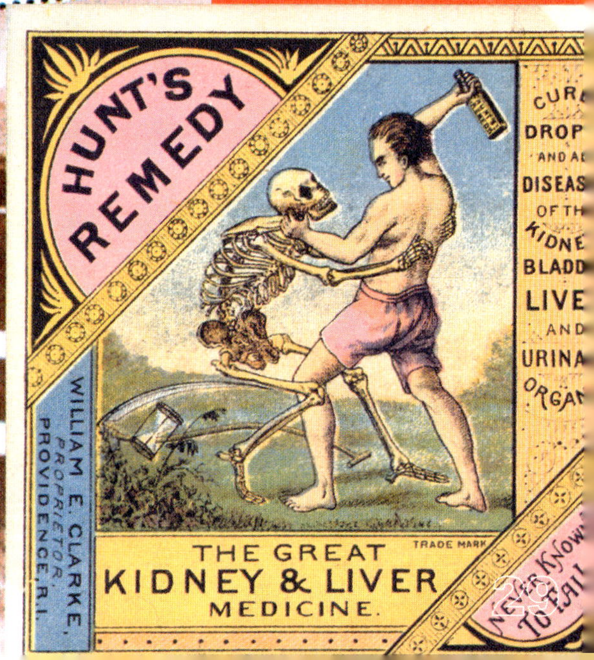

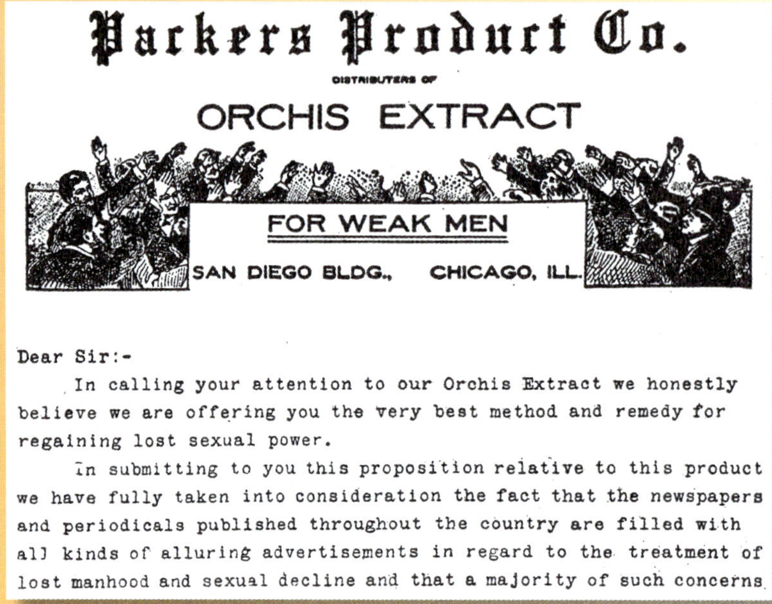

Parkers Product Co.

DISTRIBUTERS OF

ORCHIS EXTRACT

FOR WEAK MEN

SAN DIEGO BLDG., CHICAGO, ILL.

Dear Sir:-

In calling your attention to our Orchis Extract we honestly believe we are offering you the very best method and remedy for regaining lost sexual power.

In submitting to you this proposition relative to this product we have fully taken into consideration the fact that the newspapers and periodicals published throughout the country are filled with all kinds of alluring advertisements in regard to the treatment of lost manhood and sexual decline and that a majority of such concerns

# THE PRODUCTS

"We may extend our lines as a country; we may build battle ships and navies and constitute great armies; but if the health of the people is to be undermined by these concoctions of fraudulent and bogus medicines, of what avail is it?"

Weldon B. Heyburn - In the U.S. Senate, 1904

## Chapter 5

# Bitters

In a unique way, the history of bitters captures all the drama and deception of the proprietary medicine era. Under federal law bitters have always been considered to be proprietary medicine. Initially most varieties were associated with stomach maladies. The term "bitters" is generally assumed to apply to a mixture of herbs, often quinine or other herbs with a similar acrid taste. Today we know there were over a thousand different bottled brands during the bitters era.[1,2]

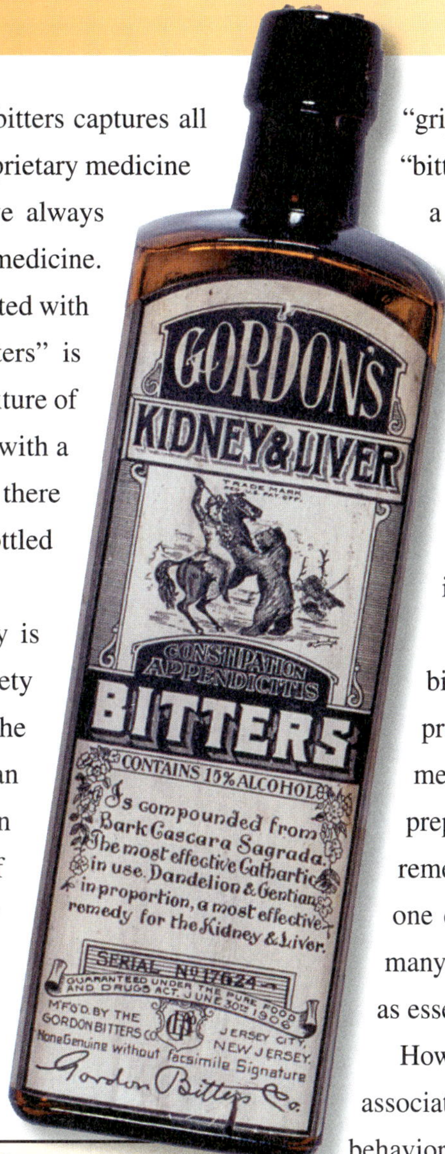


**Gordon's Kidney and Liver Bitters**
Shelf recognition became important for sales so packaging soon became more distinctive, more colorful. It is for this reason that the bottle changed from the simple square shape to the figural or ornate shape.

The story of the bitters industry is a colorful commentary on society and on the laws used to govern the consumption of alcohol. It all began in the 17th century on the European continent. Bitters consisted of various herbal mixtures usually combined with water, not alcohol. However, in England the presence of alcohol in bitters eventually became significant. It happened because of the effort to control the widespread drunkenness among the working class by King George II (1727–1760) who levied a heavy tax on gin. Gin was the cheap spirits drunk by most people. Recognizing the likely unfavorable results of their tax on gin, the liquor manufacturers responded by formulating a concoction of harsh tasting herbs in gin and calling it "gripe water," "coltick water" or more commonly, "bitters". This deception marked the beginning of a very successful saga for bitters manufacturing in England and eventually in America. Before the American Revolution the British levied heavy taxes on the consumption of rum and gin which resulted in substantial revenue from the colonies. To avoid this tax the colonist simply laced bitters with rum and gin. Following the Revolutionary period, alcohol was not taxed in the newly independent states.[1,2]

Although taxation on alcohol ceased, the bitters industry continued making its proprietary products. Many people placed their faith in the medicinal benefits thought to be contained in the preparation. The celebrated claims of a specific remedy and cure were always more enjoyed when one experienced a reassuring warm glow. Also, for many years women as well as men regarded whiskey as essential for health.

However, because of the excessive drinking and the associated antisocial behavior, there were concerns for temperance and moderation. The evils of alcohol were preached from the pulpits and formed the basis of many articles and books. In 1785 Dr. Benjamin Rush wrote an *"Inquiry Into the Effects of Ardent*

**BITTERS - ALCOHOLIC CONTENT**

| | |
|---|---|
| Warber's Safe Tonic Bitters | 75 proof |
| Drake's Plantation Bitters | 66 proof |
| Burdock Blood Bitters | 50 proof |
| Hosteter's Stomach Bitters | 88 proof |
| Parker's Tonic Bitters | 83 proof |

"recommended dose - one wineglassful three times daily"

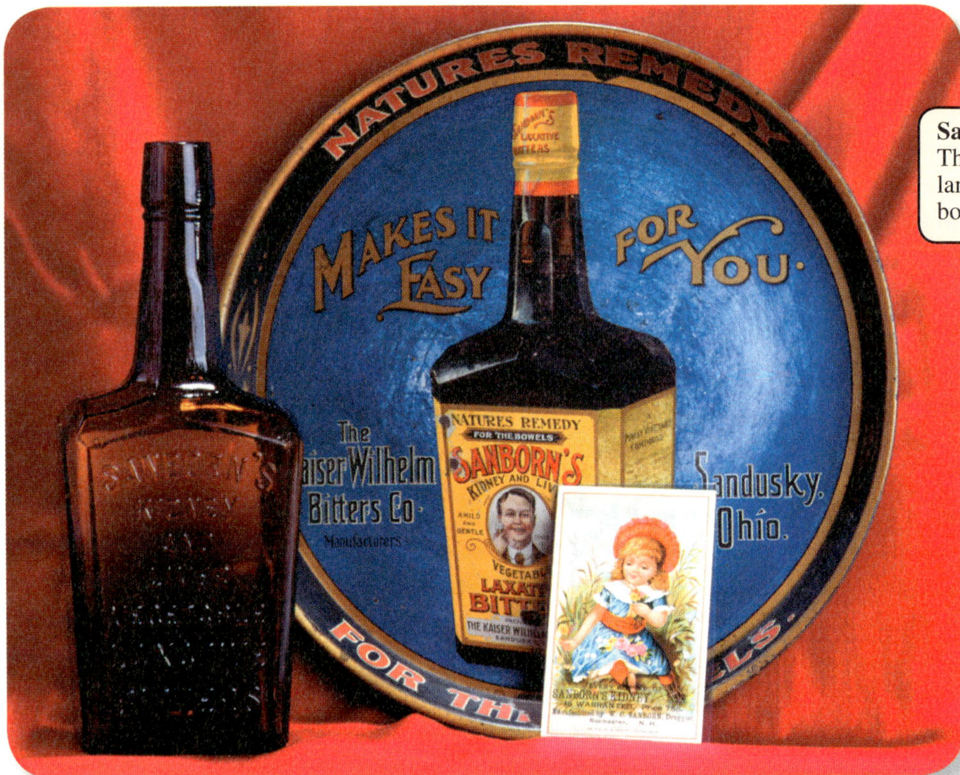


**Sanborn's Kidney and Liver Vegetable Laxative Bitters**
The titles of the medicinal products of this era reflect the flowery language in fashion in the 1800s. This extravagance was seen both in the language and elaborate art of the advertising.

*Spirits on the Human Mind and Body"* which condemned the drinking of alcohol and helped in the social acceptance of drinking bitters. The Revenue Act of 1862 further stimulated bitters consumption by heavily taxing liquor more than medicine. This successful and lengthy fraud on the American people was terminated by the vigorous protest of the Women's Christian Temperance Union (W.C.T.U.), organized in 1874. It remained, however, for the Anti-Saloon League of America, organized in 1895, to bring the final legislative pressures which led to national prohibition in 1920.[1,2,9]

Granny in her parlor, the deacon in his study, or the teacher preparing the next day's lesson by candlelight wouldn't dream of taking a swig of whiskey but "Lash's Kidney and Liver Bitters" or one of its competitors, which afforded similar health benefits, was another story. There apparently was a whisper of naughtiness about bitters since bottle diggers frequently find old bitters bottles hidden in out-of-the-way places such as attic corners, between walls studs, under barns and, apparently the most popular of all, in privies!

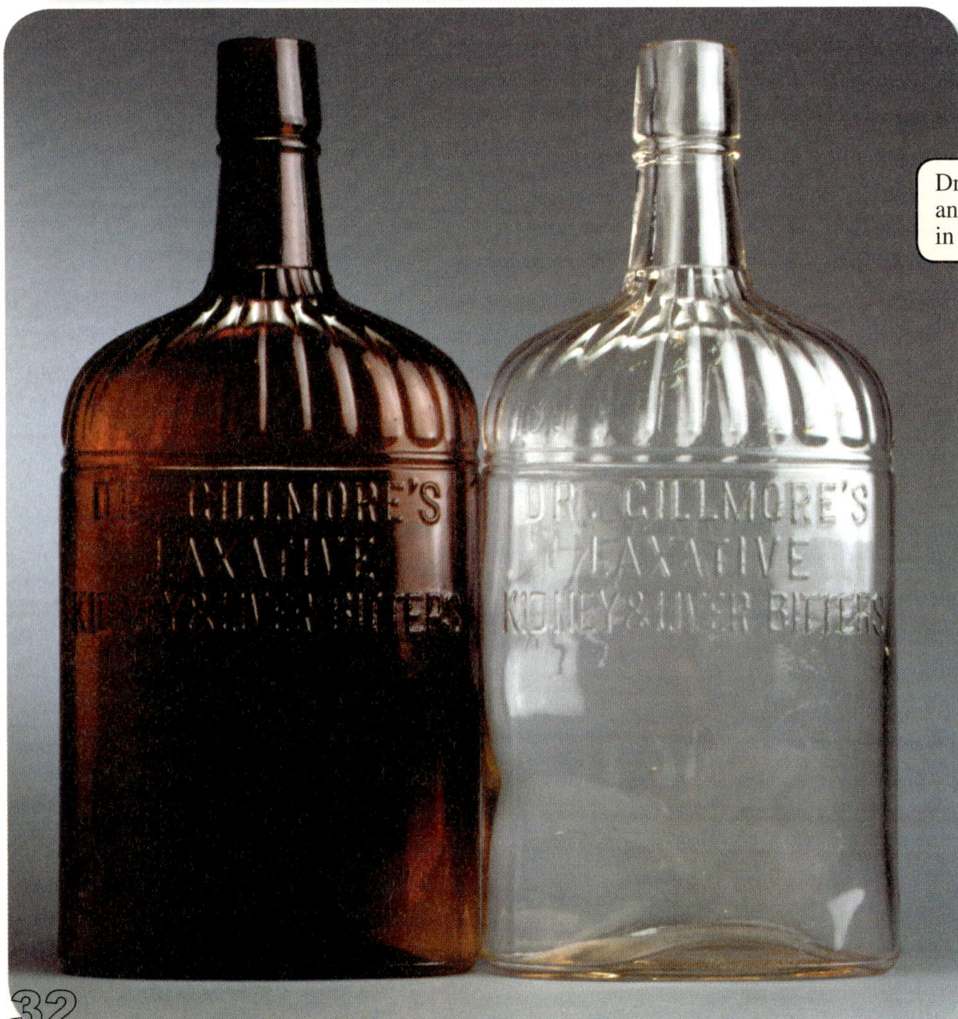


Dr. Gillmore's Laxative Kidney and Liver Bitters is a fine bottle in both amber and clear glass.

The makers of bitters made efforts to convince the teetotalers and advocates of temperance that their products were helpful. The peddlers of "Drake's Plantation Bitters" stated, "Let it be understood that Plantation Bitters is an alcoholic restorative. But mark this, it is strictly a medicine not a beverage. It is to be taken in limited quantities at its stated times, like other remedies and antidotes, and therefore its use is in accordance with temperance law, as well as with that 'higher law' which renders it incumbent upon every being gifted with reason to resort to the best possible means of accomplishing a salutary end." In addition the manufacturer

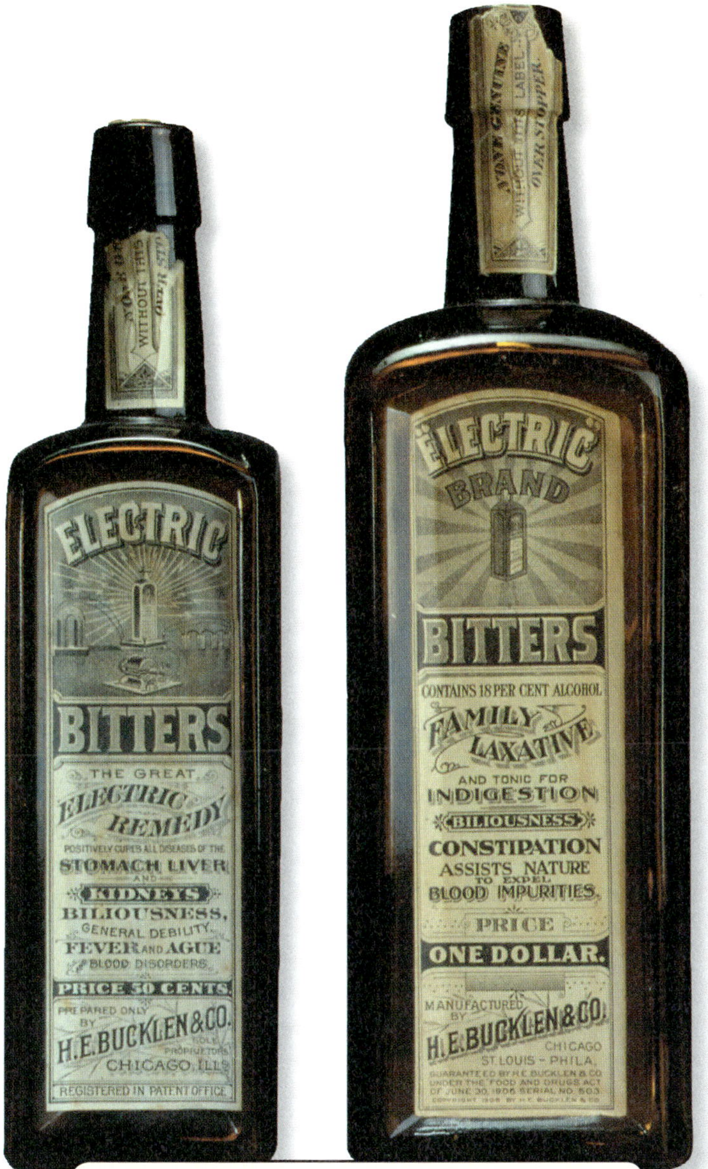


**Electric Bitters**
" When Herbert E. Bucklen, of Chicago, Ill. made application for his trademark, he claimed 'this great electric remedy positively cures all diseases of the kidney, stomach, liver and general debility.' The brand was first sold in 1880 but within ten years was one of the most popular selling bitters in the North America. The larger size bottle is much less common."(8)

tried to sell the idea that the alcohol served to intensify and preserve the described medicinal qualities of the bitters. For example: "Rush's Bitters commend themselves to the favor of temperance physicians and the leading friends of temperance everywhere. Rush's Bitters is the only general stimulant that can be freely used without danger of unduly exciting the brain, or creating a morbid thirst for spirits. Rush's Bitters, however, is a medicine, not a beverage; and derives its medical properties from the cordial juices of the tonic, alterative,—antibilious and aperient flowers, roots and herbs which compose it. These are highly aromatic in quality and have their virtues extracted and preserved by the finest spirits of wine that chemistry can produce or human skill obtain. Ten percent of these spirits is derived from the celebrated tonic Oporto grape, the balance from sound wheat, a grain that, according to the most eminent physicians and chemists, yields a more wholesome spirit than any other vegetable substance, and chemically the same with that procured from wine. The spirits used to preserve and intensify Rush's Bitters must not, however, be misunderstood as resembling ordinary brandy or whiskey. . ." Then follows a long and convoluted dissertation which attempts to inform the reader that, somehow, the whiskey and wine in "Rush's Bitters" are different from other similar bitters.[1,2]

Examination of the alcoholic content

**Star Kidney and Liver Bitters**
John Heilrath, and his brother, Robert, opened a grocery store in Sacramento, CA in 1898 after having continued in the family tradition of blacksmithing. Soon they concocted their own line of bitters and were rewarded promptly with success. William Kleinsage, a salesman for the brand, joined the partnership. As sales increased, a small factory with a bottling line was established. Desiring to expand the business to San Francisco, John and William bought Robert's interest and relocated the company in 1912. Robert remained in Sacramento to start a carriage painting shop.(6,7)

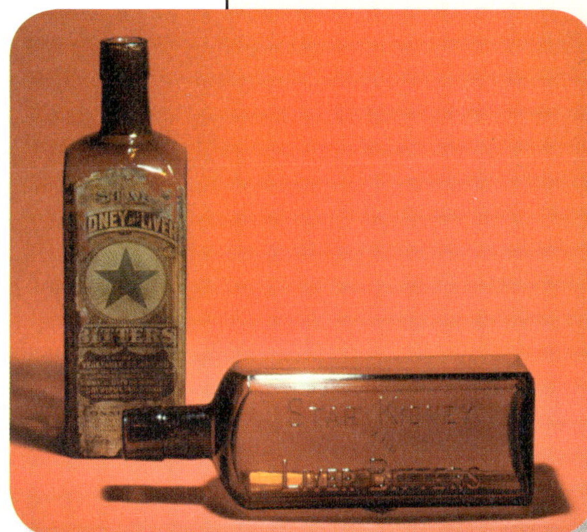


**Wait's Kidney and Liver Bitters**
George Smith Wait began his medicinal business in 1862. The Wait Bitters Company continued till 1920 under the management of sons George and Charles. George's wife lived until 1959! Maybe those bitters did work.(6,7)

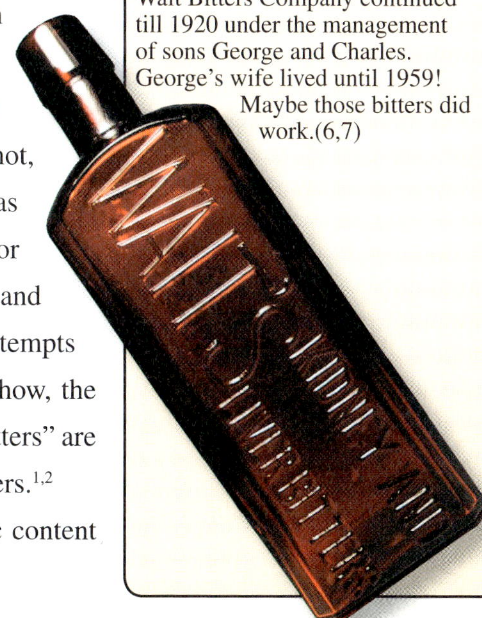

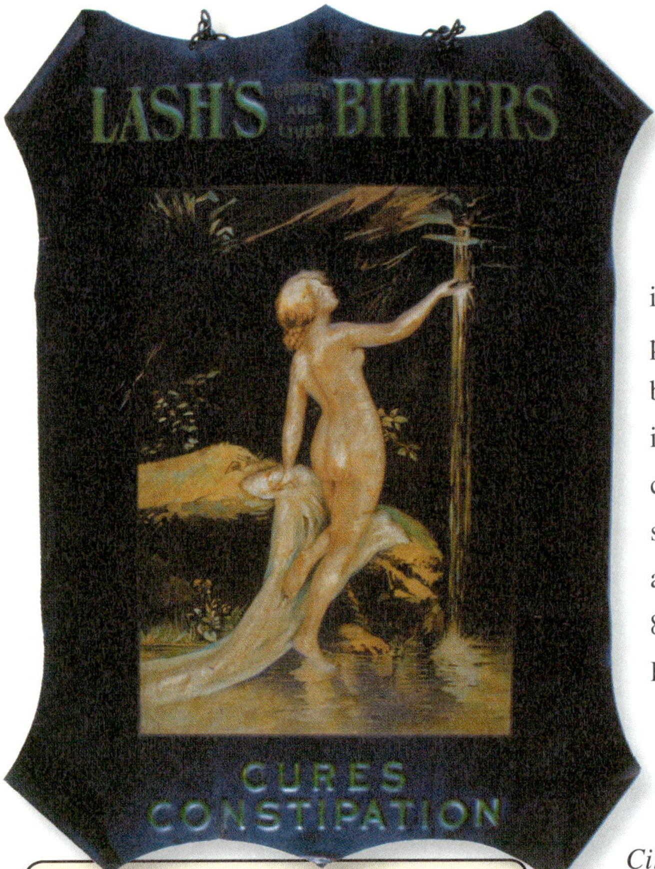


In the Victorian era a public show of nudity was particularly frowned upon. An advertising sign with such a display is certainly rare.

in most of the more popular brands of bitters of the late 1800s, illustrates how bitters could acceptably substitute for liquor, as most whiskey was 80 to 90 proof. Dr. H.W. Vaughn, State Assayer of Rhode Island, wrote in the June 1882 *Druggists Circular* that many of the popular bitters equaled or exceeded these standards. For example, "Hostetter's Bitters" was 86 proof, "Baker's" 81 proof, "Atwood's" 80 proof and "Drakes Plantation" 76 proof.[1,2,9]

Although it is realistic to believe that many Americans consciously consumed bitters as a liquor substitute for economic and social reasons, it is only reasonable to assume that many other people were convinced that they were drinking medicine. Success of the bitters business was not dependent on the product, but on excessive promotion and marketing

**Leaks Kidney and Liver Bitters**
Very similar in bottle shape and lettering to Lash's Kidney and Liver Bitters.

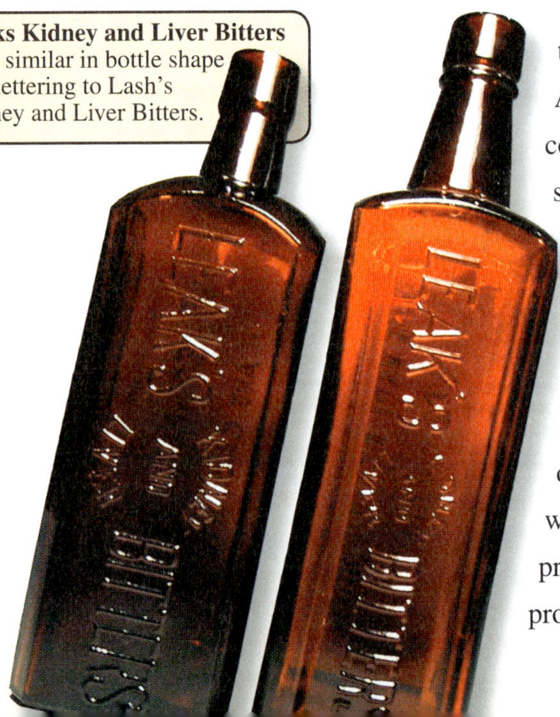

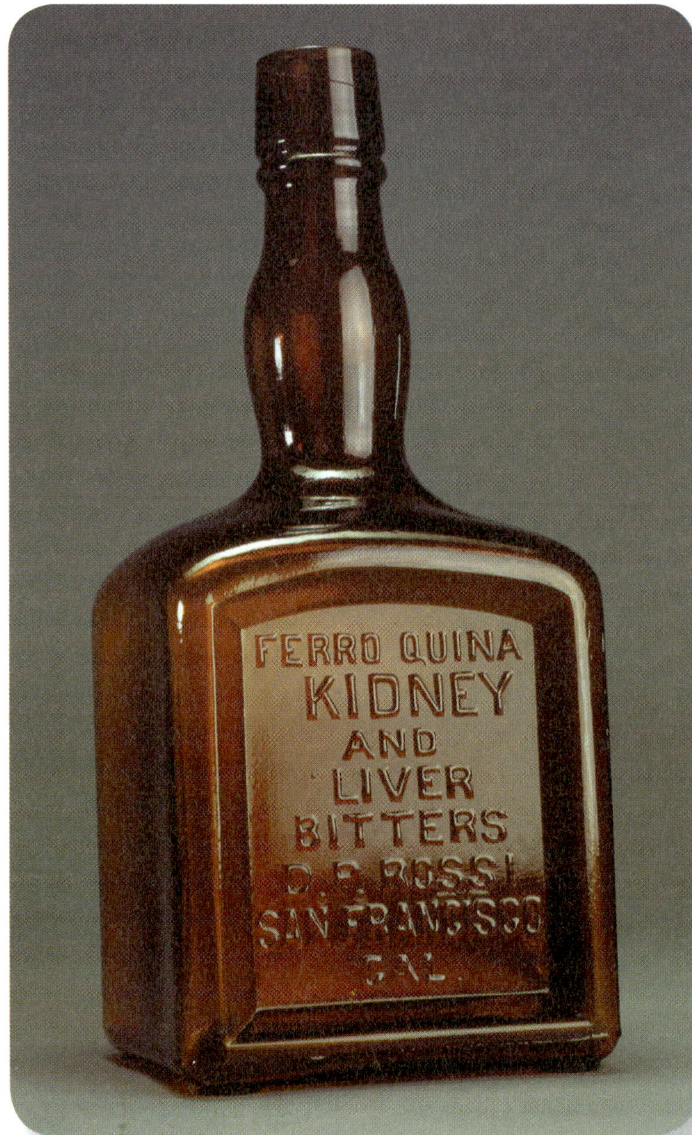


**Ferro Quina Kidney and Liver Bitters**
Angelo Rossi with his family came from Italy to San Francisco in 1875. Angelo's older son, Pietro, was educated in chemistry and became the junior partner in a drug store. In 1885 Pietro joined his brother, Domenico, to establish their own drug store on Dupont Street. They began distributing Ferro China Bisleri Bitters from Milano, Italy. It sold so well that they decided to create their own brand using ferrous sulfate and quinine as the principal ingredients. The company prospered and produced six variants of the Ferro Quina bottle. Eventually in 1906 the company was hard hit by an earthquake and the Food and Drug Act of 1906. By prohibition the Ferro Quina brand died.(6,7)

by the manufacturer. For example, because of its claims and testimonials "Hostetter's Bitters" was sold to the Federal government at the start of the Civil War as a before battle "invigorant". The government bought the bitters by the boxcar load. After the war, one historian wrote, "Hostetter's vaunted remedial properties were sadly lacking, but many a frightened Yankee at Gettysburg knew he faced Pickett's Charge as bravely as he did because of a swig of Hostetter's under his belt." Although "Hostetter's Bitters" practically guaranteed victory in battle and gold to the California prospector, it could not cure Hostetter's own kidney ailment from which he died in 1888.[1,2]

The Federal government, struggling with Civil War expenses, passed the Revenue Act of 1862 that levied an extensive system of sales taxes. However, as alcohol was taxed significantly more than proprietary medicines, the consumption of bitters increased dramatically

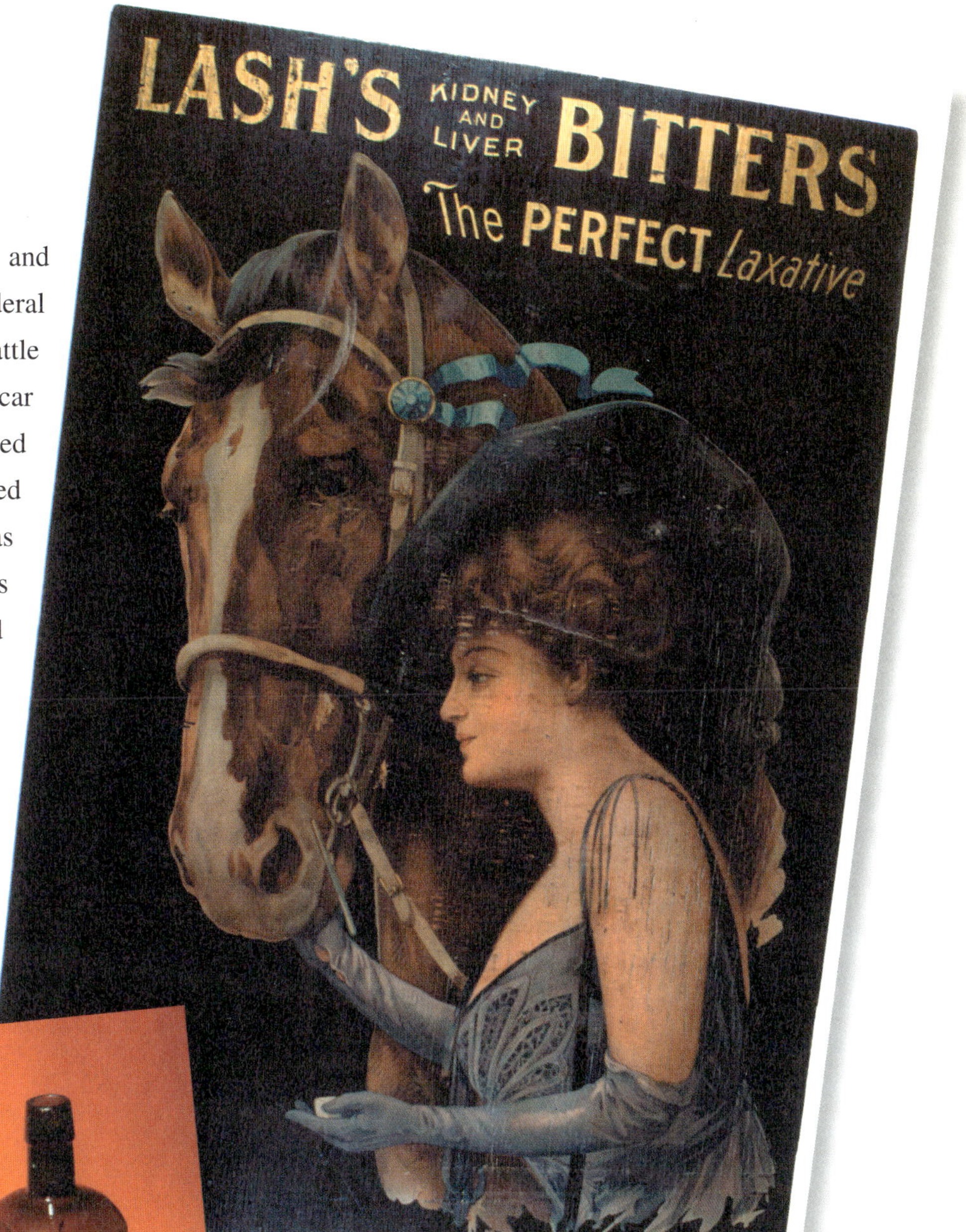


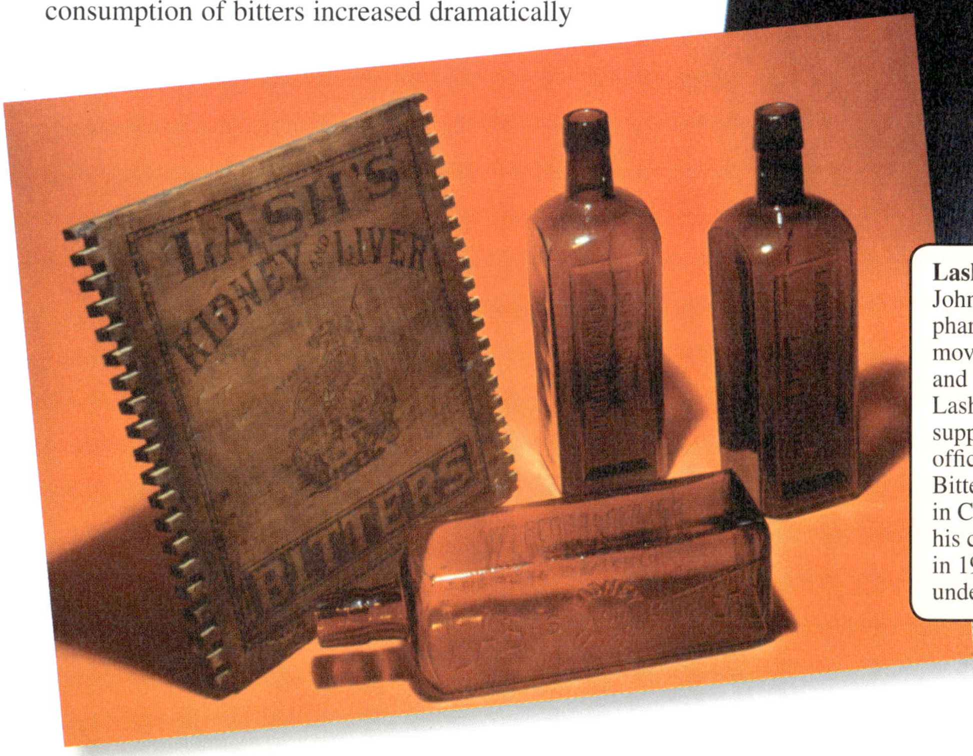


**Lash's Kidney and Liver Bitters**
John J. Spieker was born in Cincinnati, Ohio where he learned the pharmaceutical business. In 1875, as a young man of 20 years, he moved to California. He took a position in a Sacramento drug store and by 1880 he owned the place. In 1883 he partnered with Tito M. Lash in the wholesaling of proprietary medicines. Spieker was to supply the know-how and Lash the cash. Spieker and Lash opened offices in San Francisco and successfully began the sale of Lash's Bitters. After buying out Lash's interest, Spieker established offices in Chicago and New York. Spieker died a wealthy man in 1914, but his company continued successfully for many years. His wife died in 1943 after years of charitable work by providing scholarships for underprivileged students.(6,7)

since the imbibers responded to the cost advantage of bitters as well as the clever claims of the promoters. Because of this increased popularity of bitters between 1860 and 1900, the majority of collectable bitter bottles was produced during this period.[3,4,5,6,7]

In 1905 a series of revealing articles was published by reporter Samuel Hopkins Adams entitled *"The Great American Fraud."* Described were the evils and widespread presence of ardent spirits and opiates. The subsequent passage of the Pure Food and Drug Act in 1906 struck hard at the industry. The manufacturers were now required to reveal how much alcohol was present in their products. With the industry's deception now removed, the nostrum makers were fair game for the full fury of the temperance corps. Established in 1920, National Prohibition finally delivered the deathblow to the bitters business despite the repeal of prohibition in 1933.[1,2,9]

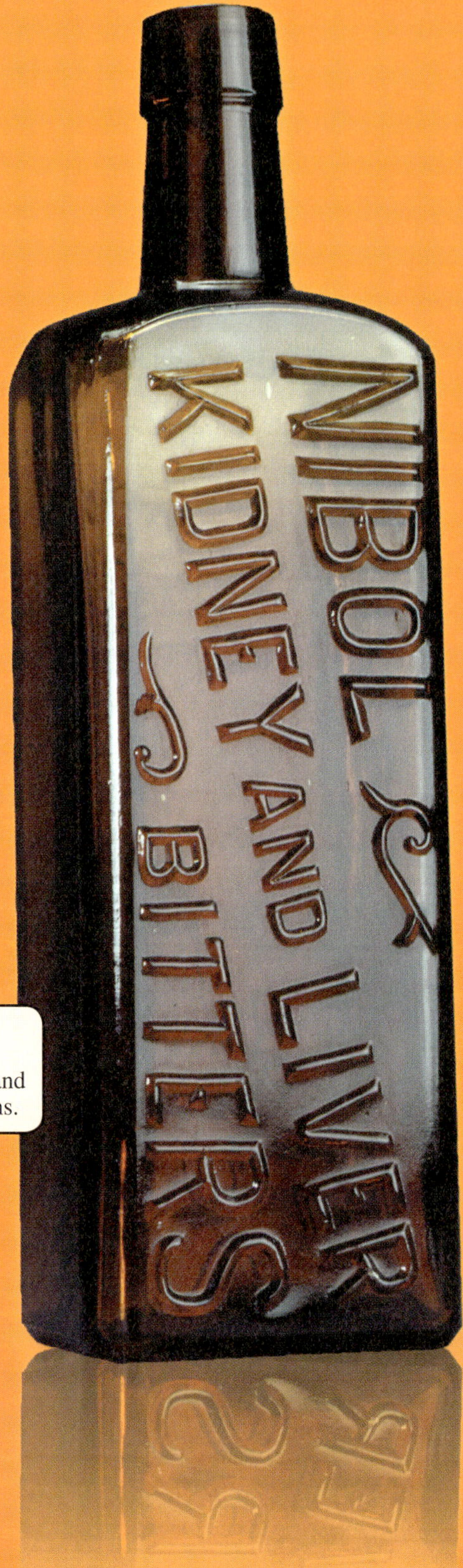


**Nibol's Kidney and Liver Bitters**
The success of the bitters industry depended on creative merchandising and not on the merit of their bottled potions.

Chapter 6

# Cures

The famous second century physician, Claudius Galen, said, “All who drink of the remedy are cured, except those whom it does not help, who will die. Therefore, it is clear that it works in all but incurable cases.” There are few things new under the sun. Certainly the word cure is not one of them.[2]

The Great Niagara Rheumatic And Kidney Cure

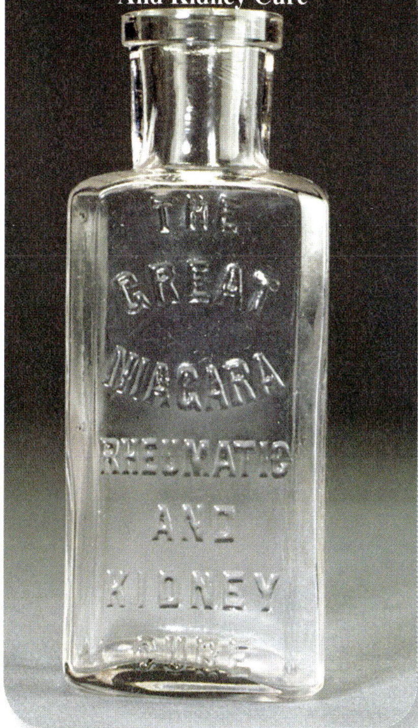


During the patent medicine era the promise of a quick cure was applied to all ailments. Magic elixirs and nostrums came with a written guarantee to cure and restore to health all helpless victims. There were no restraints on the exuberant advertiser except the limit of his imagination and a shrewd appraisal of the public’s gullibility. A disease remission was deemed equivalent to a medical healing and upon this evidence broad inclusive claims of a “cure” were made.

Embossed on the nostrum bottle were charming names with promises of cure for all types of complaints and ailments. There were “cures” for weakness, ague, cancer, colic, chill, dandruff, apoplexy, rheumatism, cholera, distemper, fits, backache, fever, diarrhea, dropsy, consumption, heart, catarrh, headache, drunkenness, Bright’s Disease, corns, mosquito bite, weak lungs, pus, cold, rupture, diabetes, la grippe, and even more.[1,2,4,6]

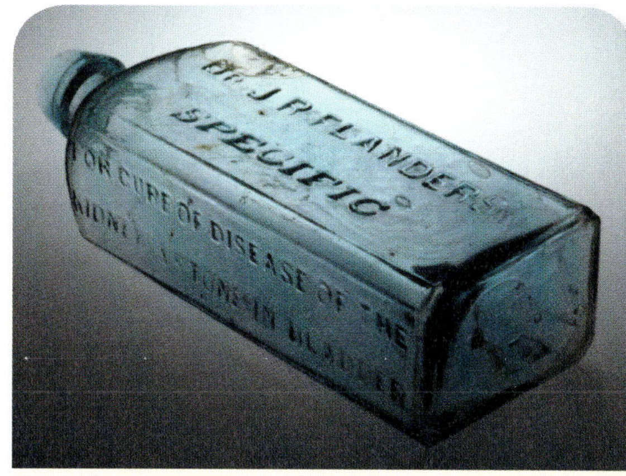


Dr. J.R. Flanders Specific for Cure of Disease of the Kidneys and Stone in Bladder. The only kidney related cure sold prior to 1850. Only two such bottles are known to exist.

To embellish the embossed title on the bottle, the word cure was modified and enhanced by these descriptive adjectives: “Sure,” “No. 1,” “Poor Man’s,” “Famous,” “Greatest,” “Magic,” “Never Fail To,” “Reliable,” “Certain,” “Wonder Worker,” “Electric,” “Safe,” “Turkey,” “Electric Mode,” “Balm,” “Imperial,” “East India,” “Instant,” “Household,” “Swedish,” “Nature’s,” “Double Chloride of Gold,” “Peruvian,” “Indian,” “Swamp Root,” “Vegetable,” “New,” “American,” “Speedy,” “Radical,” “Magnetic Oil,”

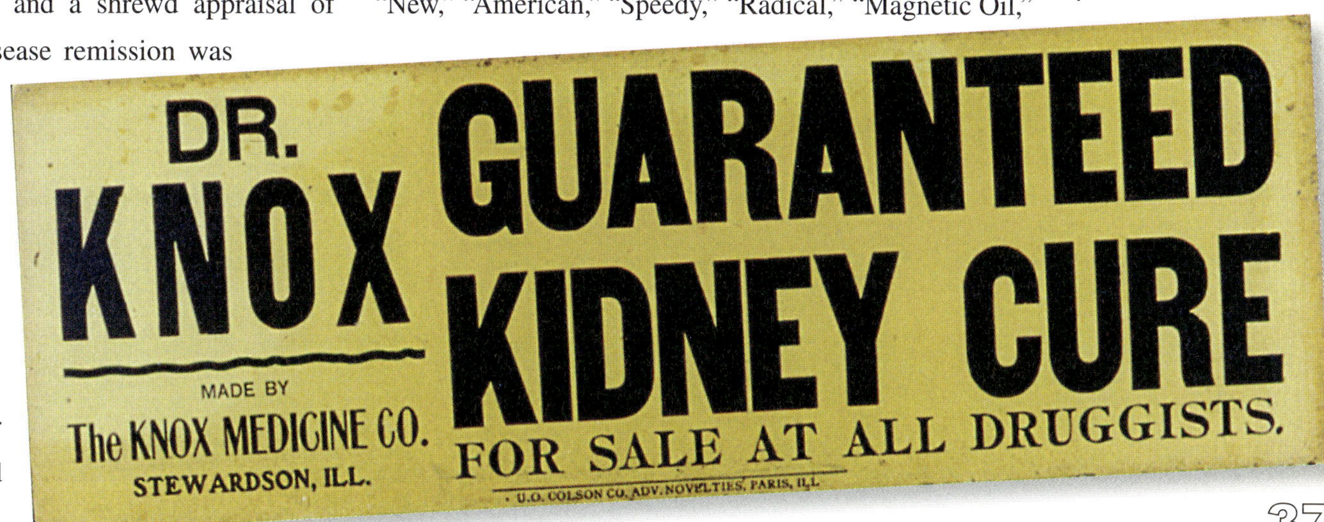

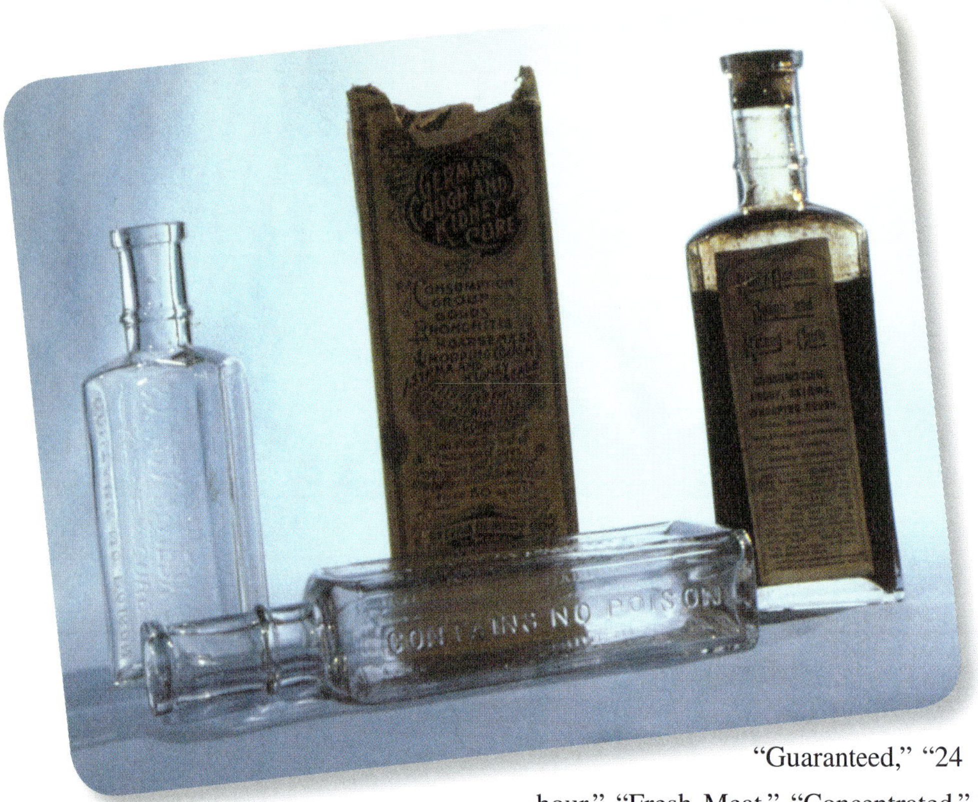


"Guaranteed," "24 hour," "Fresh Meat," "Concentrated," "Arctic Flower," "Great Peppermint," "Infallible," "Quick," "Miraculous," "Original," "Best," "Celery," "Celebrated," "Gift," "Popular," "King," "Lightning," "Tasteless," "Unk Weed," "Cherry," "African," "Restorative," "German," "Family," "White Pine," "Wonderful," "Specific."[1,2,4,6]

Prior to 1850 during the era of pontilled bottle manufacturing there were approximately sixty different "cure" medicinals. However, during this period, only one specific urinary "cure" with the pontil mark was known to exist, "Dr. J.R. Flanders Specific For Cure of Disease of the Kidneys and Stone in Bladder." After 1850 "cure" medicinals for all ailments were produced in abundance. Today over three thousand different embossed "cure" bottles are known to exist. Of these "cure" nostrums approximately one hundred relate to the genito-urinary system.[7] Titles of a few are: "Dr. J.C. Batdorf Magnetic Liver and Kidney

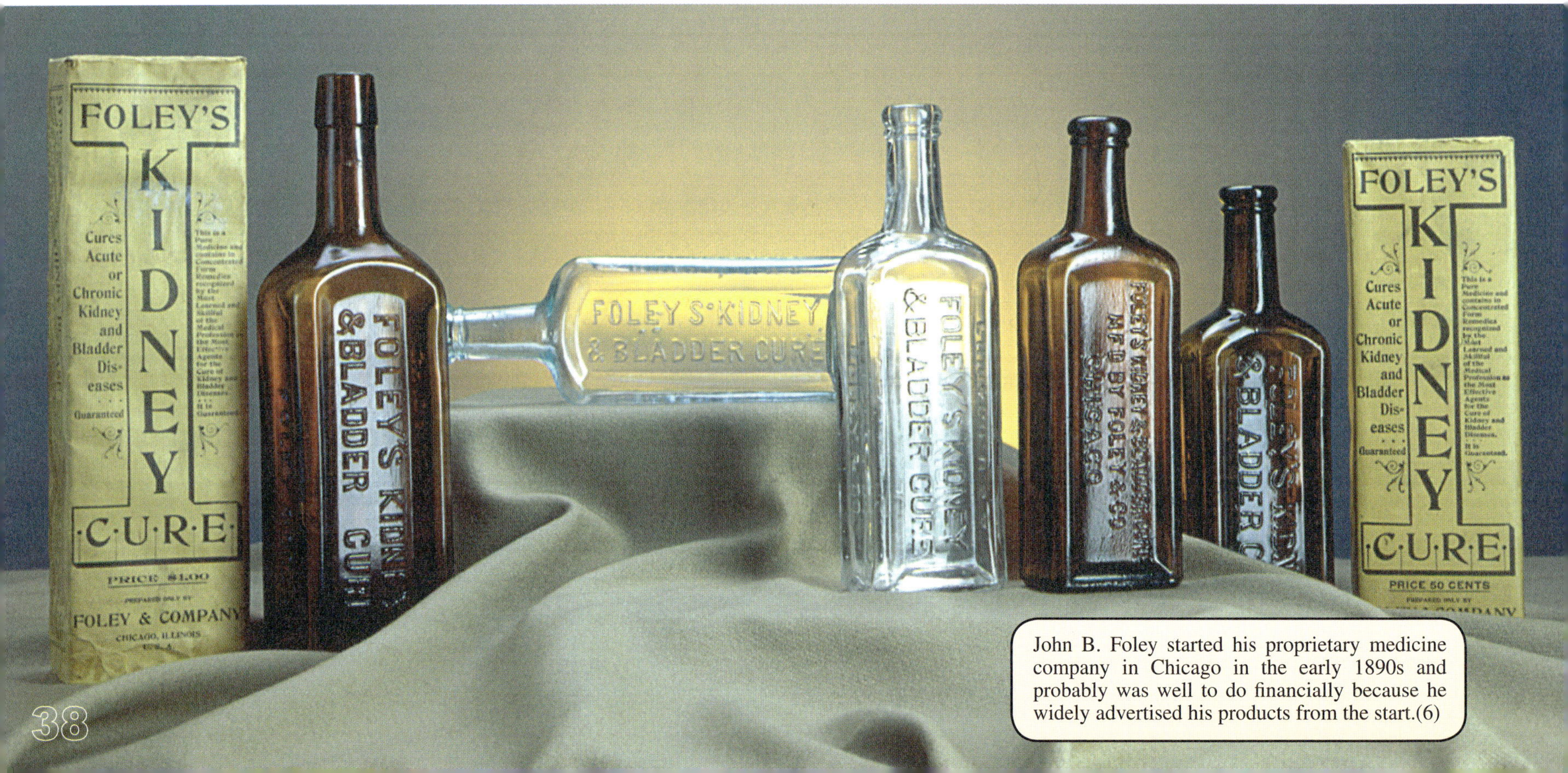


John B. Foley started his proprietary medicine company in Chicago in the early 1890s and probably was well to do financially because he widely advertised his products from the start.(6)

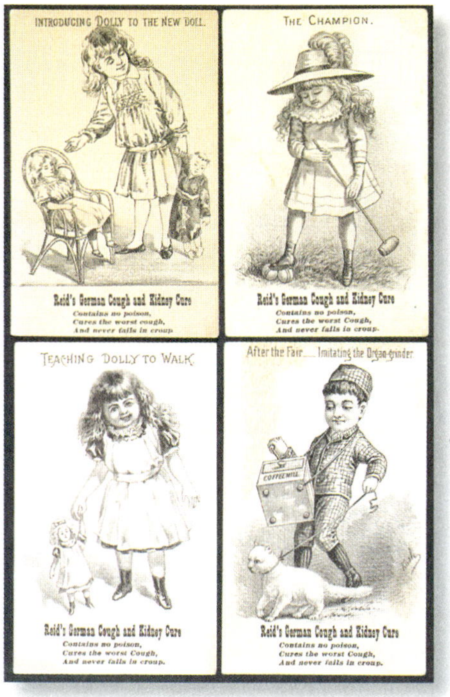


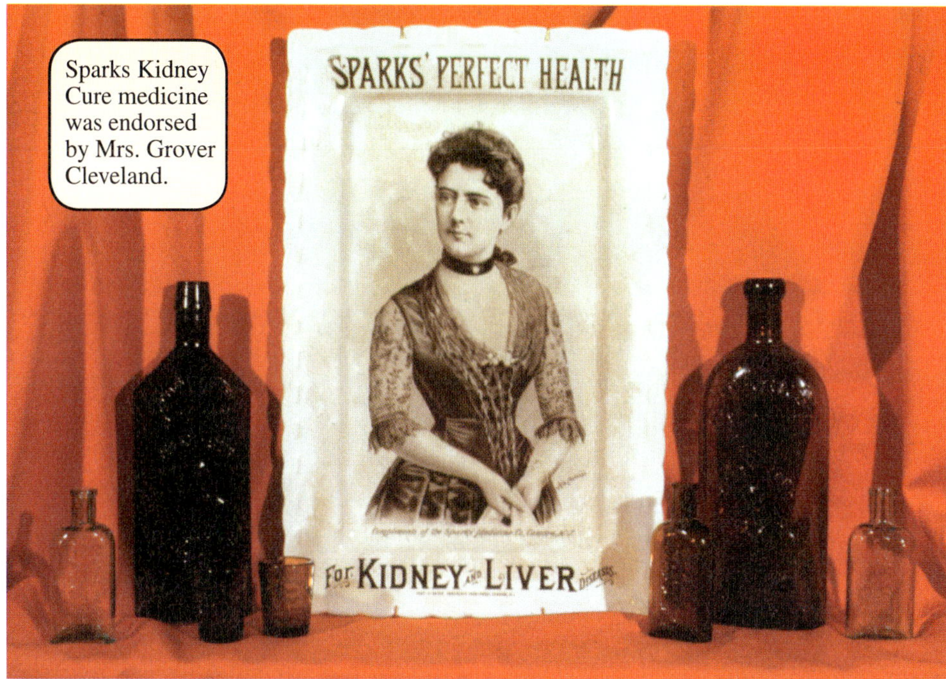


Sparks Kidney Cure medicine was endorsed by Mrs. Grover Cleveland.

Cure," "Brightbane the Great Kidney and Stomach Cure," "The Great Niagara Rheumatic and Kidney Cure," "The HKB Sure Cure for Heart, Kidney and Bladder."

Some of the most desirable of all "cure" bottles to collect are the Dr. Craig's Kidney Cures. They are rare beauties, and to collect all five types is very difficult. The most coveted of this group is the bottle that displays the embossed kidneys. From its label we read that the contents of the bottle were supposed to cure dropsy, jaundice, impotency, and diseases of the urinary organs, and that it was the only remedy known to cure Bright's disease. The bottle sold for one dollar. The last in the series of Dr. Craig's Kidney Cures was entitled "The Original Craig's Kidney Cure." Today only eight such desirable bottles are known to

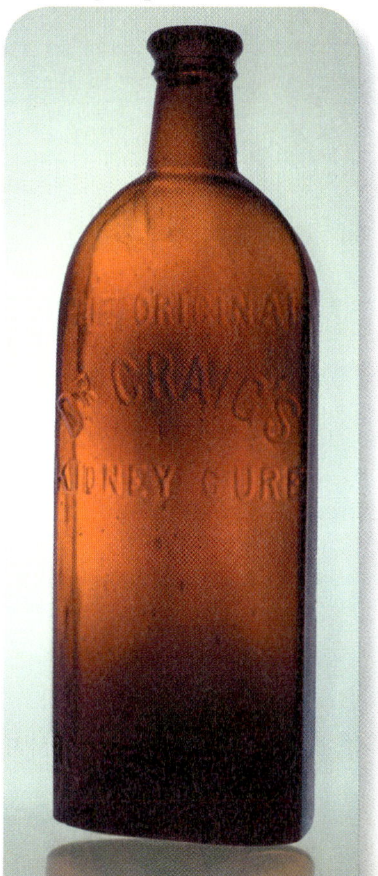


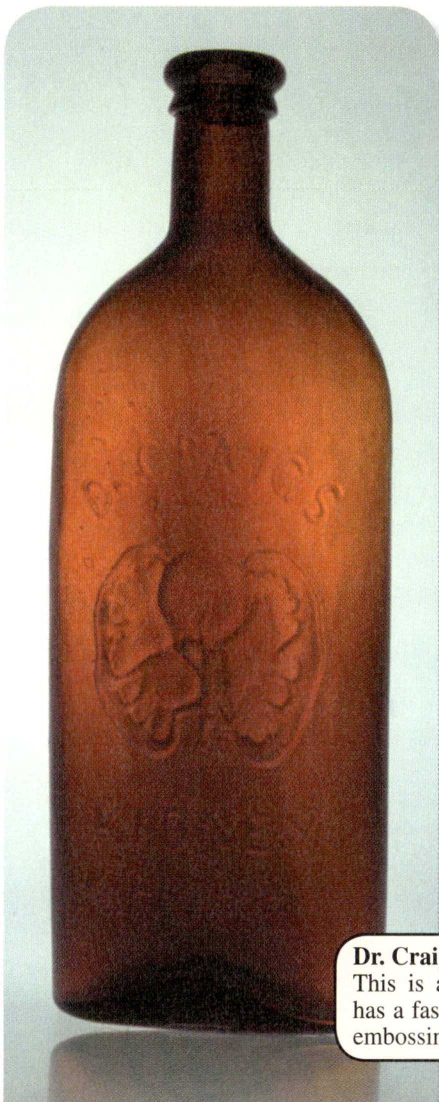

**Dr. Craig's Kidney Cure**
This is a fabulous cure bottle. It has a fascinating history, has great embossing and is very rare.

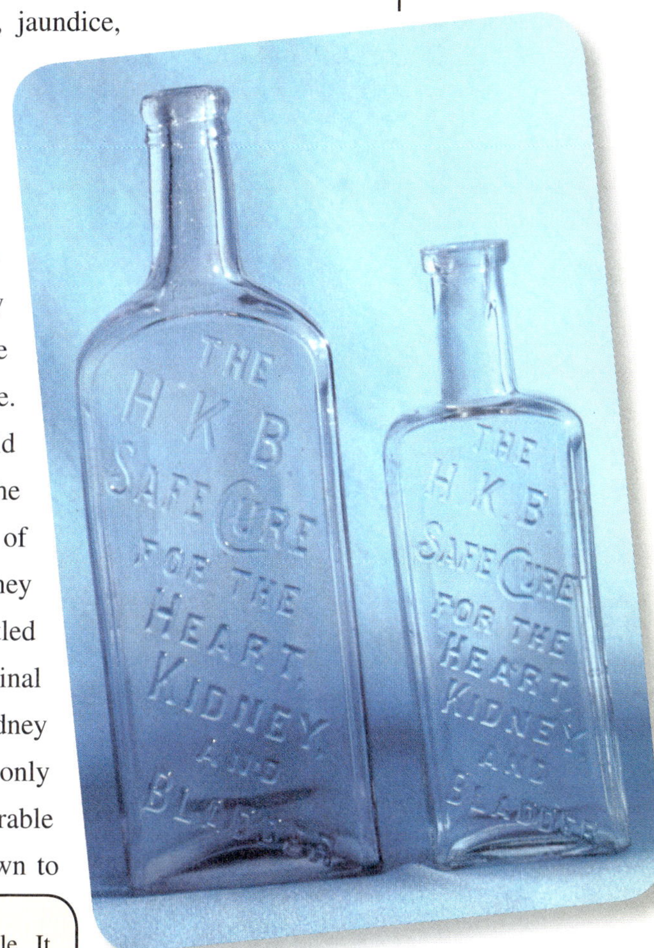

exist. Doctor Craig sold his patent medicine formula to Mr. H.H. Warner, who then peddled it as "Warner's Safe Kidney and Liver Cure." H.H. Warner, the ex-safe manufacturer, followed with a long line of other "safe" nostrums and fashioned the largest patent medicine empire ever to exist.[5]

After the passage of the Pure Food and Drug Act of 1906, shocked Americans learned that these nostrums contained liquor and opiates. The medicinal manufacturers were forced to disclose the bottle's ingredients and to substitute for the word "cure" less utopian words such as "remedy," "elixir," "alterative," "renovator," and "balm."[3]

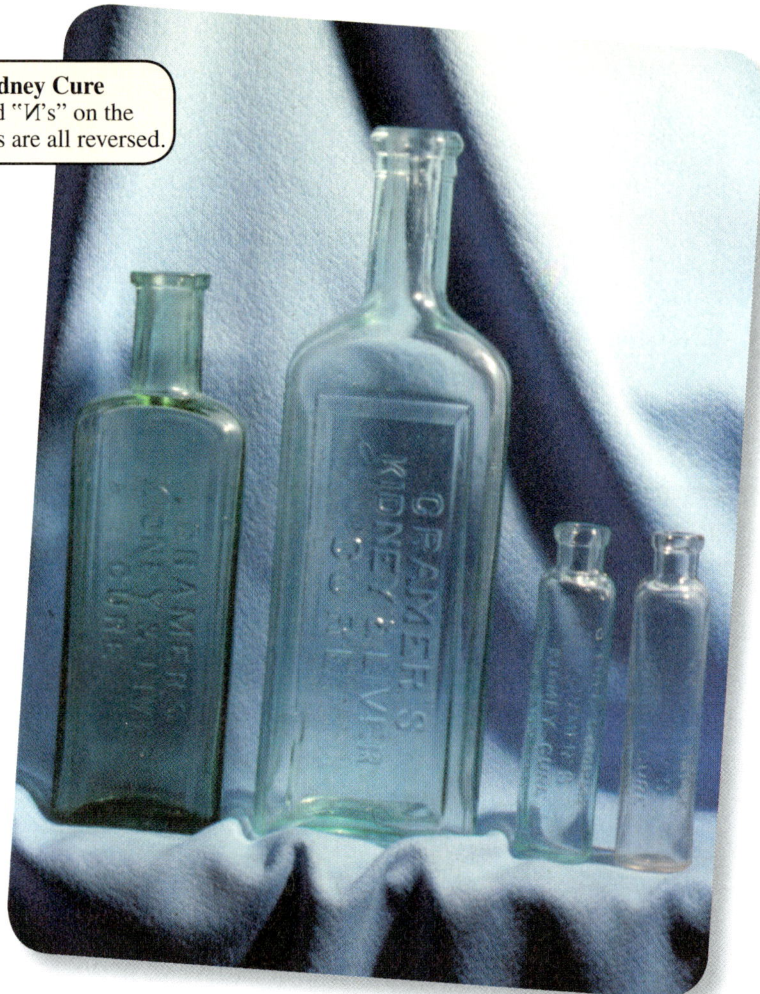


**Cramer's Kidney Cure**
The embossed "И's" on the sample bottles are all reversed.

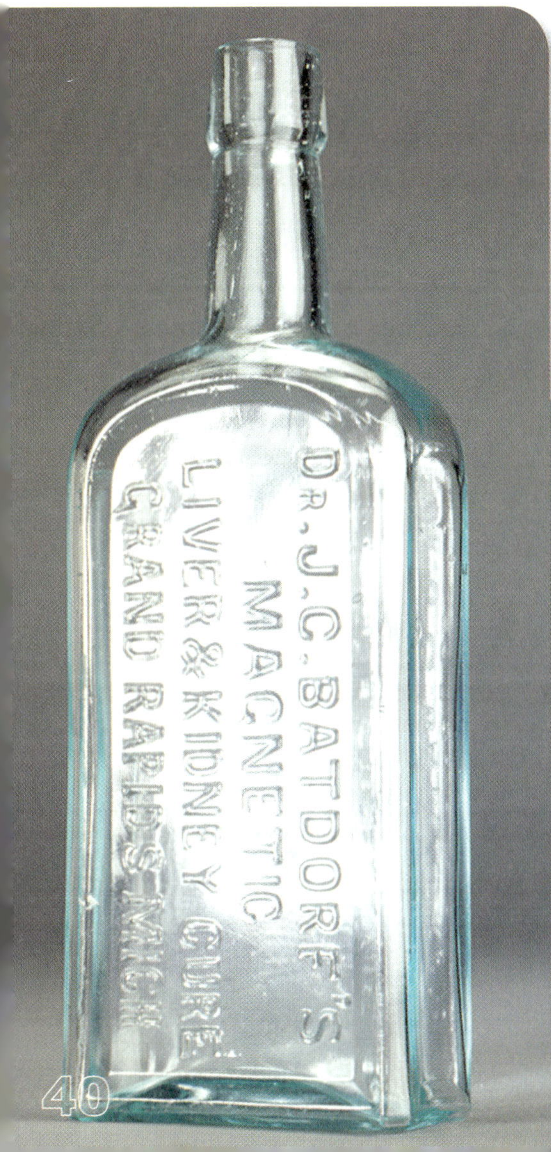


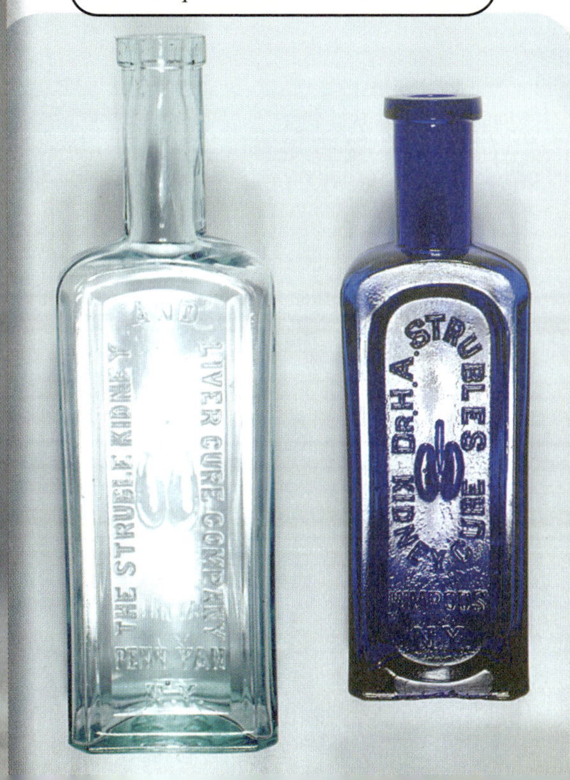


Two fantastic cure bottles. Note the embossed kidneys. Dr. Struble's Kidney Cure in aqua and cobalt blue.

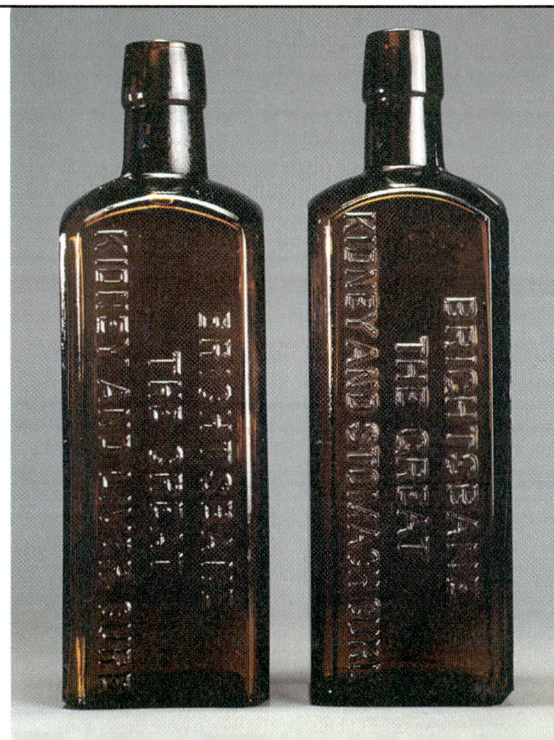


A pair of "great" western cure bottles. Brightbane the Great Kidney and Liver Cure, Brightbane the Great Kidney and Stomach Cure.

# Teas

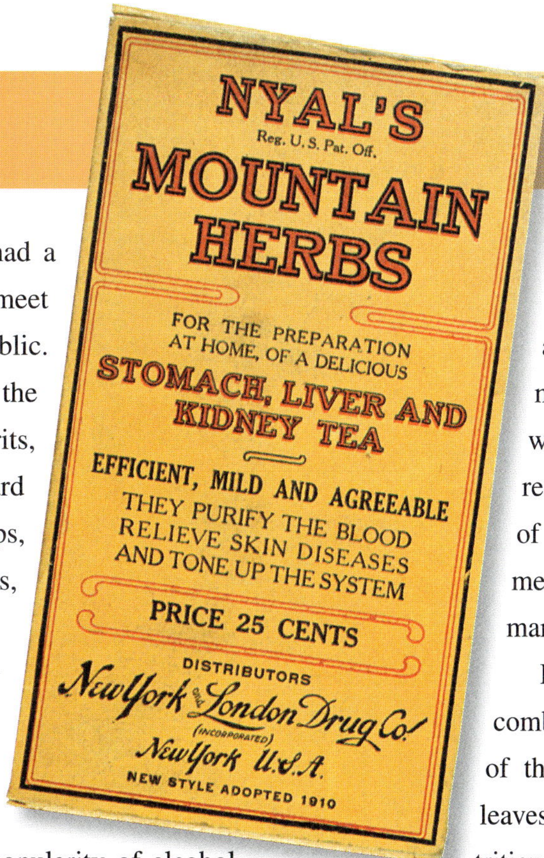


The nostrum peddler had a variety of medicines to meet the needs of the gullible public. He offered quick cures in the form of medicinal spirits, mineral waters, Wizard oils, diuretic pills, syrups, kidney plasters, liniments, and teas.

During the proprietary era commercial medicinal teas never attained a large sales volume. This was in part due to the great popularity of alcohol based nostrums. These ardent spirits continued to have a significant hold on the habits of the imbibers. Also, the consumption of alcohol was less expensive when drunk as a medicine.

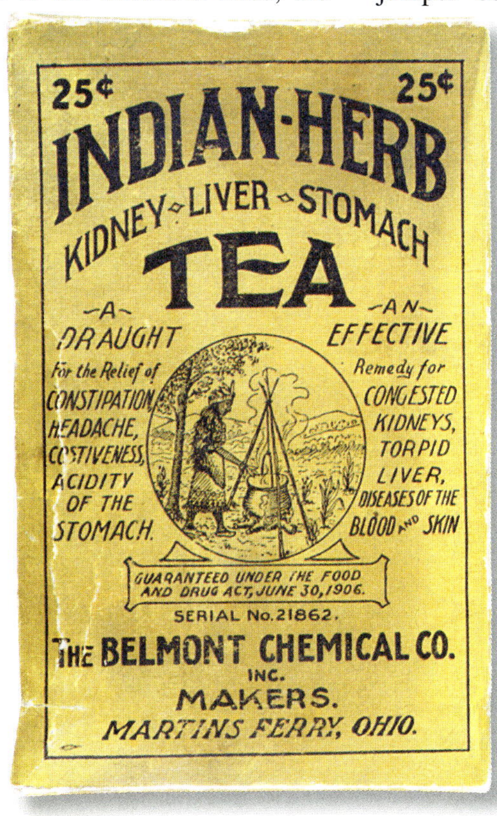


During the era of the doctorless countryside many people turned to herbs for all their "doctoring" needs. Many teas were concocted by local people, who dosed themselves with the herbs all around them. They didn't have to go much farther than their backyard for the "beneficial herbs." Being rooted in the soil in the best folk tradition, country medicine endured for several generations. Since the ingredients of herbal teas were limitless and readily available, the use of medicinal teas was widespread with grandparents passing on their recipes to their offspring. Because of the availability of homemade medicinal teas, there was a limited market for a commercial brand.[1]

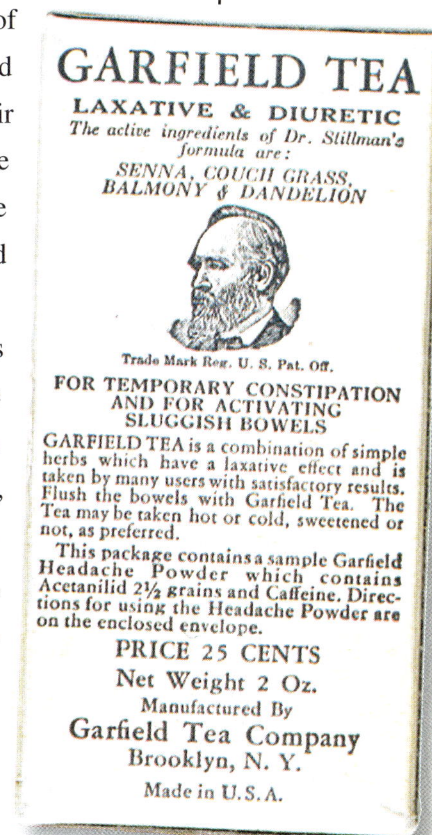


Herbs were selected in various combinations. The list of some of the herbs used included: senna leaves, mandrake root, uva ursi leaves, triticum, witch hazel leaves, bonset and wintergreen leaves, sarsaparilla root, juniper berries, cough grass, balmony, dandelion, buchu, alexandria senna, licorice, broom tops, and parsley piert.

Although the medicinal tea was labeled "kidney tea," the list of maladies to have been benefitted from the concoction was lengthy. Most included such urinary complaints as congested kidneys, tortured kidneys, gravel and bladder afflictions. Also listed were sluggish bowels, torpid liver, headache, costiveness, biliousness, constipation, dropsy, and backache. The tea was described as a laxative and a blood purifier having a diuretic effect.

Since medicinal teas were a proprietary medicine, they became regulated in 1906 when Congress passed the Pure Food and Drug Act.

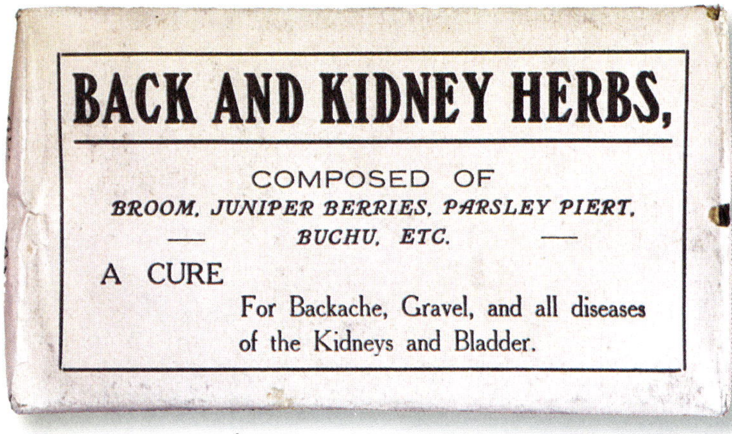


The law required disclosure of the names and amounts of all ingredients and denied the use of the word cure.[2,4]

Interest in tea drinking has never really decreased. Because of fine and exotic teas, tea sipping today is a burgeoning industry. Since 1990, tea sales have more than doubled to $4 billion a year in the United States. Tea had been regarded by most Americans as a bitter tasting second choice to coffee. But in the mid 1990s, interest perked up when studies suggested that green tea could ward off some cancers, deliver large amounts of vitamin C and even fluoride to the teeth. Another study suggested that a cup of black tea a day cuts the risk of heart attacks by 44 percent. Others point out tea's Zen appeal and calming effect.[3]

With all these gourmet delights and beneficial hopes, tea drinking will certainly go on forever. As a result the teacup runneth over, with purveyors only planning to offer more.

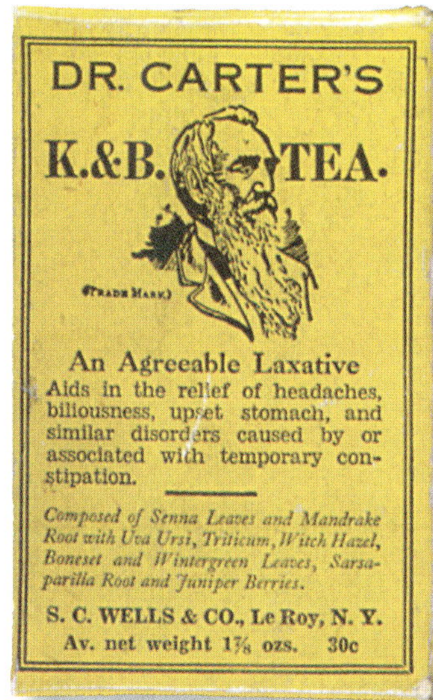


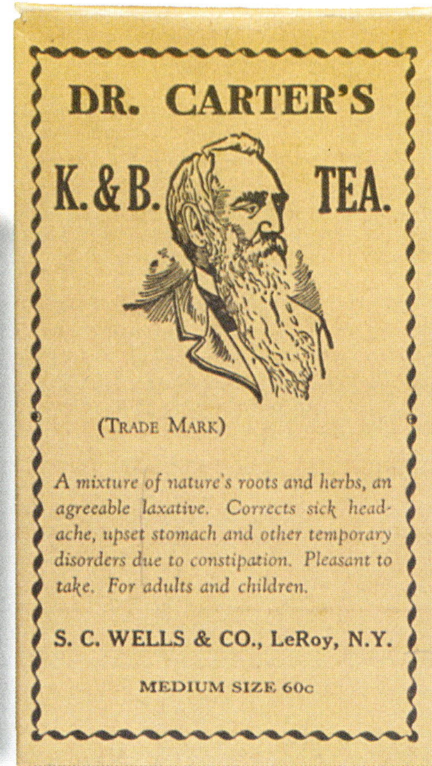


**Carter's Kidney and Bladder Tea**

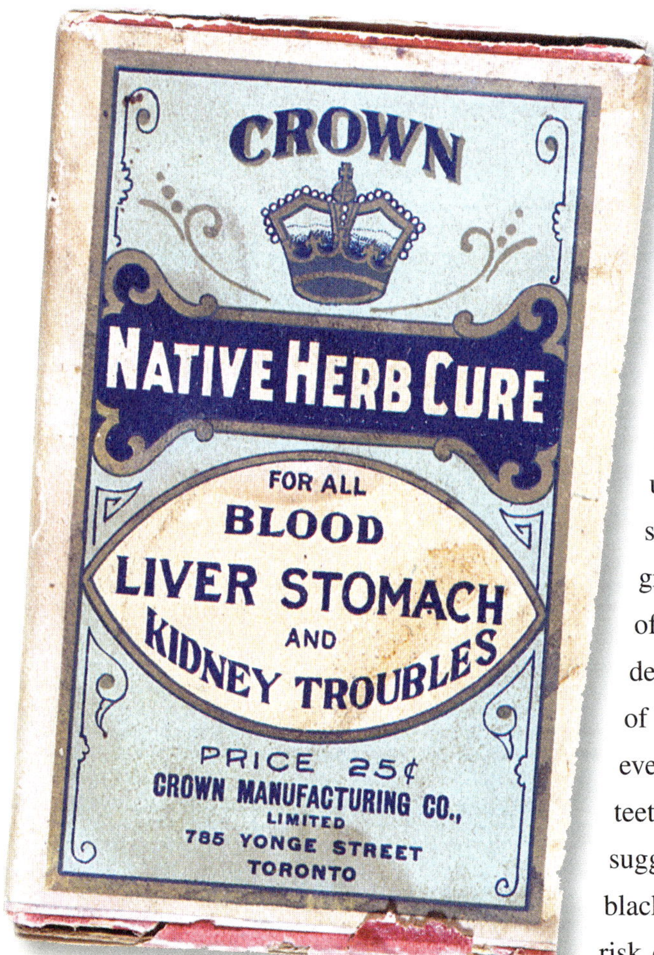


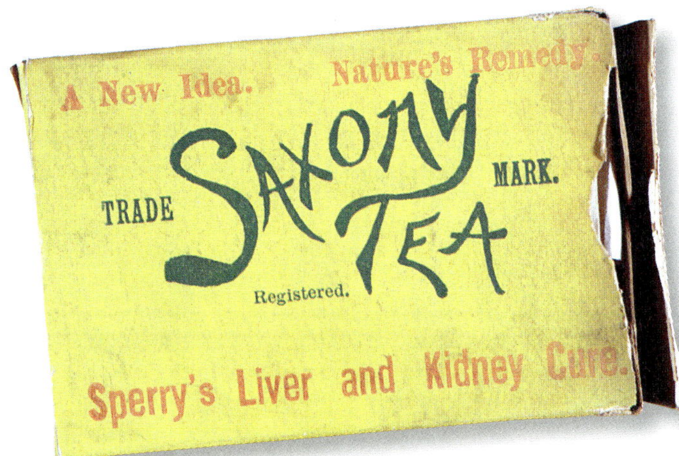

# Pills

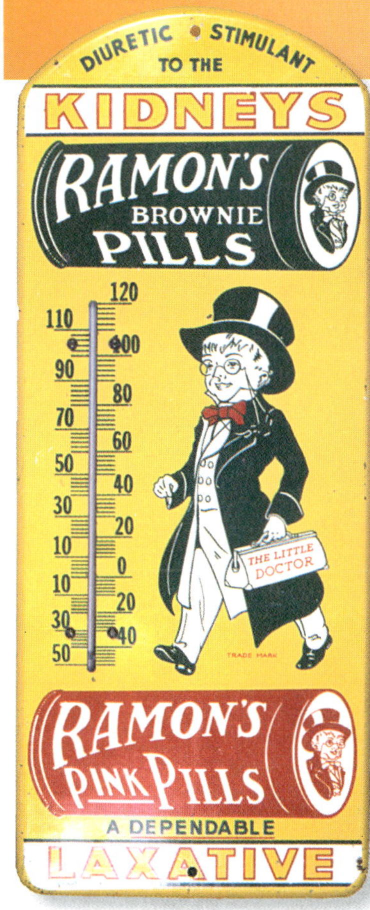


During the colonial period the services of the pharmacist as we know him today were practiced by several different practitioners: pharmacists, apothecaries, druggists and chemists. Also, many apothecaries practiced medicine and physicians often practiced pharmacy.[2]

In the early medicine shops in this country the prescription laboratory was usually a small room, or sectioned area, at the rear of the store. It was here that the pharmacist used ware and apparatus to prepare and package medicines. He would use the pill rolling slab and later, the pill mass mixer, to satisfy the public's demand for pills and capsules. He ground crude drugs and herbs, rolled pills, sifted powders, mixed and bottled liquids, and measured ingredients.[2]

Druggists often compounded one or two patent nostrums under their own names. One choice piece of labeled material from such a container reads, "Harrigan's Onagin—A swell dressing and tonic for the hair. As long as you have hair to put this on, you'll never be bald. Hair denotes strength; Samson was not bald headed, else Delilah would not have fell for him. Blondes prefer gentlemen. Delilah was a blonde. To be up and comin' and look it, wash your head once a week and apply this tonic twice as often. While this is prepared for men, no women will go wrong using it. Concocted in the rear and sold in the front."[1] As P.T. Barnum said, "there's a sucker born every minute."[3]

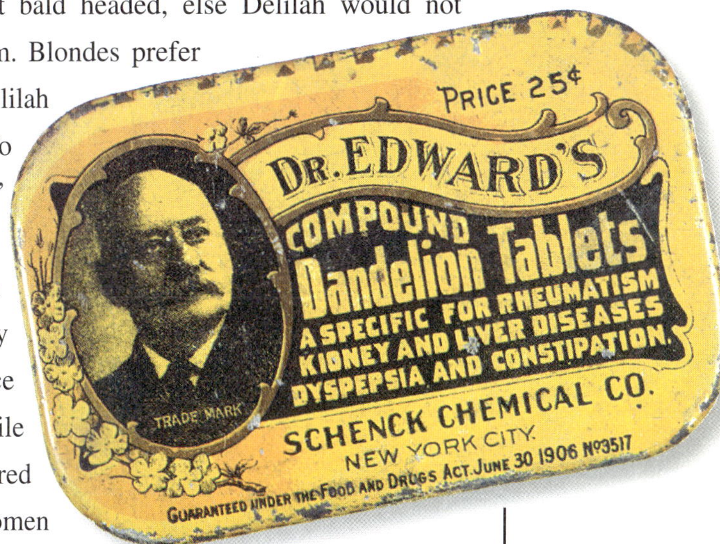


In time the emphasis of the botanic practice of medicine changed. Before, the pharmacist used his knowledge of herbs and crude drugs in the preparation of medicines for dispensing. Later, pharmaceutical factories and chemical works became involved in the manufacture of these nostrums, which were attractively packaged and reasonably priced. The patent medicines that were sold in drug stores

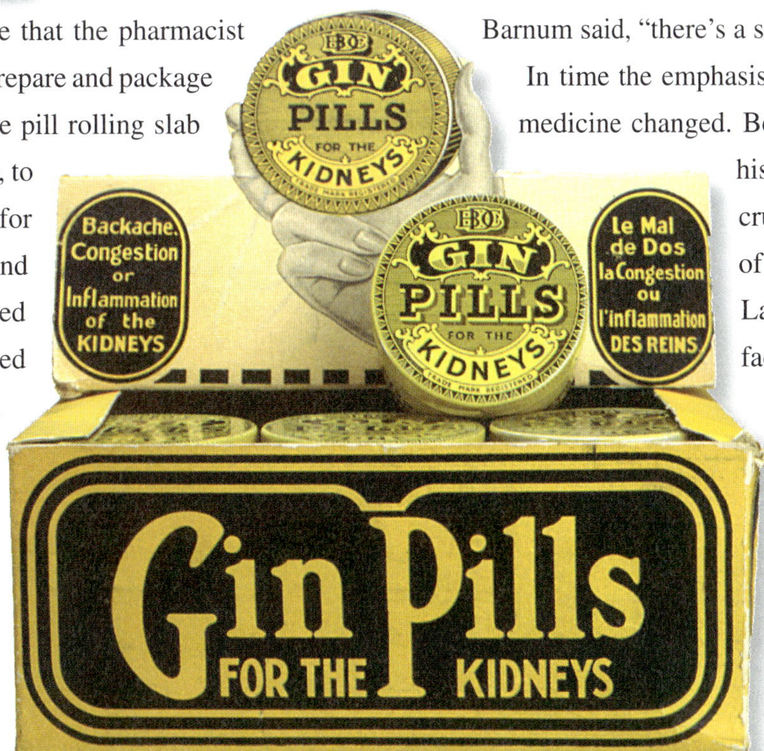

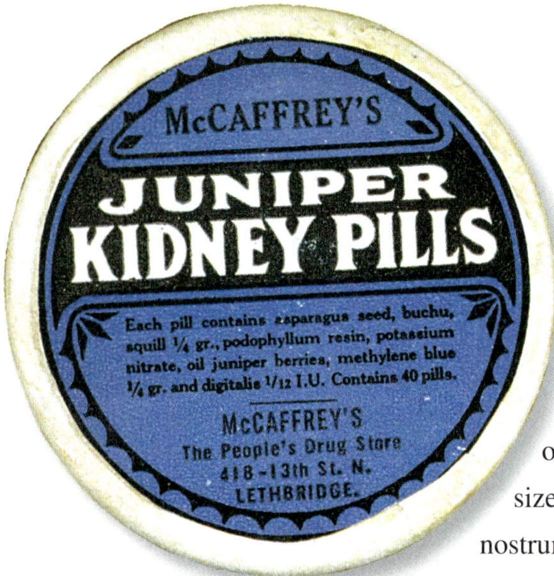


were those that were well known and well advertised. The patent medicine and home remedy section of the old-time drug store became sizeable. Consequently, the sale of these nostrums accounted for a large volume of the pharmacy business particularly during the years of folk medicine and self-dosage.[1,2]

Pills were sold as patent medicine in small containers of wood, glass, tin, and paper-card board. Pills for every ailment were available as a cure, stimulant, regulator, corrective, remedy or specific. Available for urological needs were such medical miracles as "Pettingill's Kidney-Wort Tablets," "Dr. Hobb's Sparagus Kidney Pills," "Dr. Pierce's A-Nuric Tablets," "Hill's Kidney Kaskara Tablets," "Blackburn's Victory Kidney Pills," and many more. The convenience of taking medicine in pill form certainly enhanced the popularity of the pill as a patent medicine.

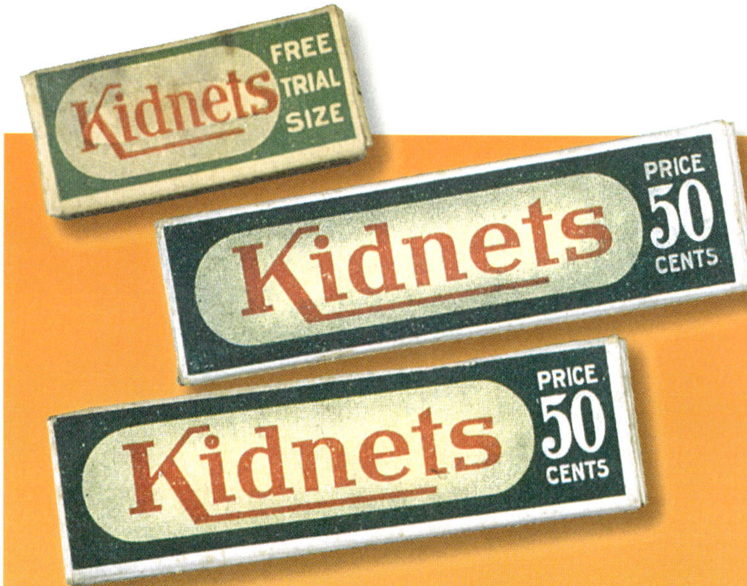


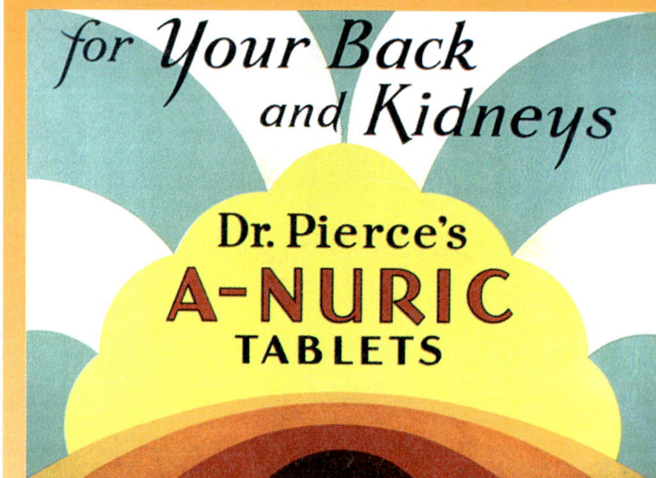


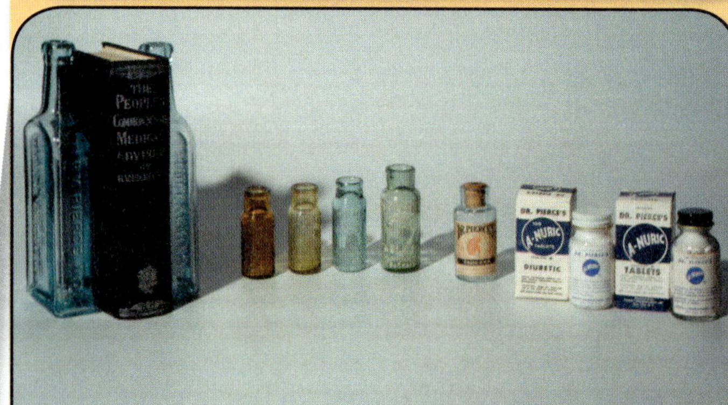

Dr. R.V. Pierce was a man of varied talents. He built the Invalid's Hotel and Surgical Institute in Buffalo, New York, as well as headed the World's Dispensary Medical Association. He would patent medicines under the name of Dr. Pierce and Dr. Sage. It was a bleak farmhouse indeed that did not contain a copy of "The People's Common Sense Medical Advisor in Plain English," Dr. Pierce's crowning work. First published in 1875, it contained 1,008 pages of advice on biology and the human body. Included were recommendations for patent medicines, pages of testimonials, and a map of downtown Buffalo.

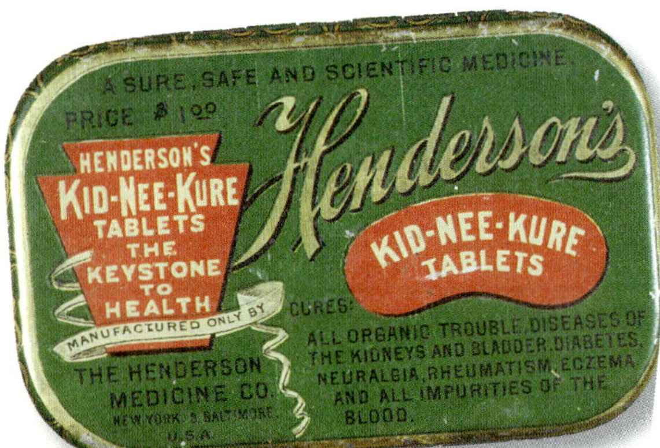


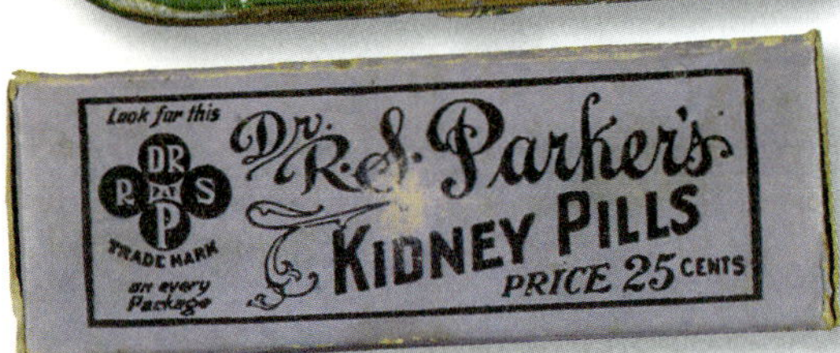


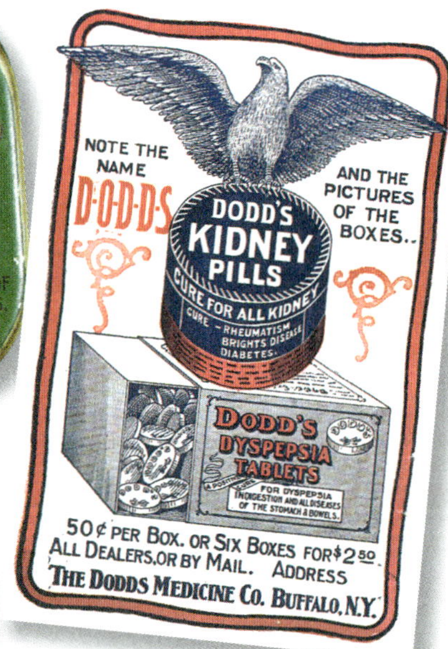

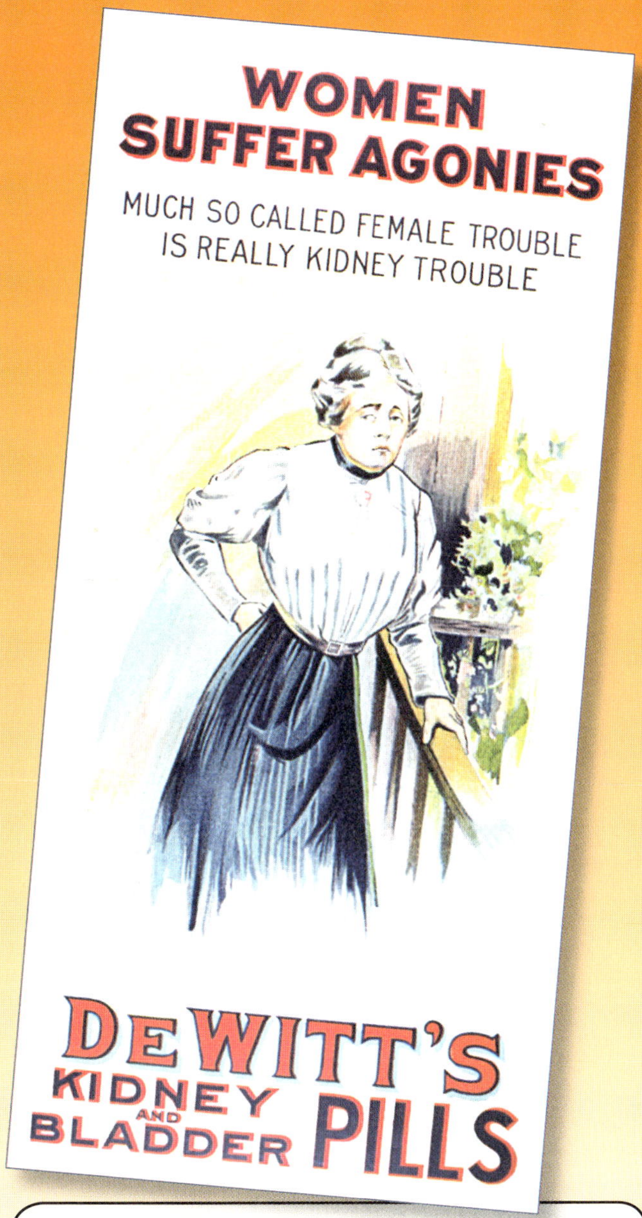


**DeWitt's Kidney and Bladder Pills -**
"Reported to contain methylene blue, potassium nitrate, and plant material including a volatile oil such as juniper oil."
*Nostrums & Quackery. Vol.III, p.69, 1936.*

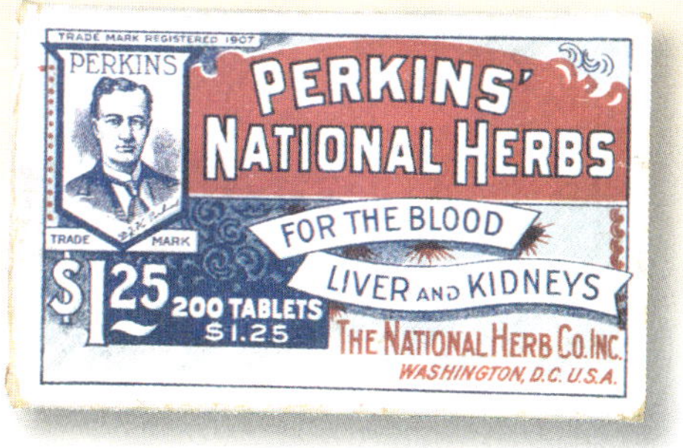


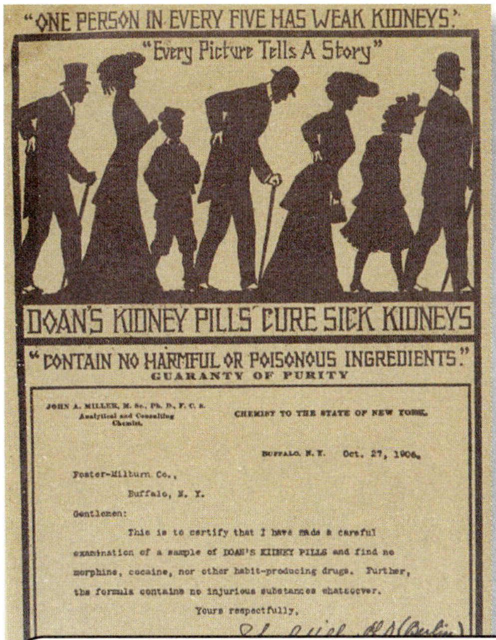


**Doan's Kidney Pills**
One of the methods by which Doan's Kidney Pills were advertised was to publish testimonials given by those living in the locality in which the newspaper was published. The Blackwell (Okla.) NEWS for August 24, 1910 contained a testimonial of one Mrs. Charles Butcher of Blackwell. She testified that she suffered from kidney disease - had taken Doan's Kidney Pills - enjoyed "prompt relief". Unfortunately, Mrs. Charles Butcher was dead and buried 2 months before the ad appeared; and she died from kidney disease!
*Nostrums and Quackery. Vol.II, pg.188, 1921.*

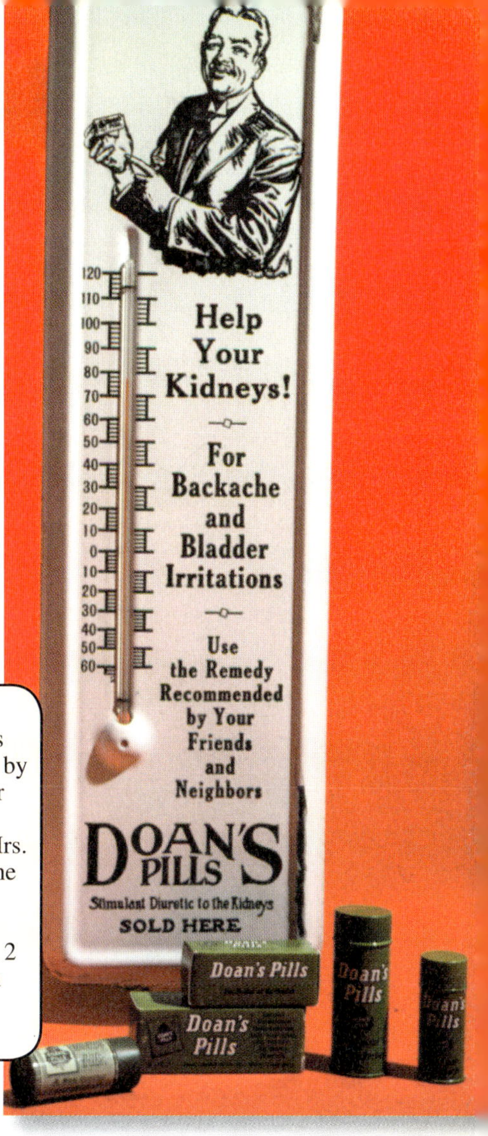


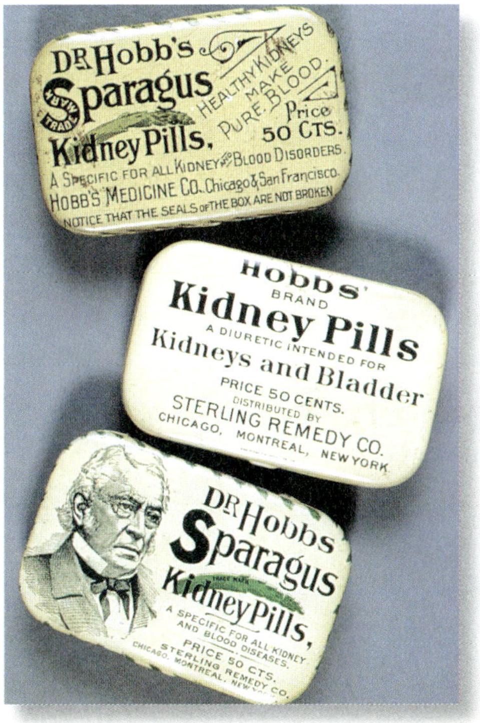


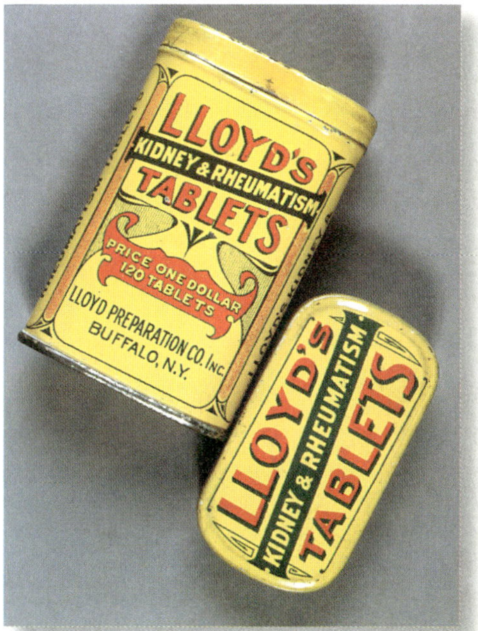

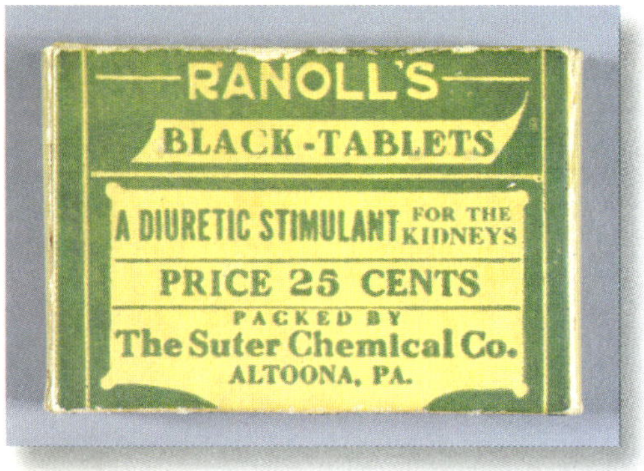


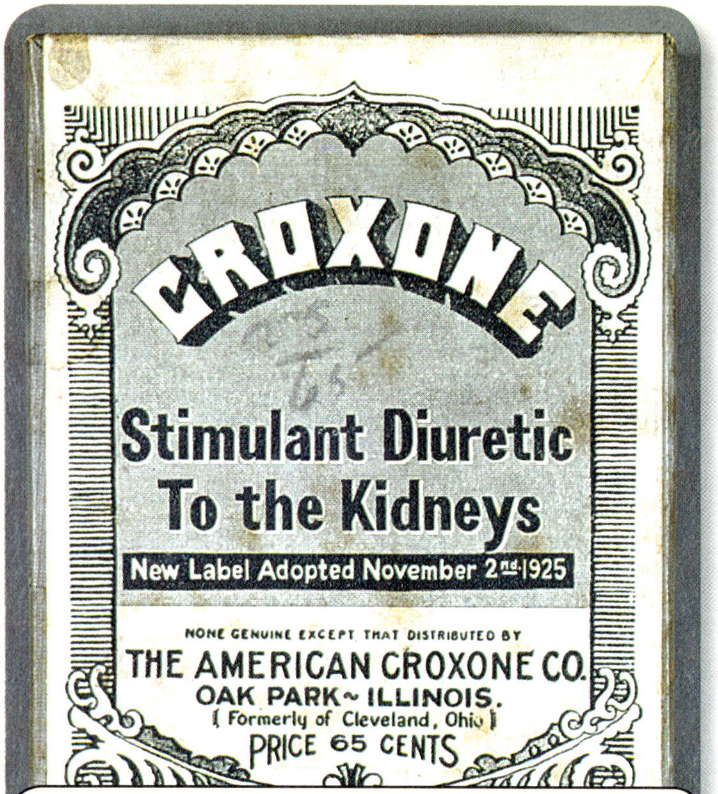


**Croxone -** "The pill consisted essentially of strychnine, a trace of brucin, aloin, hexamethlyenamin, lithium carbonate, potassium nitrate and a trace of atropine."
*Nostrums & Quackery. Vol.II, p.214, 1921.*

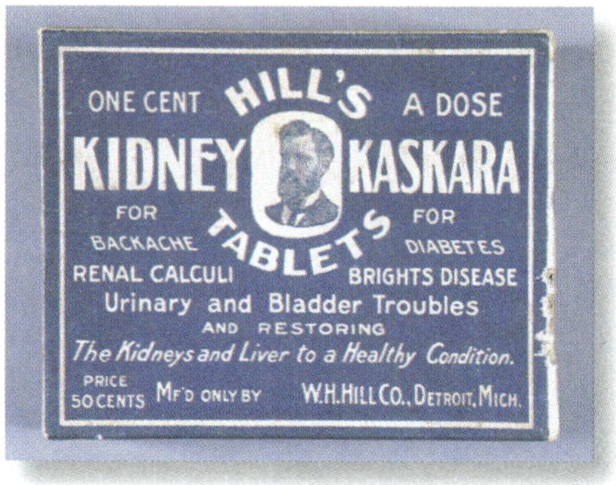


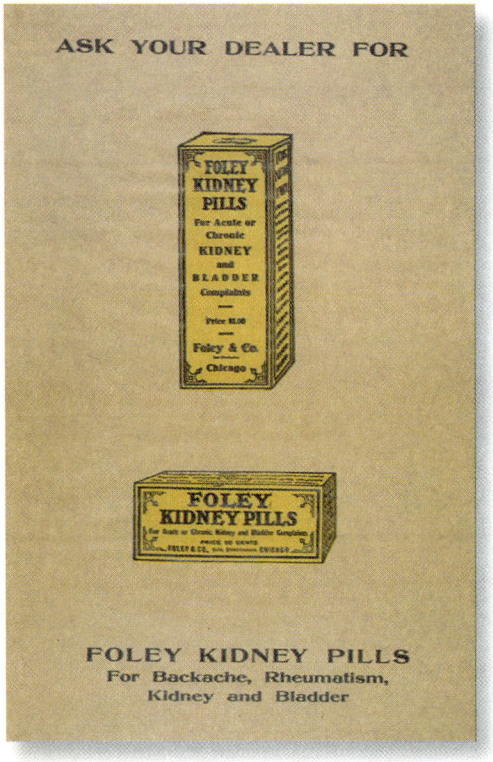


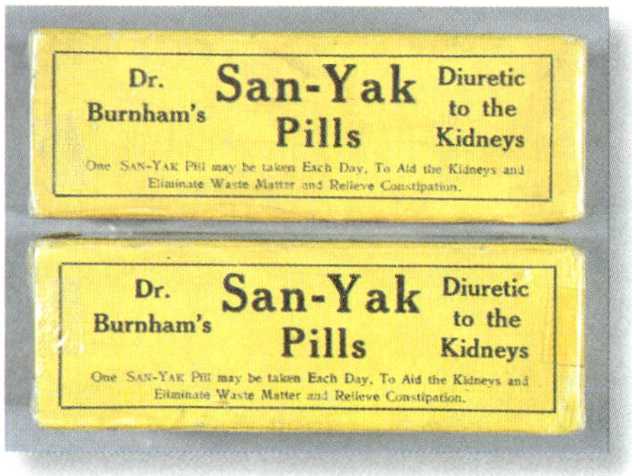


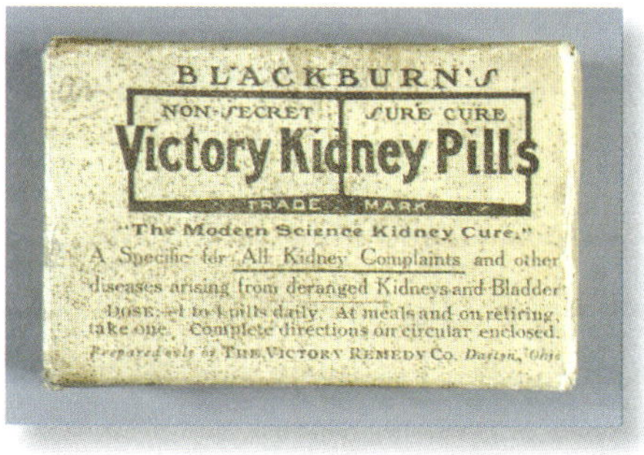


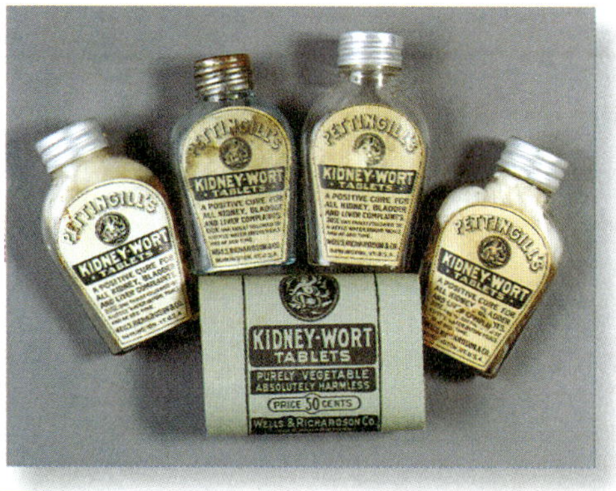


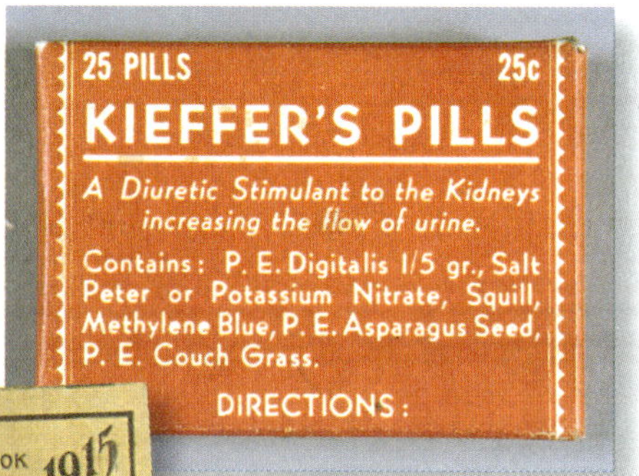


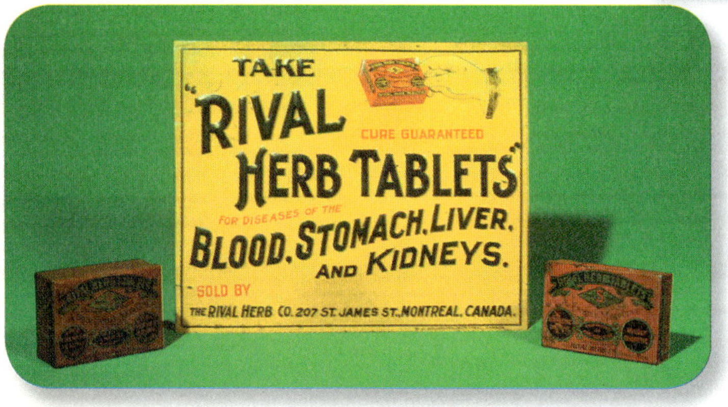


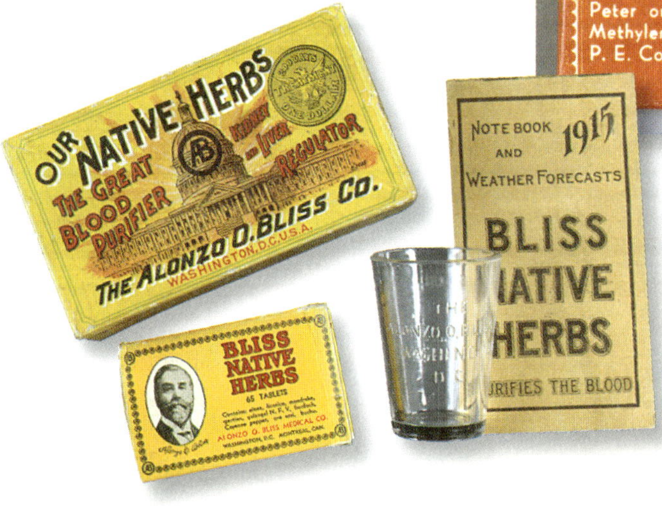

Chapter 9

# Venereal Disease

The historical awareness of venereal disease or sexually transmitted disease is age old. From antiquity there is the recorded description and treatment of the urethral discharge. An early writing of the problem is found in *The Bible*. In Leviticus 15:3 it states: "When any man has a discharge issuing from his member, he is unclean." It is further noted that when he becomes cleansed of his discharge, "he shall count seven days for his cleansing; he shall wash his clothes, and bathe his body in fresh water, and he shall be clean," (Leviticus 15:13).

Similar ancient records make mention of urethral discharge which is believed to have been gonorrhea. It is significant that we find it referenced in the writings from the Egyptian papyruses, early Hindu literature, Indian Samhitas, and Mesopotamian tablets. Subsequently, Hippocrates knew of it and mentioned the flow of pus seen with the disease. Aristotle and Plato described what undoubtedly must have been gonorrhea. Of interest is Epicurus who developed a post gonorrheal stricture and finally committed suicide while in urinary retention.[4,5]

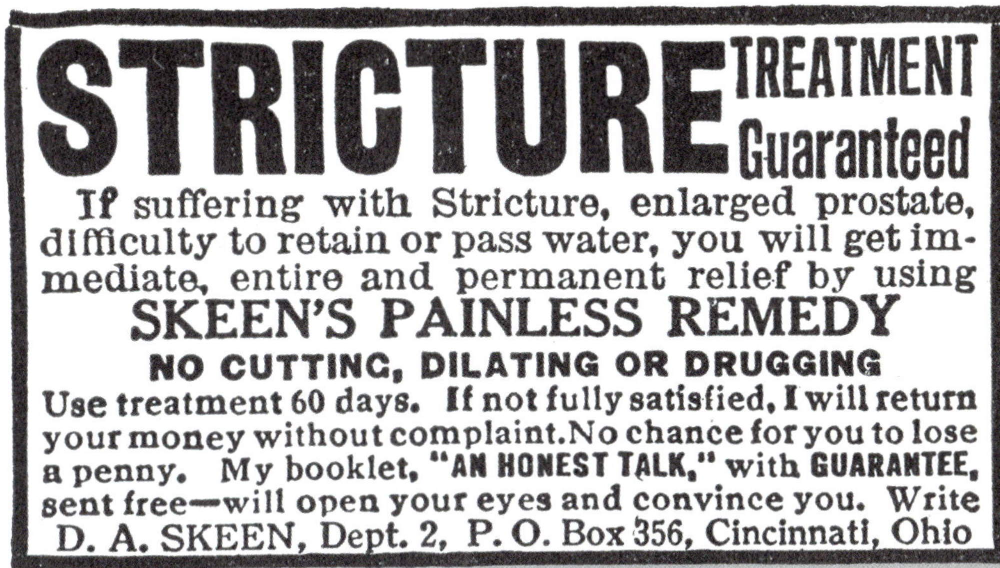


**Stricture**
Stricture and scarring of the urethra commonly resulted from the improper treatment of gonorrhea.

The outstanding Roman physician, Claudius Galen, was the first to name the purulent urethral discharge as gonorrhea. The name was mistakenly given, since he thought it was a leakage of semen. The misnomer is now commonly accepted. Other common names besides gonorrhea were "gleet", "whites", and "clap." Clap was probably derived from the name of the red light district in Paris, known as "Le Clapier."[4]

Before the sixteenth century gonorrhea and syphilis were known as separate diseases, until a group called the Identists claimed that the diseases were one and the same and interchangeable. The English physician, John Hunter,

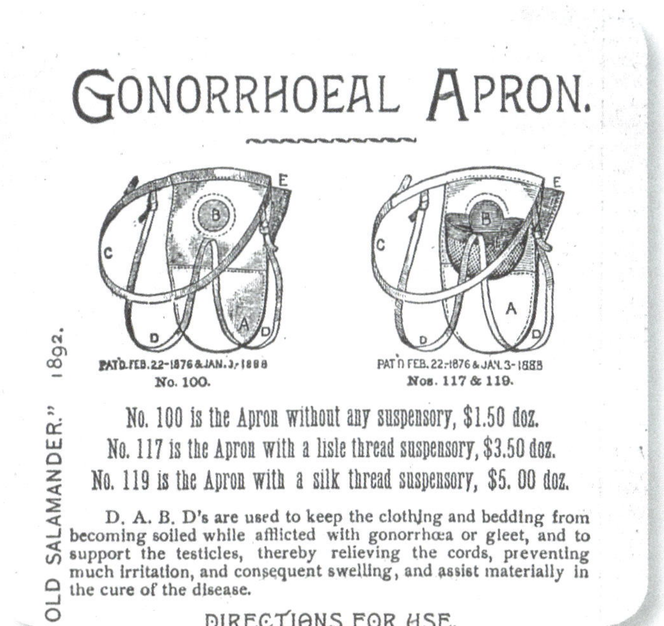


**Gonorrheal Apron**
An apron was advertised as an aid for "mucus discharge care" and to speed recovery.

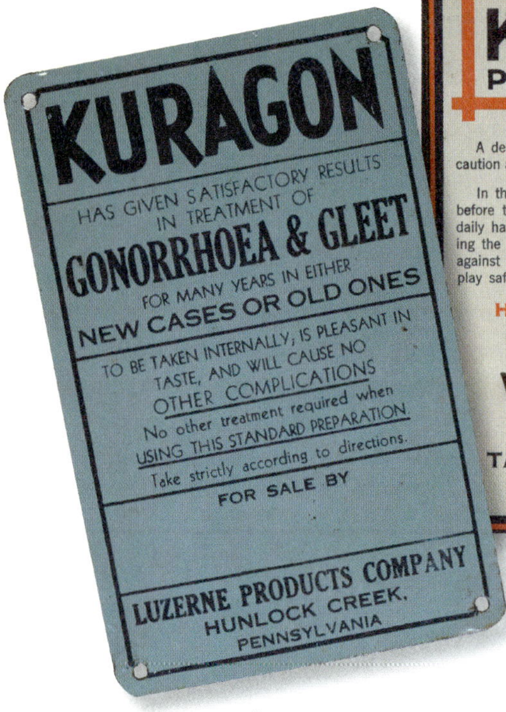


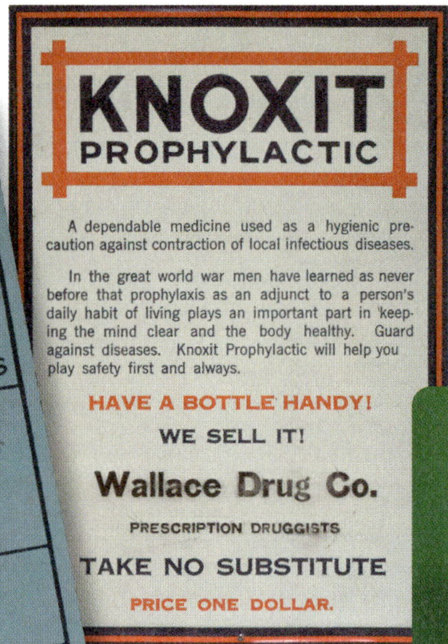


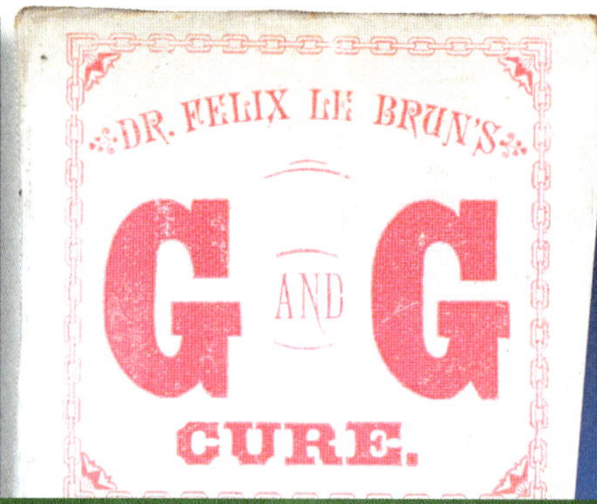


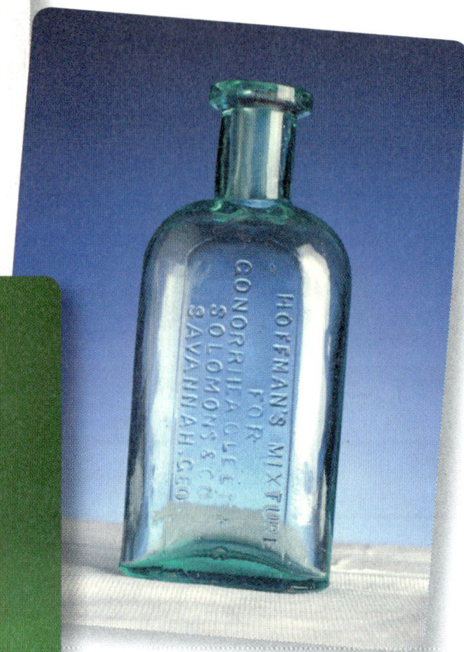

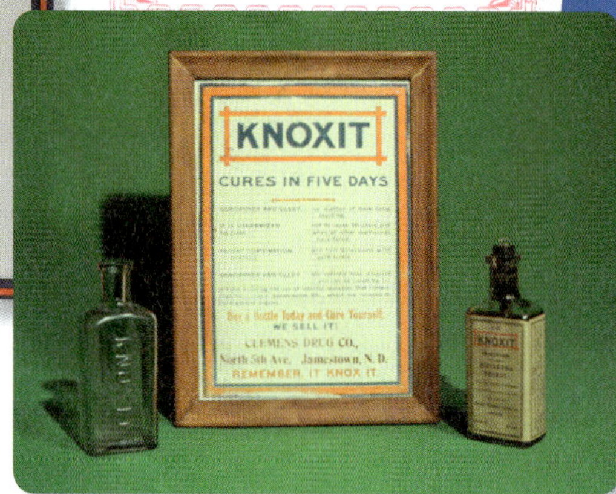


a famous man held in high esteem, inoculated himself with what he thought was only gonorrheal pus. However, he contracted both gonorrhea and syphilis. This was proof to him that they were the same disease. His hypothesis was fallacious, but it remained the rule for the next 100 years. It wasn't until the 1800s that scientists were able to demonstrate that they were indeed separate diseases. In 1872 Haller identified microorganisms in the pus of gonorrhea; in 1889 Albert Neisser specifically described the gonococcus and proved it to be the causative organism. The germ theory and its treatment were thus born.[4,5]

An understanding of microbes, including pathogenic bacteria, became widespread only in the last quarter of the nineteenth century. The germ theory was not even accepted by many physicians when patent medicine peddler, William Radam, began to capitalize upon popular gullibility with his Microbe Killer, a pink fluid composed of very weak sulfuric and hydrochloric acids, plus a trace of red wine. This nostrum, which sold in the millions of gallons, could kill some germs in the test tube, but to take these acids internally for an extended period was hazardous to one's health. It did, however, float William Radam from his Texas acres to a New York mansion overlooking Central Park.[7,8]

Since "symptoms equal disease" in the Mathematics of Credulity, the quack could go a step further in tampering with the equation. He could, through his promotion, substitute false symptoms as harbingers of syphilis and

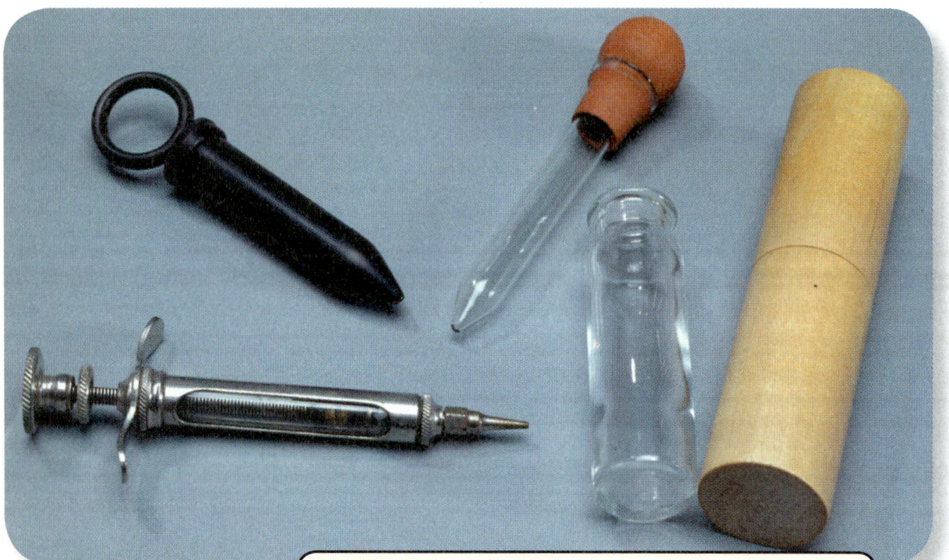

**Syringes**
Used to inject topical solutions directly into the urethra.

insanity. By adding a measure of guilt to any indiscretion, the nostrum peddler became more effective with his miracle medicines.[3,7] He hawked such medicines as "Gonor," "Kuragon," "Gonosan," and "Dr. Felix Le Brun's Guaranteed Cure for Gonorrhea and Gleet." Medicines like "Nichol's Infallible Injection," "Knoxit," "Hoffman's Mixture," "Dr. Moore's Venereal Antiseptic," "Jaynes Gonorrhea and Gleet Injection," "Big C," "Gon-Kure," were to be injected directly into the urethra. The ingredients of most injectable nostrums were not listed. Of those that did reveal the contents, a typical example is "Pabst O.K. Special."

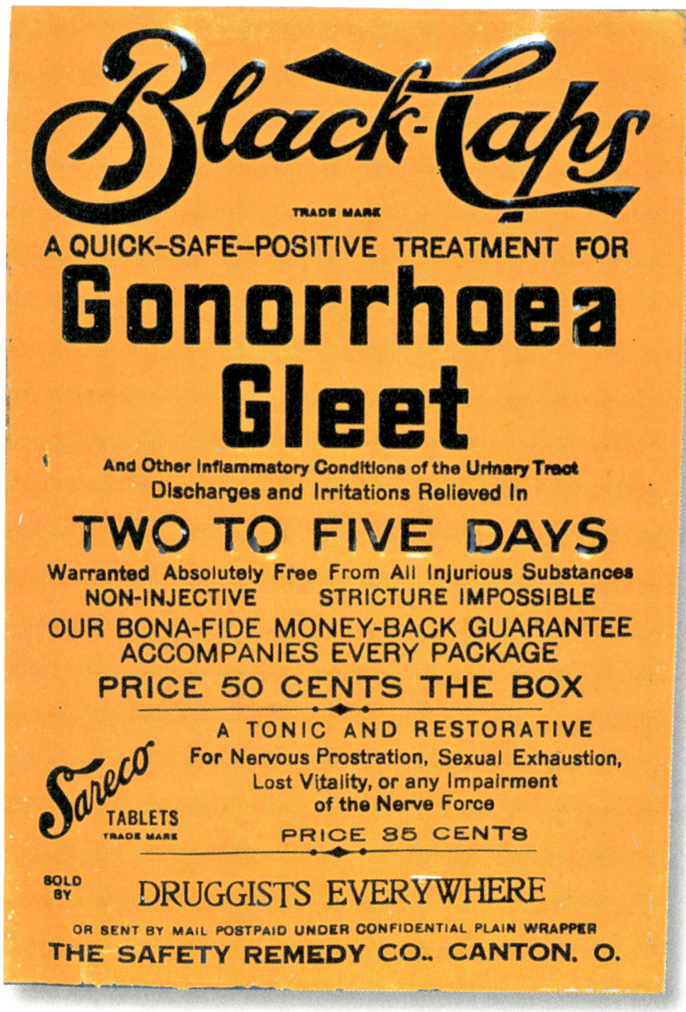


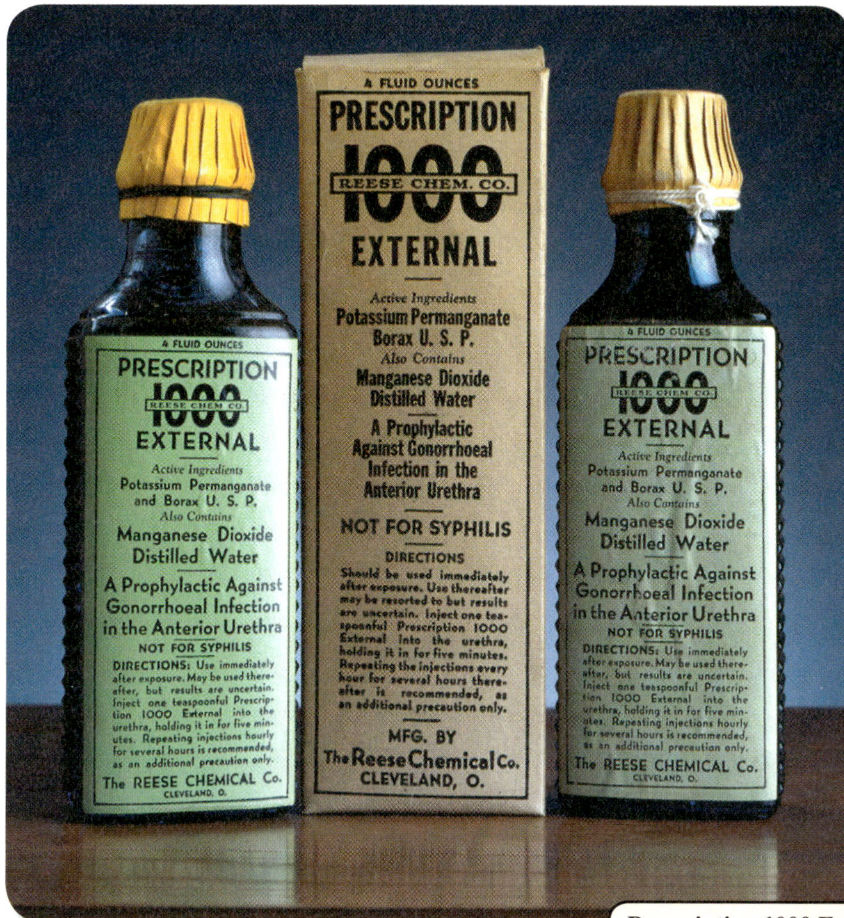


**Prescription 1000 External**
A solution to be injected into the urethra that contained the purple colored medicine, Potassium Permanganate.

The active ingredients were Balsam Copaiba, Oil Sandalwood, Oil Copaiba, Cubebs, Uva Ursi, Buchu, Juniper Berries, Matico, and Sweet Spirit Nitre.

Before the antibiotic era, medically trained urological physicians also treated the infection with the use of topical solutions that were injected directly into the urethra. The solutions used were specific antiseptic medicines made with Acriflavine or Mercurochrome or Potassium Permanganate (the latter was referred to as the "purple passion plunge").[4]

The sordid saga of syphilis is unclear. Researchers suggest that syphilis was identified in China as early as the Ming Dynasty (1368–1644 A.D.). It is also thought that syphilis was present in Europe long before the time of Christopher Columbus, but diagnosed by different names. In 1530 pathologist Hieronymus Fracastorius of Verona is credited with naming the contagion, syphilis. However, the story that

**Sarsaparilla**
Sarsaparilla is generally considered as an alterative, although stated by some to possess diuretic, diaphoretic and emetic properties. This agent possesses a high reputation as an alterative in the treatment of chronic rheumatism, scrofulous affections, cutaneous affections, inveterate syphilis, pseudo-syphilis, syphiloid diseases generally, and struma in all its forms. It possesses the power of purifying the blood, regulating the secretions, and comporting as a general alterative. It will be found to be highly advantageous in the treatment of that shattered state of the system which oftentimes follows an imprudent use of mercury in syphilitic affections, as also in that depraved condition of the general health to which it is difficult to apply a name. It has also been advised in chronic rheumatism, cutaneous diseases, passive and general dropsy, gonorrheal neuralgia, and other conditions of the system, where an alterative is required.
*From: Bill and Betty Wilson, "19th Century Medicine In Glass" p.40.(6)*

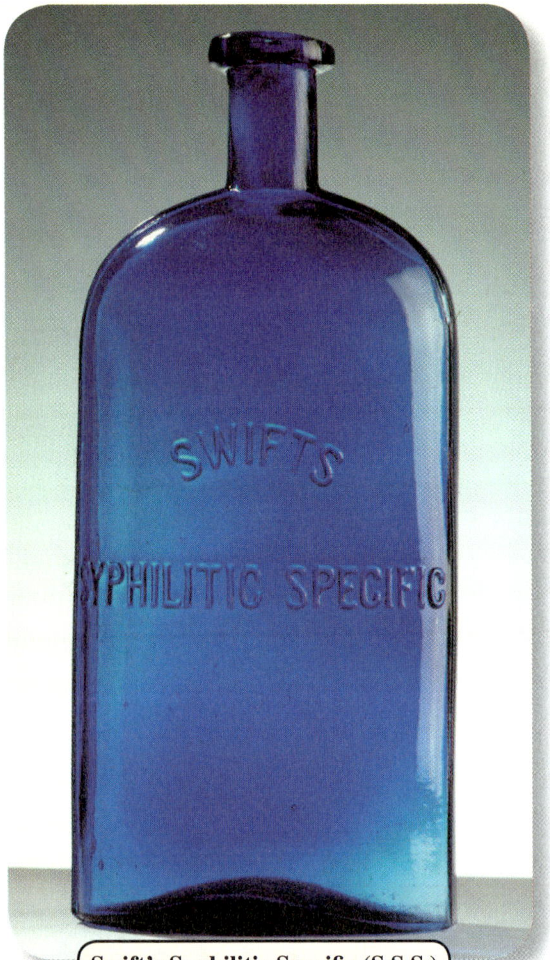


**Swift's Syphilitic Specific (S.S.S.)**
May be the best smooth based medicine bottle. It is a cobalt blue, 9¼" tall, rare beauty.

Columbus' sailors introduced syphilis into Europe will probably remain tradition. It struck Naples in 1494 when the city was under siege—a battle between the French and the Spanish. Some of the latter had sailed with Columbus. They reputedly had picked up a strange disease in the Indies, which they then passed on to the democratic ladies of Naples. The ladies relayed it in turn to the French when the city changed hands. The French eventually returned home, but not before they left "the calling card of civilized man" at every port they chanced to visit. Soon syphilis spread throughout all of Europe with each country passing on the blame from the scourge. However, it was Philippe Record who later stated that "Paris is the capital of the syphilized world."[4]

The triumphant march of syphilis throughout Europe instilled a collective fear of the infection. Although gonorrhea was more common, together with syphilis, they were directly responsible for the suppression of communal baths. In many areas this meant loss of the only convenient means of personal hygiene. In the wake of the disease Guaiac wood was the miracle drug of the Renaissance in spite of its questionably helpful properties. Physicians also used mercury, championing this metallic remedy in defiance of Galen who sponsored the herbal tradition.[5]

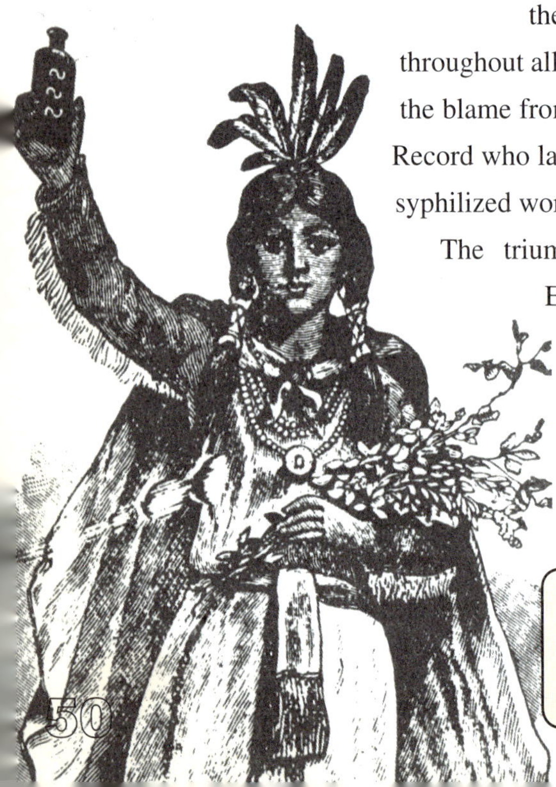

**S.S.S.** - The concoction contained roots of an old man's beard, sarsaparilla, prickly-ash, red and white sumac, copper sulfate and alcohol, 15-17%.

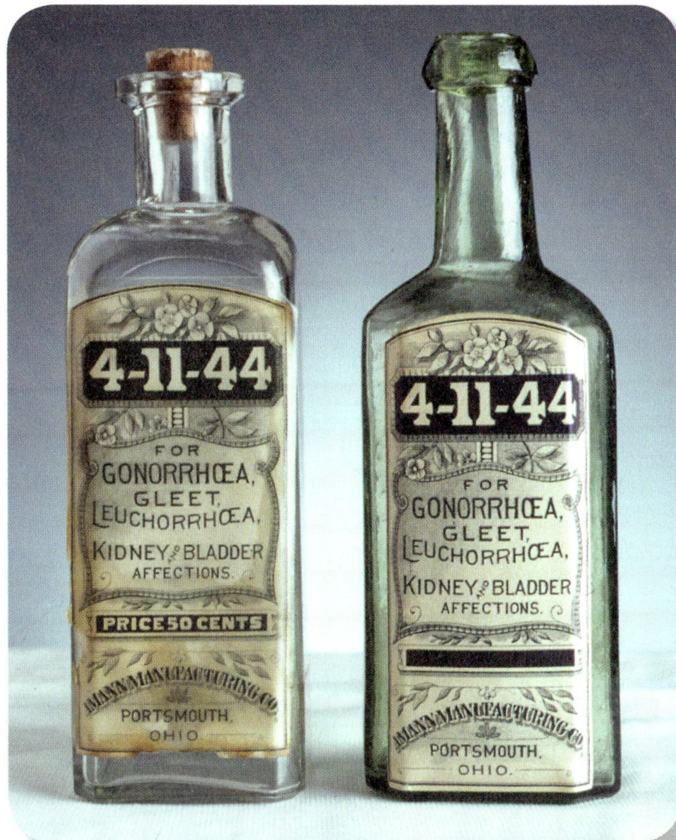


In 1905 Schaudinn proved the cause of syphilis to be the pathogen, Treponema pallidum. Ehrlich in 1910 developed Salvarsan, the first synthetic antimicrobial. For the first time in history the patient with syphilis had a good chance to not only survive the treatment, but also to be cured of his disease. Three decades later sulfonamides and penicillin were introduced.[4,5]

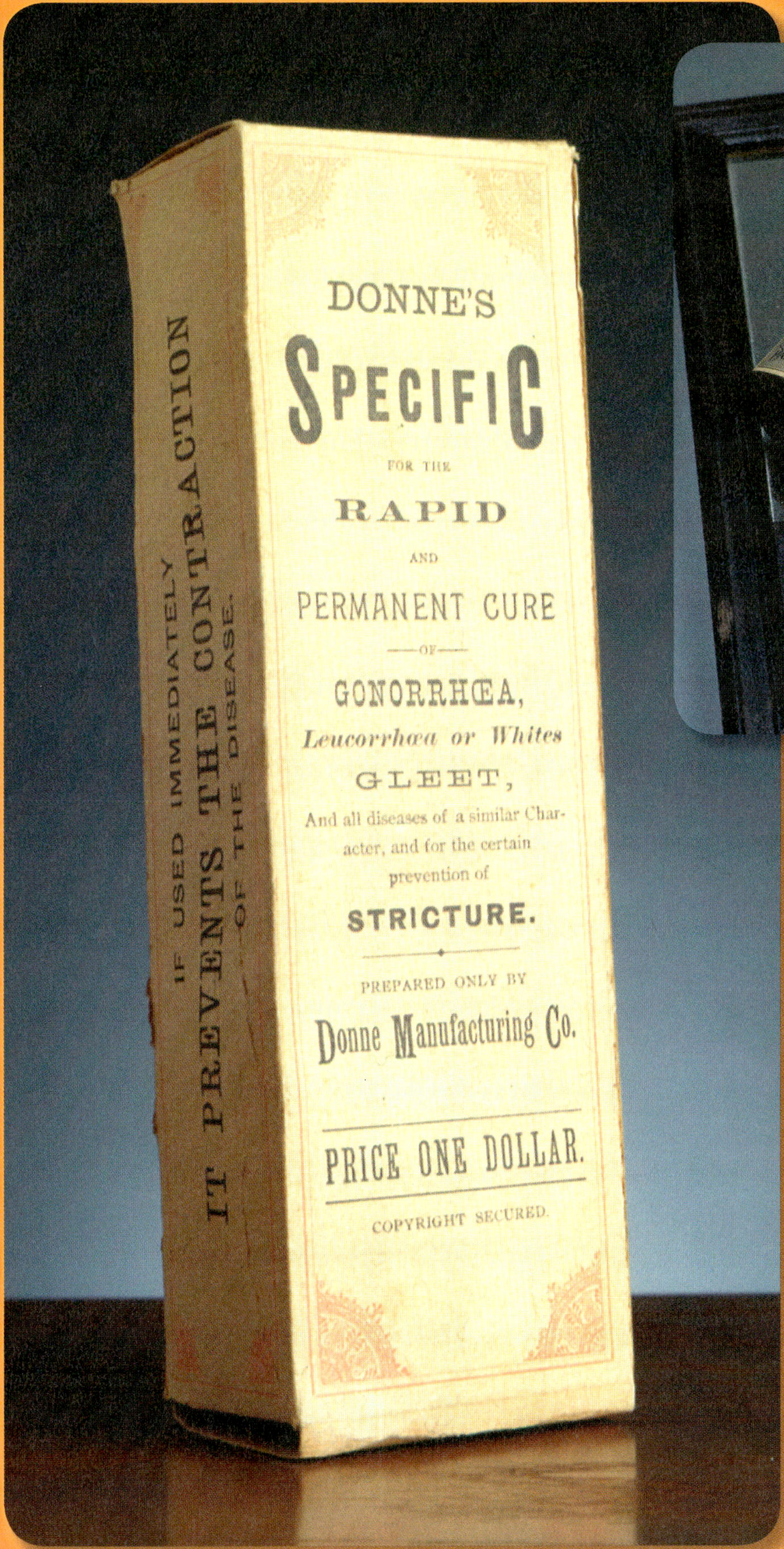
DONNE'S
SPECIFIC
FOR THE
RAPID
AND
PERMANENT CURE
OF
GONORRHŒA,
Leucorrhœa or Whites
GLEET,
And all diseases of a similar Character, and for the certain prevention of
STRICTURE.
PREPARED ONLY BY
Donne Manufacturing Co.
PRICE ONE DOLLAR.
COPYRIGHT SECURED.
IF USED IMMEDIATELY
IT PREVENTS THE CONTRACTION
OF THE DISEASE.

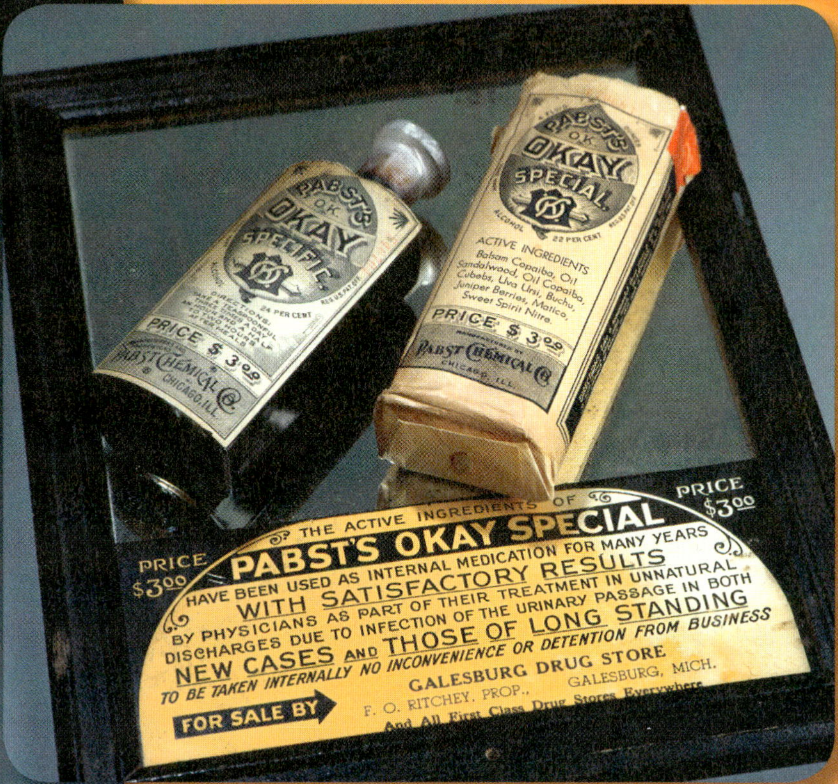
PABST'S O.K. OKAY SPECIFIC
PRICE $3.00
PABST CHEMICAL Co. CHICAGO, ILL.
PABST'S O.K. OKAY SPECIAL
ACTIVE INGREDIENTS
PRICE $3.00
PABST CHEMICAL Co. CHICAGO, ILL.
PRICE $3.00
THE ACTIVE INGREDIENTS OF
PABST'S OKAY SPECIAL
HAVE BEEN USED AS INTERNAL MEDICATION FOR MANY YEARS
WITH SATISFACTORY RESULTS
BY PHYSICIANS AS PART OF THEIR TREATMENT IN UNNATURAL DISCHARGES DUE TO INFECTION OF THE URINARY PASSAGE IN BOTH
NEW CASES AND THOSE OF LONG STANDING
TO BE TAKEN INTERNALLY NO INCONVENIENCE OR DETENTION FROM BUSINESS
FOR SALE BY
GALESBURG DRUG STORE
F. O. RITCHEY, PROP., GALESBURG, MICH.
And All First Class Drug Stores Everywhere
PRICE $3.00

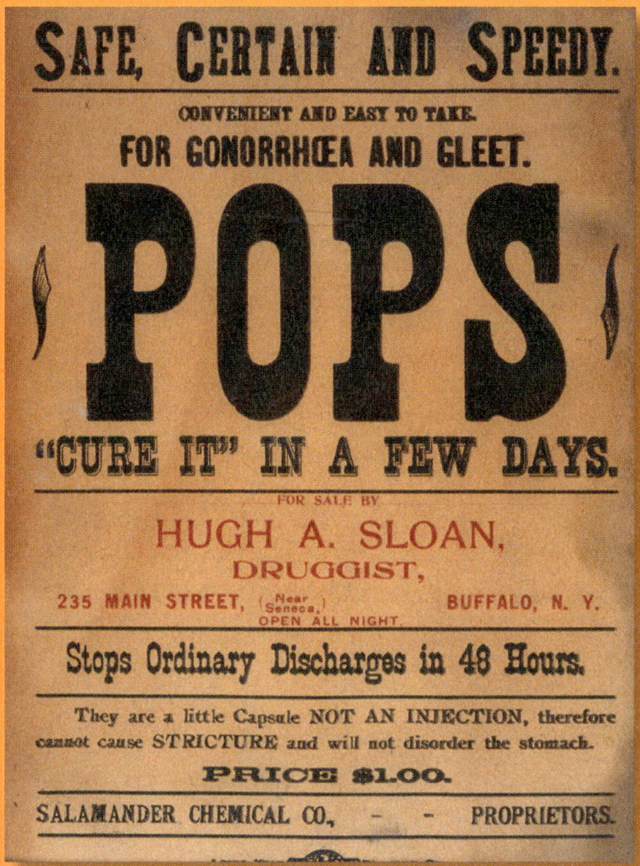
SAFE, CERTAIN AND SPEEDY.
CONVENIENT AND EASY TO TAKE.
FOR GONORRHŒA AND GLEET.
POPS
"CURE IT" IN A FEW DAYS.
FOR SALE BY
HUGH A. SLOAN,
DRUGGIST,
235 MAIN STREET, (Near Seneca.) BUFFALO, N. Y.
OPEN ALL NIGHT.
Stops Ordinary Discharges in 48 Hours.
They are a little Capsule NOT AN INJECTION, therefore cannot cause STRICTURE and will not disorder the stomach.
PRICE $1.00.
SALAMANDER CHEMICAL CO., - - PROPRIETORS.

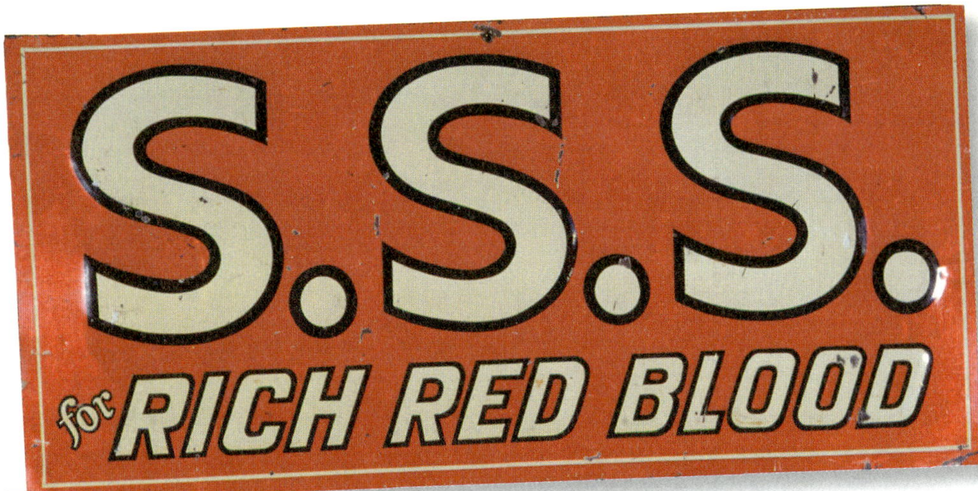


C.T. Swift, of Atlanta, Georgia, registered his trademark on April 16, 1878.

The contagious disease of syphilis, America's gift to Europe, "returned" to America as a significant scourge. Great growth in patent medicine products for self-treatment took place during the same decades that saw a revolution in the science of medicine. Quacks were just as quick to exploit advances in the physical sciences as they were to discredit biological achievements. Nostrums from the sarsaparilla root were hawked as being curative for syphilis, especially for the cutaneous manifestations. Another proprietary medicine was "Swift's Syphilitic Specific" from Atlanta, Georgia. The impact of repetition was enhanced if the product name was memorable. Some peddlers turned to the alliteration and familiarity of signage with S.S.S. in bold letters all over the countryside.[7]

Device quackery preyed on the same widespread credulity, fear, and desperation which permitted all other forms of quackery to flourish. Gadgets could possess certain kinds of persuasiveness denied to drugs. James H. Young describes in his book, the *Medical Messiahs*, the power to shock. A New York "clinic" early in the nineteenth century treated young men who were led to believe they might be suffering from syphilis or the dire consequence of self-abuse. The patient sat naked upon a sort of toilet throne, his bare back resting against a metal plate, his scrotum suspended in a whirling pool. The plate and pool were linked by wire to a battery. No frightened sufferer could question the rigor of this therapy.[8]

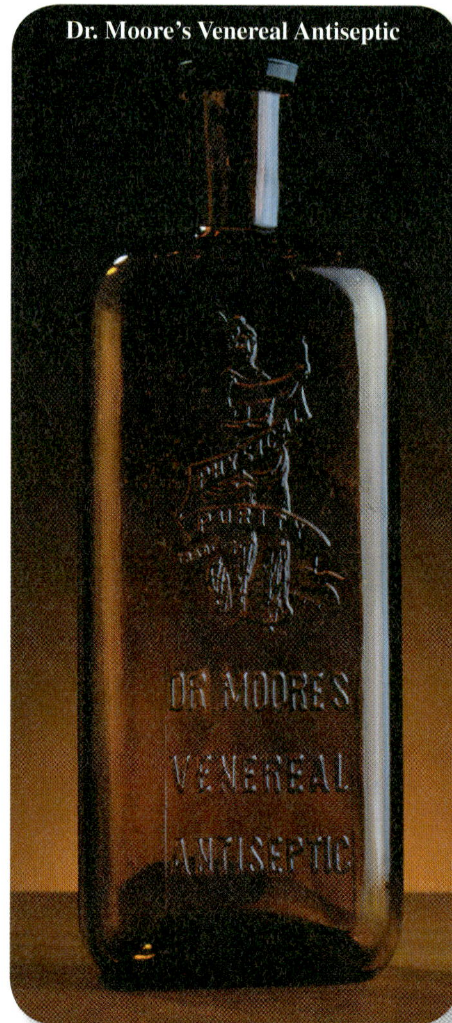

Dr. Moore's Venereal Antiseptic

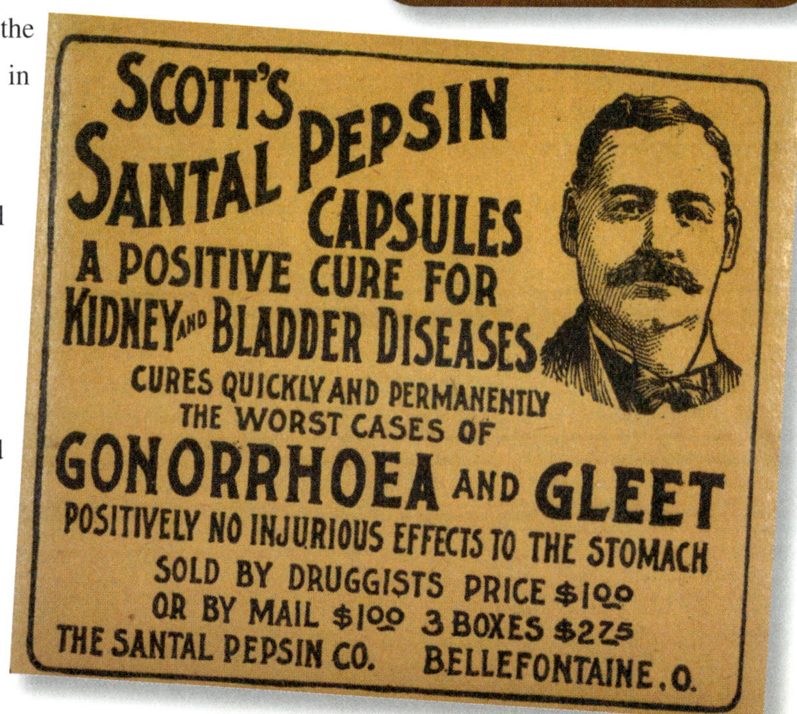

# Virility Aids

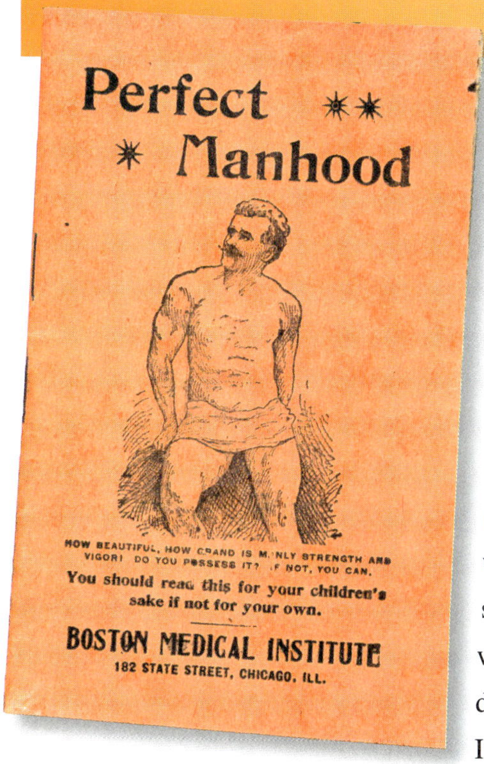


In the 1800s, the Victorian era, the public mention and discussion of sexual matters was frowned upon. Medical problems that were considered sexual in nature were discreetly dealt with in private. Imaginative names and euphemistic titles were used to describe the malady of erectile dysfunction. Impotence or erectile dysfunction was referred to as lost manhood, failure at marital duties, impairment of the nerve force, or sexual exhaustion. The perceived need, combined with a burning desire, gave rise to creative solutions. The advertiser played upon the guilty apprehensions of all who secretly knew that they had sinned. Guilt or the "loss of manly power due to indiscretions" was corrected, appropriately, by "natural remedies." The desire for a miracle invariably brought forth miracle workers.[1,3]

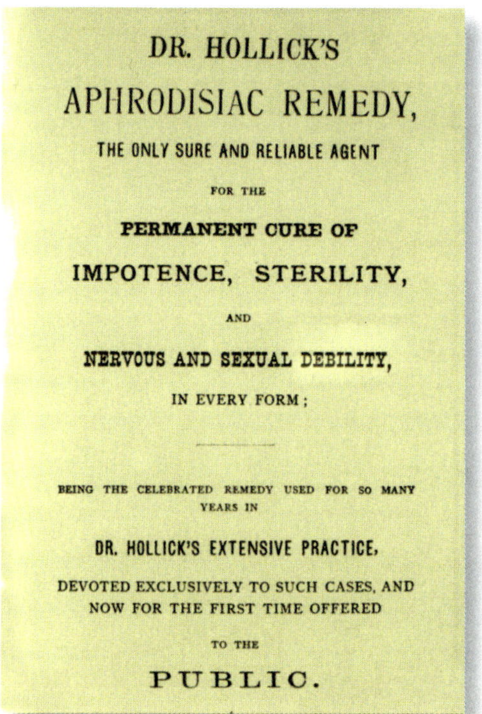
DR. HOLLICK'S
APHRODISIAC REMEDY,
THE ONLY SURE AND RELIABLE AGENT
FOR THE
PERMANENT CURE OF
IMPOTENCE, STERILITY,
AND
NERVOUS AND SEXUAL DEBILITY,
IN EVERY FORM;
BEING THE CELEBRATED REMEDY USED FOR SO MANY YEARS IN
DR. HOLLICK'S EXTENSIVE PRACTICE,
DEVOTED EXCLUSIVELY TO SUCH CASES, AND NOW FOR THE FIRST TIME OFFERED
TO THE
PUBLIC.

Man's age-old pursuit of a cure for impotence seems eternal. From antiquity mandrake root *(Mandragora officinarum)* had a significant reputation for qualities of sexual stimulation. It was mentioned in *The Bible* for its enhancement of fertility (Genesis 30: 14-17). A number of ancient writers such as Pythagoras, Plutarch, and Columella record their belief that mandrake had powers as a love philter or love potion to aid fertility. It was used to "excite the amorous propensity, remedy female sterility, facilitating conception and prolificness." Throughout history the romantic qualities of mandrake were exaggerated in fictional accounts by many authors. In the fifteenth century Machiavelli wrote a play about *"La Mandragora,"* using the scientific name for mandrake.[4]

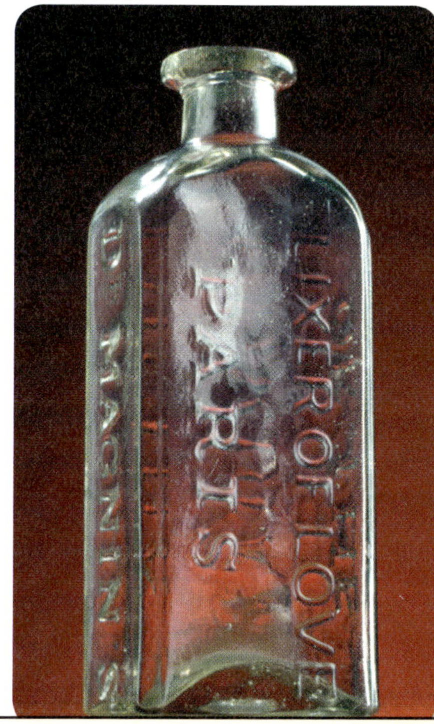


**Magnin's Elixer of Love**
John Winters Holderwell was the first U.S. agent for this medicine beginning in New York City in 1839. He sold his medicine business to Mortimer Harrison in 1845 who continued it until 1856.
The Elixer of Love was a supposed cure for sexual debility.(5)

The problems of impotence have been discussed in writings from almost all civilizations. The oriental writing *Nei-Ching* discussed the philosophy of impotence. The *Aqrabadhin of Al-Kindi*, an Arabian text, recommended

Piuma's Sexvitor

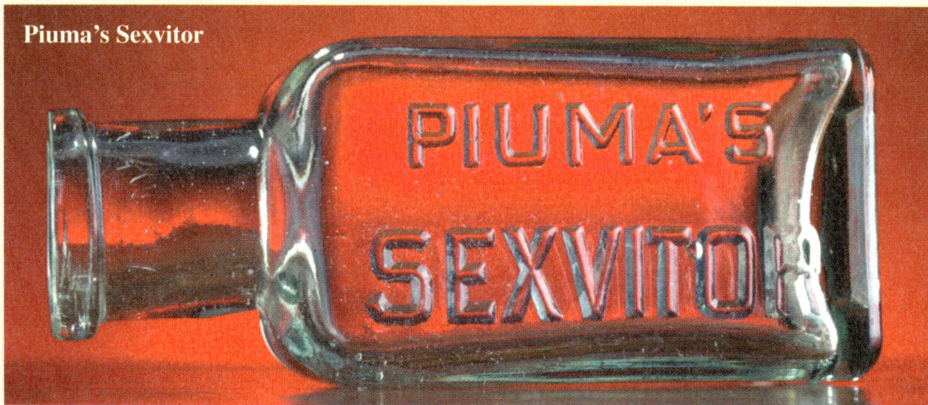


Sexine Pills

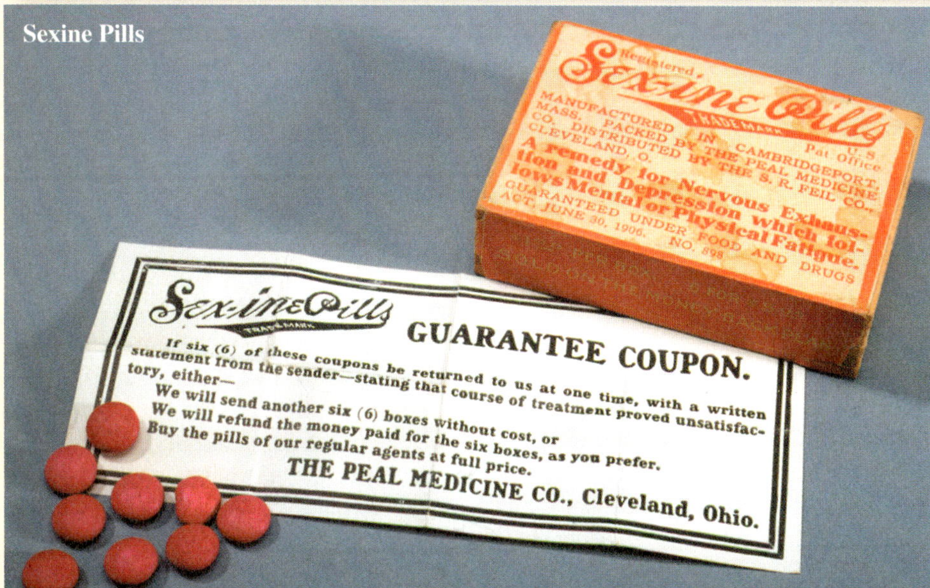


Steven's Sexual Vitalizer

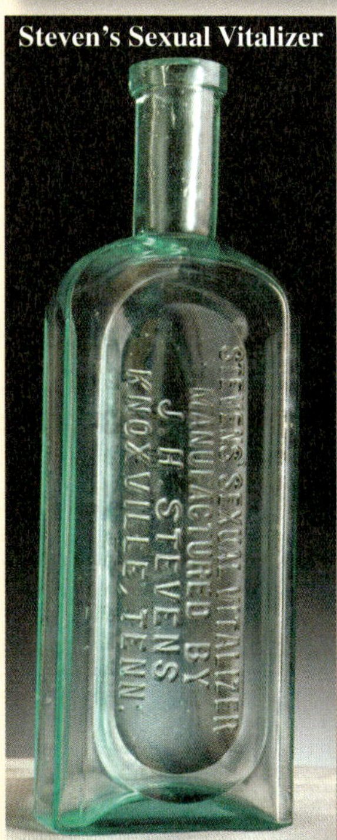


Dr. Murphy's Elixir of Life

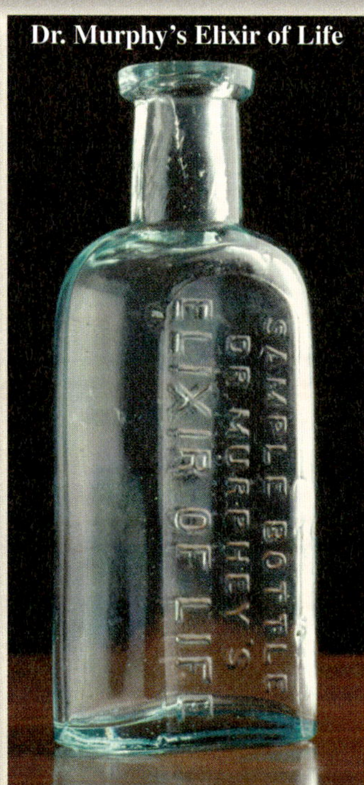


Natasha's Russian Root

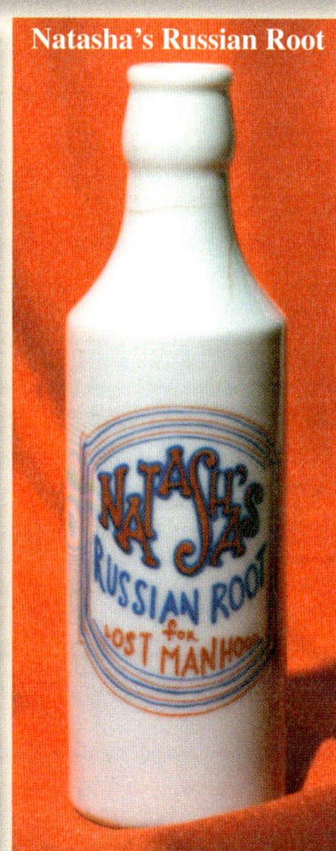


Orchotine

**Fatigue, Nervous Exhaustion, Sexual Apathy and Sub-Efficiency—**

indicate a lowered state of total metabolism in a male organism. A treatment of this sexual inadequacy that is scientific and effective is the restoration of the whole metabolism. This is best accomplished with such an association of glandular substances as are contained in

**ORCHOTINE (H. P. C.)**

Prepared in the Laboratories of The Hudson Pharmacal Co.
Orchotine (H. P. C.) contains the active principles of the Testes (interstitial cells of Lydig) with the other vital glands of the Testicular Cycle reinforced with Lecithin, Neuclein and one-eighth grain Nux Vomica.

Put up in bottles of 50 five-grain tablets or in units of 500 or 1000

**Send This Coupon for Free Clinical-Trial Sample**

The Hudson Pharmacal Co.,
Union Hill, N. J.

Without cost or obligation please send me one bottle of 50 five-grain tablets Orchotine (H. P. C.) for clinical trial.

Name . . . . . . . . . . . . . . . . . . . . . . . . . . . . . . . . . . . .

Address . . . . . . . . . . . . . . . . . . . . . . . . . . . . . . . . . . . .

prescriptions of oil of jasmine and asafetida. The *Sushruta Samhita*, probably originating in India more than 3000 years ago, contained an entire section devoted to the Vagi-Karana (aphrodisiac) remedies. Various causes of impotence were described and different remedies were given. Powders, juices and herbs were ingested as well as preparations made from the testes of a he-goat or alligator.[4]

In 1869 John Davenport wrote the following: "when it is considered how strongly the sexual desire is implanted in man, and how much his self-love is interested in preserving or in recovering the power of gratifying it, his endeavors to infuse fresh vigour into his organs when they are temporarily exhausted by over-indulgence or debilitated by age, cannot appear surprising."[4]

During the patent medicine era the nostrum peddler, whose ethics were still in the formative stage, offered a variety of treatment options for impotence. He hawked pills, wafers, tonics, elixirs, lotions, rays, pods, belts, packs, and plasters. In the hope of turning back the clock the public sought the elixir of life in sexual renewal nostrums as did Dr. Faust, who made a pact with the devil to gain a few more frisky years.[2] Various medicines were offered such as "Natasha's Russian Root for Lost Manhood," "Sexine Pills," "Orchotine," "Dr. Murphy's Elixir of Life," "Piuma's Sexvitor," "Steven's Sexual

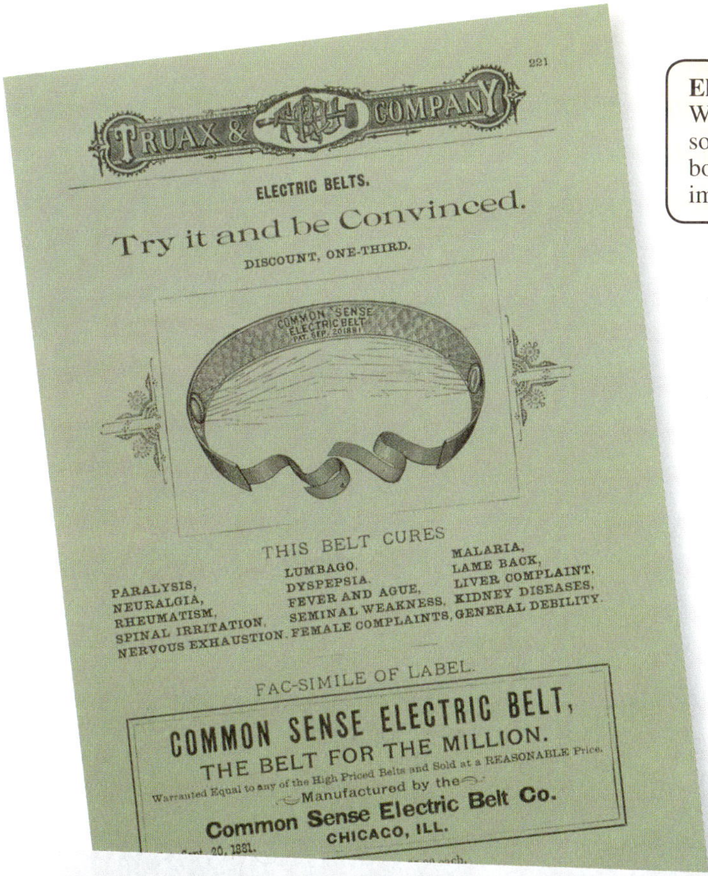


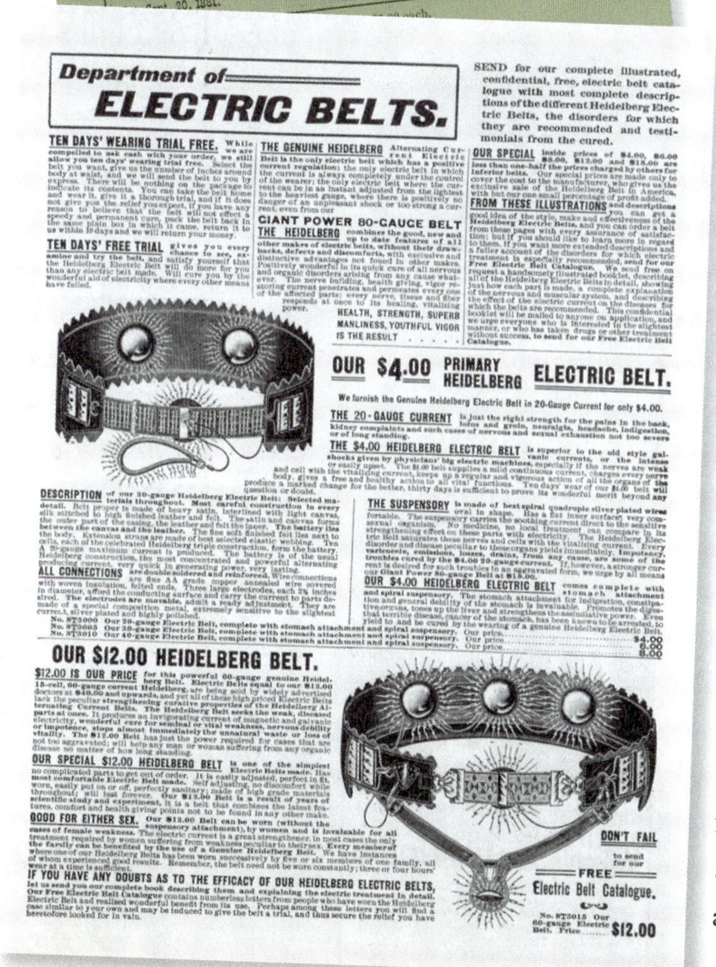


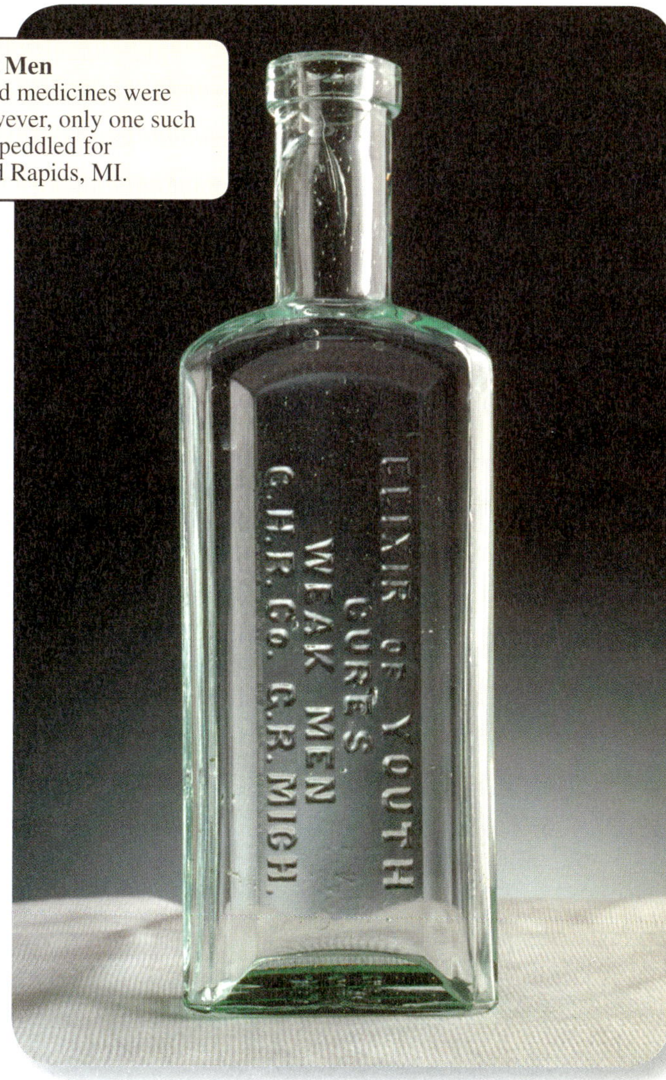


**Elixir of Youth - Cures Weak Men**
Well over 3000 different bottled medicines were sold as "cure" medicinals. However, only one such bottled "cure" concoction was peddled for impotency. It came from Grand Rapids, MI.

Vitalizer."

The public had a voracious interest in science and glands. The advertiser promised gadgets that were health giving, vigor restoring, and power vitalizing to the debilitated sexual organs from whatever cause. The advertiser offered an electric belt that gave genuine self regulating 80 gauge alternating current for a cure of "weakness peculiar to man." The cost was $18.00—or about two weeks pay for the average man. Other ploys that were available were electromagnetism and even radium.[2]

Physicians have long been involved in the treatment of impotence. Around the turn of the century vasectomy was advised to increase sexual potency. It was usually performed on one side only, but occasionally on both. The theory was to save all the male "juices" usually discharged with orgasm and to recycle them into the body to make it stronger and more virile. In addition monkey "glands" and goat testes were used as a favored form of treatment for many years. These men of science also used the psychrophore. They believed that prostatic atony was a cause of impotence.[4] The psychrophore was

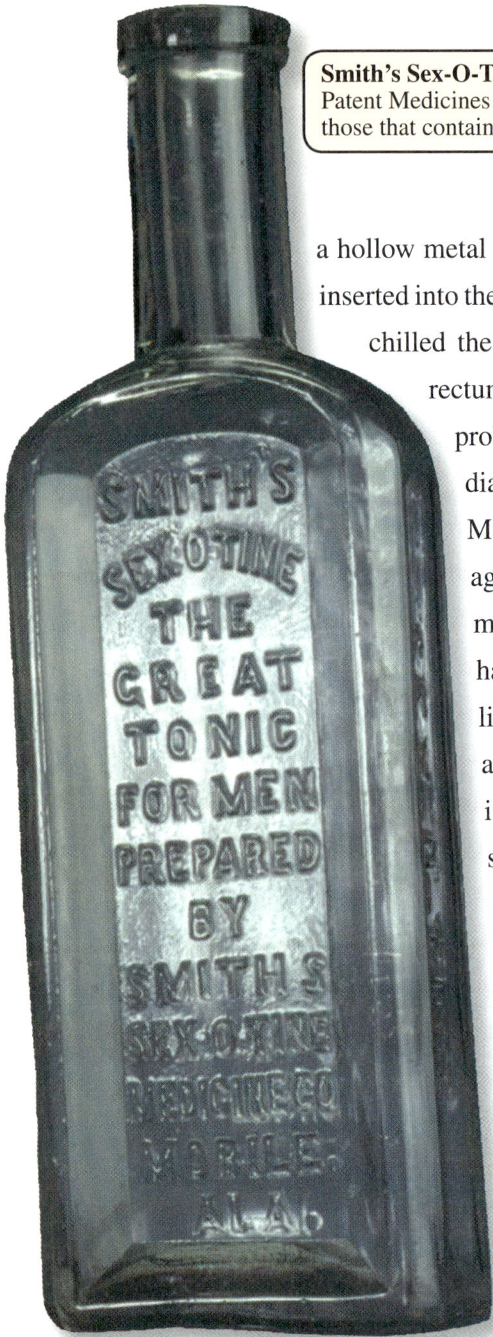


**Smith's Sex-O-Tine the Great Tonic For Men**
Patent Medicines for impotency are rare especially those that contain the word SEX in the label.

a hollow metal finger-like instrument that was inserted into the rectum. Cold water instillation chilled the prostate as well as the entire rectum supposedly to correct the problem. They also used electric diathermic insertions.

Mankind has traveled through the age of gods and witchcraft into modernity but, as Henry Sigerist has wisely said, "Impotence….. like other nervous disorders and particular sexual neurosis, is still the playground of superstition and quackery."[4]

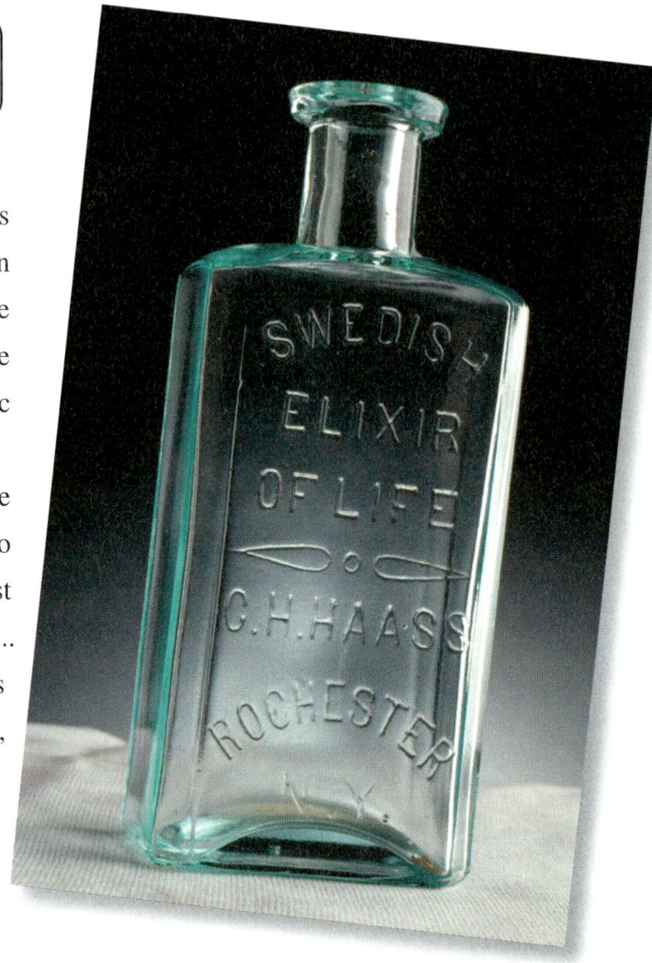


Dr. Wade's Golden Specific for $3.00

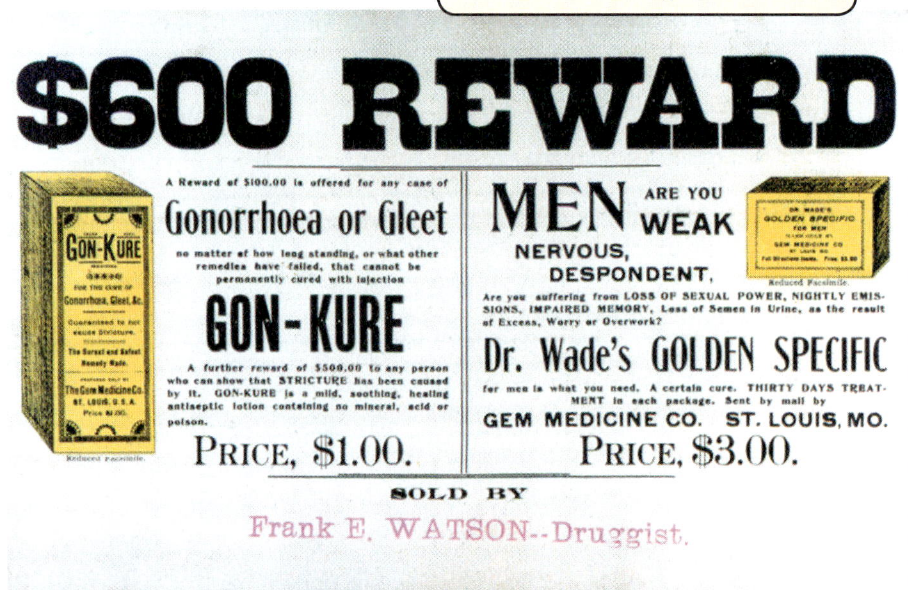

Chapter 11

# Urinary Stone Dissolvers-Lithontriptics

The history of medicine is also the history of human fallibility and error. From primitive man's knowledge of therapeutics to today's advancement of medical science, the narrative of discovery and invention has never been continuous nor even progressive. Inspired scientific ideas at times were lost due to human indifference or accidental circumstances. This dilemma was never better illustrated than by the history of the treatment of urinary stones. The story of man's suffering from urinary stones both in illness and in treatment is known to have existed since 3000-4000 B.C. During these centuries the success of a scientific contribution usually depended upon the time of its appearance.

Bladder stones are no respecters of persons. Those known to have suffered from stone disease include such notables as Leopold I of Belgium, Napoleon III of France, the saintly Ignatius of Loyola, diarist Samuel Pepys, philosopher Francis Bacon, physicist Isaac Newton, and author Horace Walpole. Among statesmen were Peter the Great of Russia, Louis XIV of France, Oliver Cromwell, and George IV of England. Thomas Sydenham, a pioneer of internal medicine, made the compassionate observation from his own experience that "the patient suffers until he is finally consumed by both age and illness, and the poor man is happy to die."[2,4]

Man's first accounting of the surgical treatment of bladder stones is found in Hindu writings, that date well before Christ. In the fifth century A.D. the *Susruta Samhita*

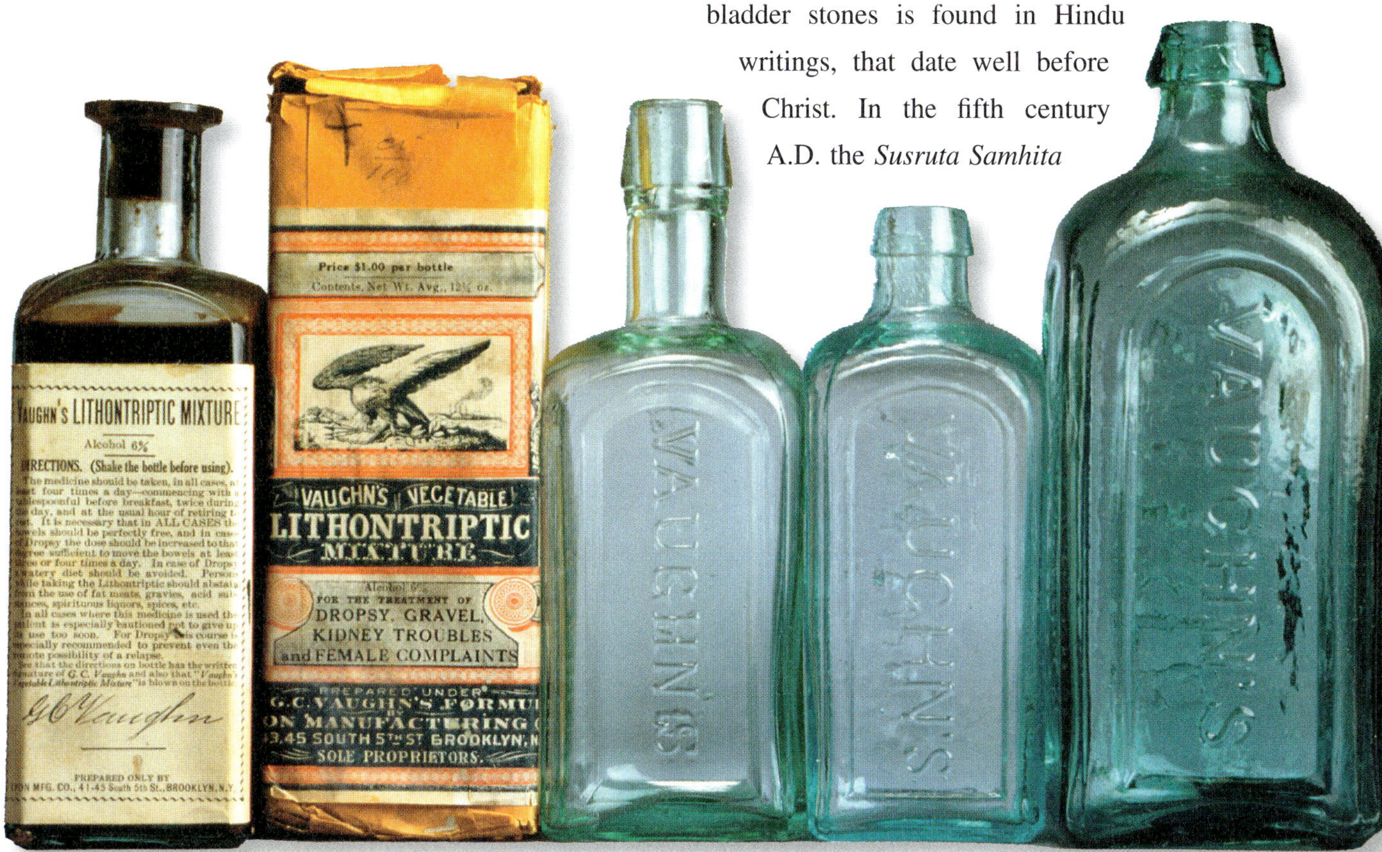

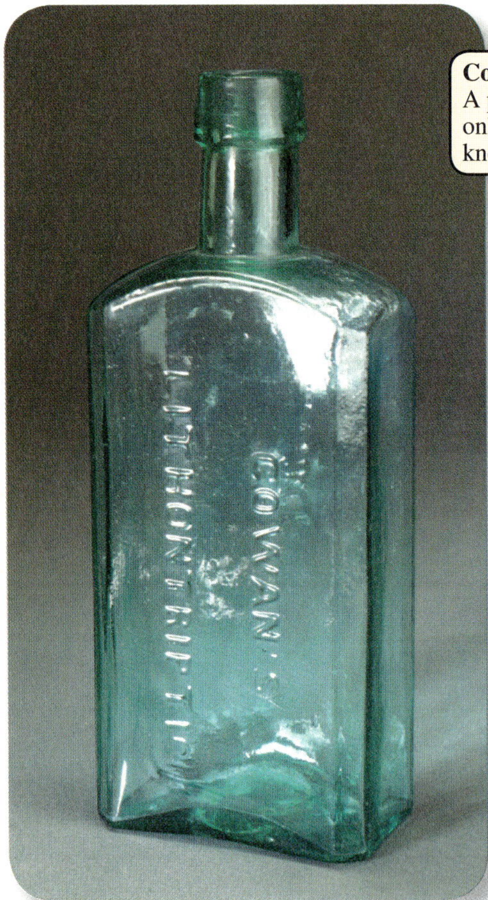

**Cowan's Lithontriptic**
A pontilled medicine - only two such bottles are known to exist.

Lithotomy Instruments(7)

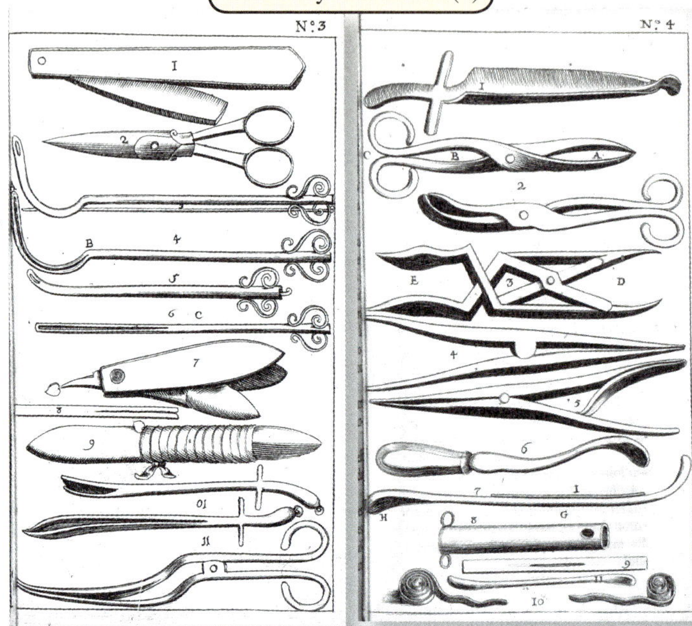


gives the first known description of a lithotomy or "cutting for stone" procedure. A perineal lithotomy between the genitalia and rectum afforded access to a bladder stone. A sizable stone could be located by inserting a finger into the rectum and feeling it through the intestinal wall. The "stone cutting" was relatively simple and required only a knife and tweezers .[2,4,5,7]

The Father of Medicine, Hippocrates (460-370 B.C.), although himself a daring surgeon, recommended that cutting for stone was to be performed by specialists. In the famous Hippocratic Oath the operation was only for the capable. In subsequent years lithotomists continued to perform the operation with unfortunate problems of incontinence and a significant mortality rate.[2]

Of those who performed lithotomy, no one received greater recognition for his mastery of the lithotomy procedure than British surgeon, William Cheselden (1688-1752). He was the personal physician to Queen Caroline. As an outstanding anatomist he learned to protect the blood vessels of the pelvis and preserve structures for continence. Prior to the age of anesthesia, stone cutting was scarcely a pleasant event. Therefore, the speed of the surgeon was prized all the more highly. On this point, Cheselden could offer good service, indeed. Usually he completed the entire procedure in less than sixty seconds.[4,5]

Many ingenious methods were used to diagnose and remove bladder stones. The presence of a stone was determined by sounding with a curved metal rod or sound. A straight rod that was hollow permitted the introduction of sharp penetrating points, drills, hammers, and chemicals. Adaptations of forceps were also used.[4,5]

Dr. Henry J. Bigelow (1816-1890), a Boston urologist, made a significant advance towards safe lithotripty. He developed a metal lithotrite with strong intercepting jaws that could

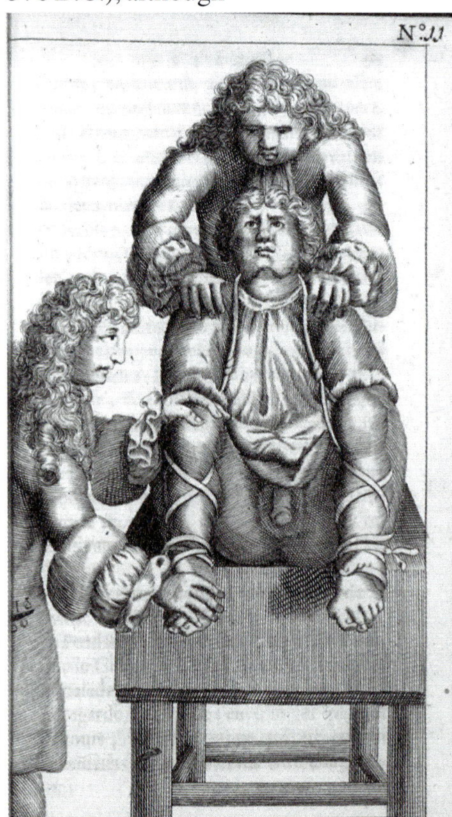


**Lithotomy Position(7)**
The operative position of the patient when "cutting for stone." *Lith* means stone; *otomy* means cutting for.

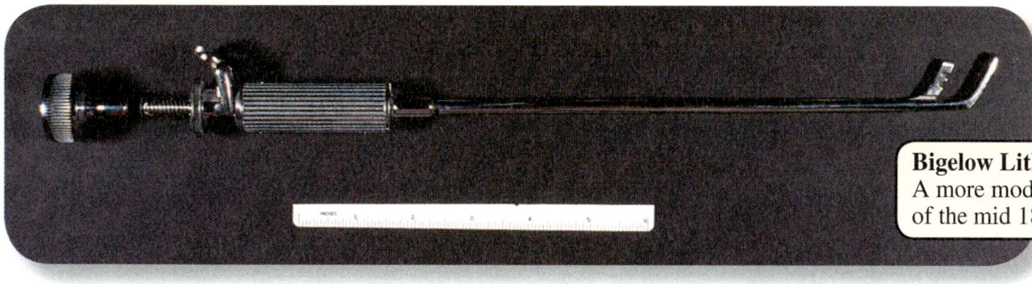

**Bigelow Lithotrite**
A more modern version of the mid 1800s original.

grope for and crush large stones. The use of evacuators facilitated the removal of all fragments. Although the procedure was performed "blind," it was very successful with a low mortality rate.[1]

In spite of significant progress in medical science which marked the eighteen and nineteenth centuries, this period may also be considered a Golden Time for Charlatanism. Over the years it was only natural for man to hold out hope that a miraculous medicine could be ingested which would dissolve stone. Various concoctions were offered such as the one by a prominent physician, Richard Lower (1631-1691). A leading physiologist of his day, he proposed that "To alleviate a stone-attack and the usually consequent retention of urine, take snail shells and bees in equal quantities, dry them in a moderately hot oven, and grind them to a very fine powder. Take as much of this as a sixpence holds, dissolve it in a quarter-mug of bone-meal water, and give it on an empty stomach, followed by two hours of fasting, every day for three days in a row. It has often been found to break down the stone and drive the urine forth."[4]

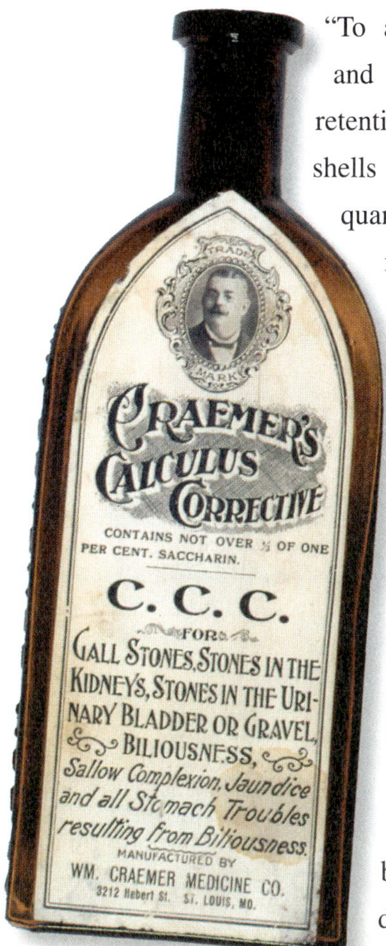


Probably the most notorious of all the "stone solvents" was the quack remedy of Joanna Stevens, a remedy actually purchased by an Act of the British Parliament in order that it might be made public for "the good of the people." Even the great English surgeon William Cheselden believed that Stevens had discovered a sovereign remedy for dissolving urinary stones, with the result that the gullible public paid five thousand pounds for the secret formula of this worthless concoction. The recipe was published in the London Gazette of June 19, 1739. The ingredients consisted of powder from old tobacco pipes, egg shells, snail shells, soap, white onions, saxifrage, burdock seed, hips and haws, and a few other common vegetable extracts.[2]

Other "infallible" medicines offered were "Craemer's Calculus Corrective," "Cowan's Lithontriptic," "Hayden's Uric Solvent," "Dr. Haskin's RE-NU," "Vaughn's Vegetable Lithontriptic Mixture." George C. Vaughn (1812-1863) started employment as a Buffalo, New York watchmaker. In 1844 his "Vegetable Lithontriptic Mixture" came into being and was manufactured and marketed successfully until the 1880s.[3]

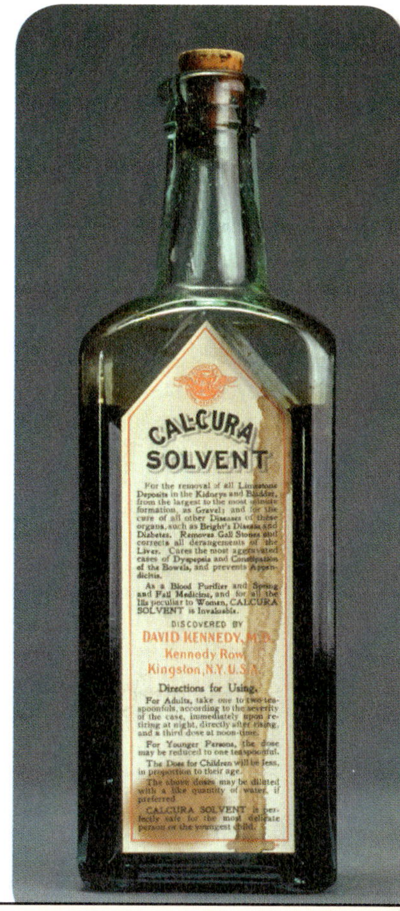


**Cal-Cura Solvent & Dr. Haskins' RE-NU**
These medicines were advertised as solvents for kidney and bladder stones and as a cure for Bright's Disease and diabetes.

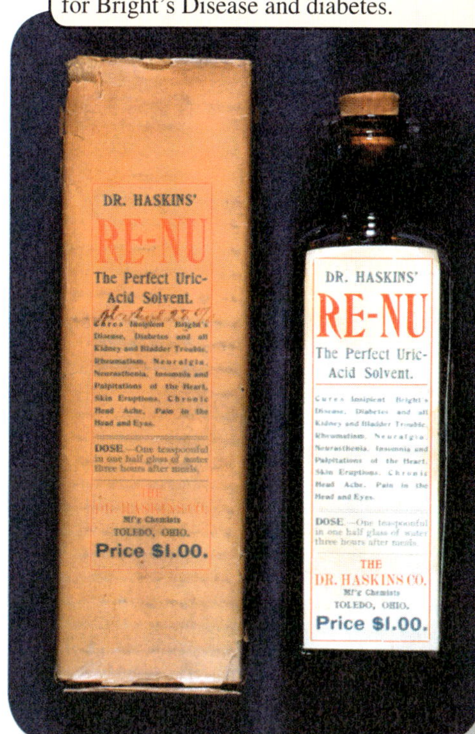

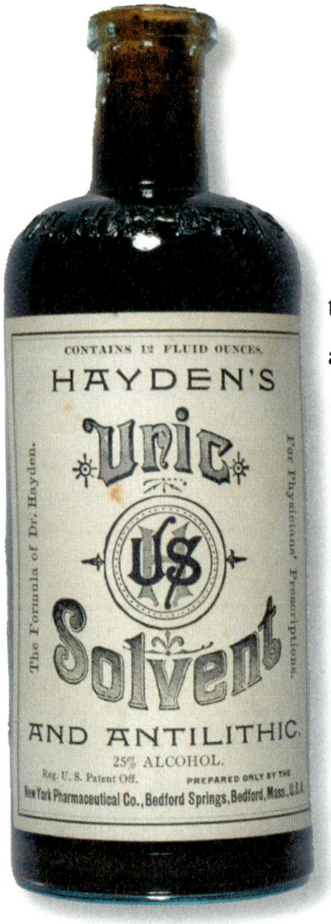


Despite the profusion of quackery at that time, there were earnest efforts being made to add information to the subject of stone disease. Some of the knowledge gained emphasized the importance of determining the basic cause, composition, and structure of the various types of stones and their relationship to different forms of therapy.

However, today we still have practitioners of botanical medicine who use herbs in combination "to help facilitate the passage of small kidney stones and to help prevent their formation." Currently, herbal diuretics also are given as teas to further increase fluid intake as well as deliver the medicinal herbs. Herbal over-the-counter correctives for stone disease include: Horsetail *(Equisetum arvense)*, Java tea *(Orthosiphon stamineus)*, Stinging nettle *(Urtica dioca)* as well as Asparagus root, Birch leaf, Couch grass, Goldenrod, Lovage, Parsley, and Spiny restharrow.[6]

Despite the progress of today's science man continues to be afflicted by urinary stone disease. It is estimated that about 10 percent of all men and four percent of women suffer from stones at some time and half will experience a recurrence. Older methods of "open surgery" will be increasingly replaced by new percutaneous and endoscopic methods of fragmentation and removal. Shock wave lithotripsy has revolutionized urinary stone management.

While one awaits the event of his first stone attack, pondering the following may help to develop a philosophic mind.

"**Stones Unturned**

I never saw a bladder stone
I hope I never see one
But, I can tell you here and now
I'd rather see than pee one."

(Author unknown)

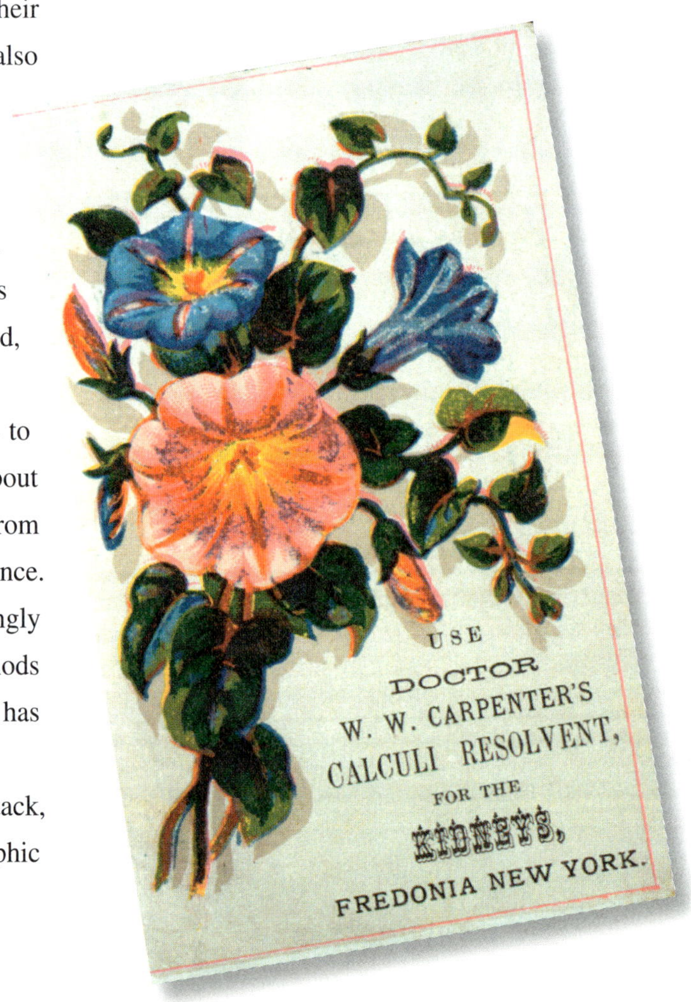

Chapter 12

# Mineral Spring Waters

Throughout history, natural mineral waters were regarded as beneficial to one's health. Europeans believed in the invigorating properties of mineral baths and health spas. The rich would frolic in the cure-all waters, while the less fortunate could only dream of its taste. By 1880 there were many mineral spring resorts across America. Soon bottled mineral spring waters, either imported from Europe or produced in the United States, added up to an impressive amount of drinking. Such waters were spring waters with or without natural carbonation. However, the waters contained minerals and lithia, which tweaked the fertile imagination of the hucksters, who fancied a new product to be promoted and peddled. The bottle labels described miraculous cures and remedies for all of man's ailments. There were "Gettysburg Katalysine Water, Nature's Great Remedy for Gout, Rheumatism, and All Kidney and Bladder Troubles," "Bethesda Mineral Spring Water, Cures All Kidney Diseases, Bright's Disease, Diabetes, Torpid Liver, Insomnia, Calculi,

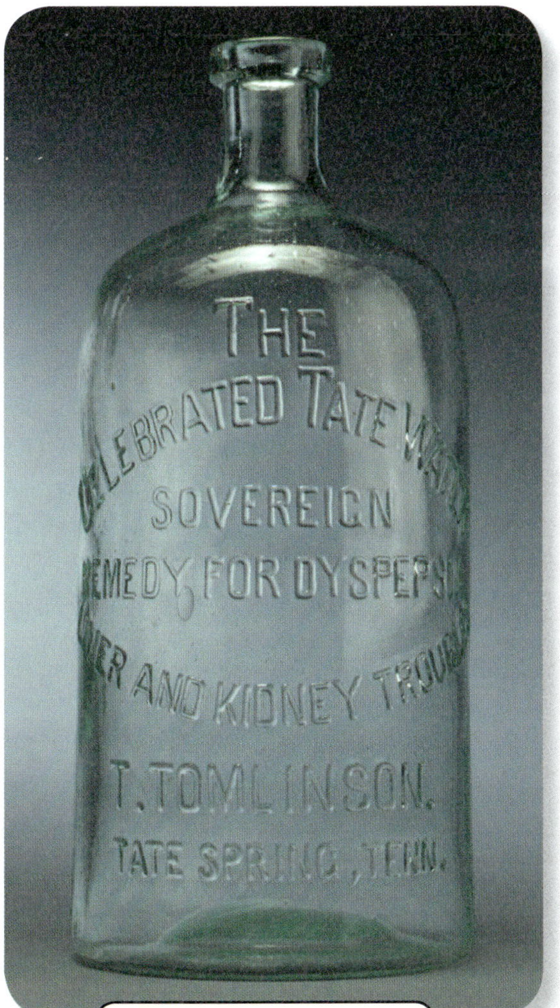

The Celebrated Tate Water

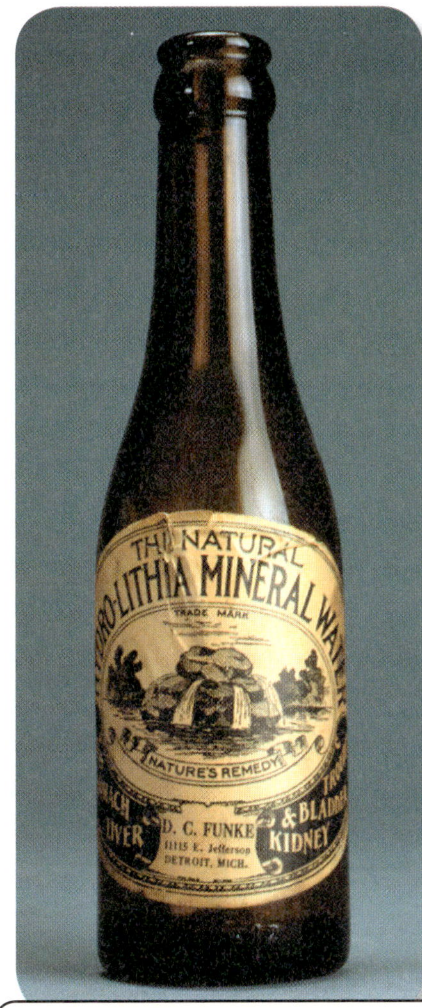

The Natural Hydro-Lithia Mineral Water

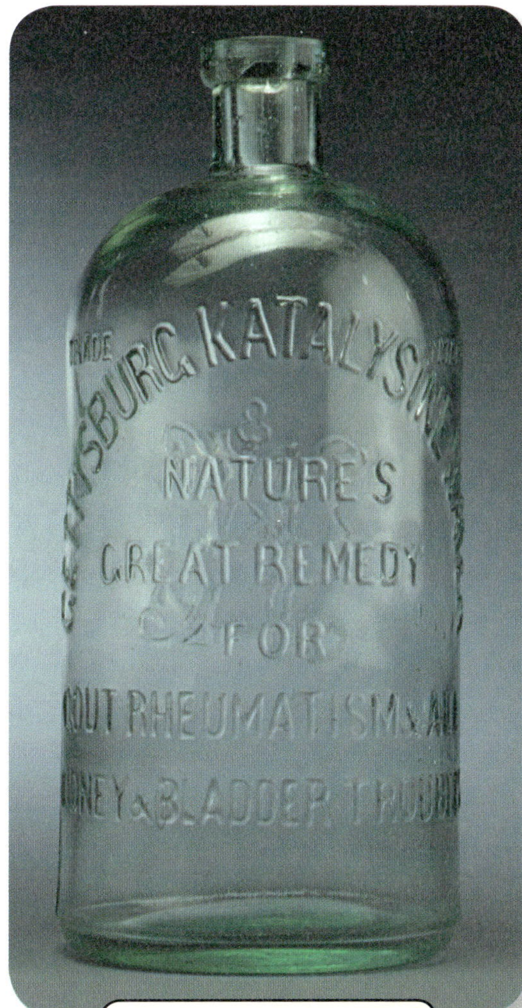

Gettysburg Katalysine Water

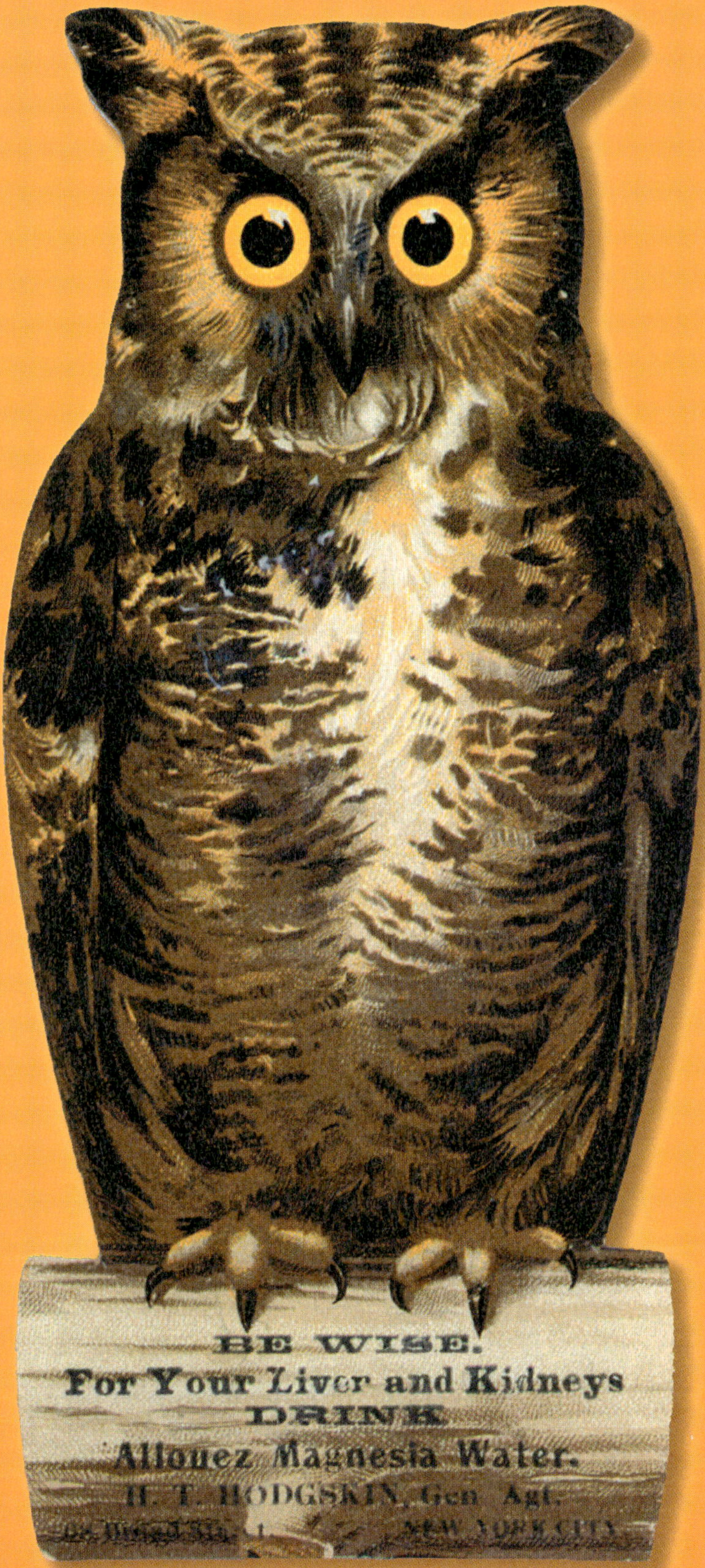
BE WISE.
For Your Liver and Kidneys
DRINK
Allouez Magnesia Water.
H. T. HODGSKIN, Gen. Agt.
NEW YORK CITY

and Nervous Prostration," "Londonderry Lithia Spring Water Co., Cures Gravel, Bright's Disease, Diabetes, Dropsy, and Diseases of the Kidney and Bladder," and more.[1,2,3]

Eventually the medicinal waters were artificially carbonated, sweetened, and then flavored to improve the taste. In the late 1800s many new "soda" beverages were produced for medicinal purposes. And so, the soft drink or soda beverage industry of today had its beginnings producing patent medicines.[3]

Today bottled water is regulated by the FDA and the International Bottled Water Association. A water product, such as spring water, must be water that is derived from an underground formation from which water flows naturally to the surface of the earth. It must be collected only at the spring. Mineral water, by definition, must contain not less than 250 parts per million total dissolved solids that come from the water source. No minerals can be added. Regulations have dramatically changed the bottled water industry so that today, according to the Beverage Marketing Corporation, it is the fastest growing beverage segment in the United States.[4]

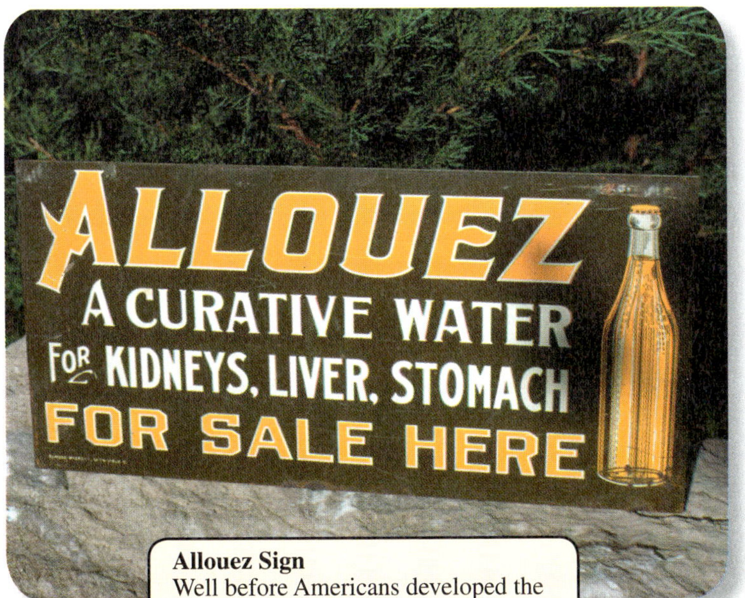


**Allouez Sign**
Well before Americans developed the health spa business, Europeans were "taking the waters" both by the way of bathing and drinking.

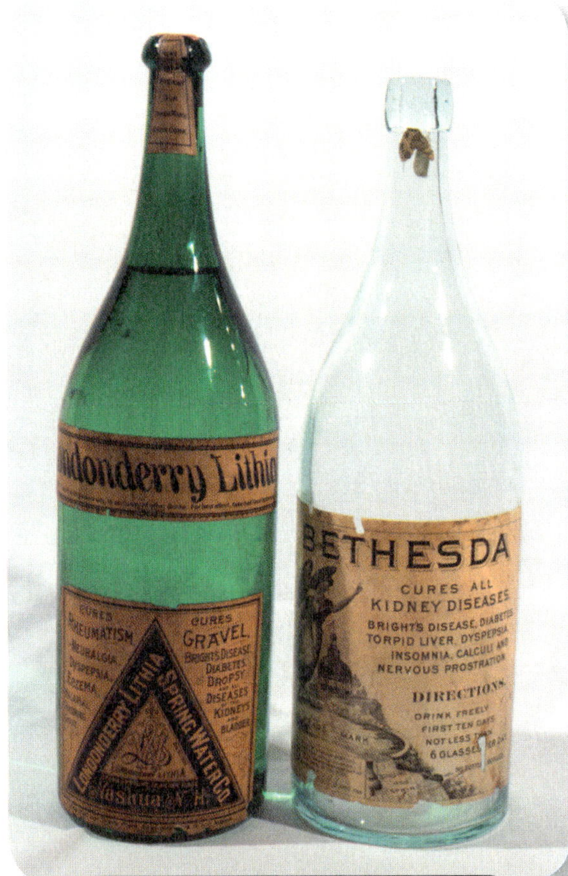


**Bethesda Mineral Spring Water**
**Londonerry Lithia Spring Water Co.**
The bottling of mineral spring water developed from the mineral spring health spa business on the theory that what is good for the outside of the body, must also be good for the inside.

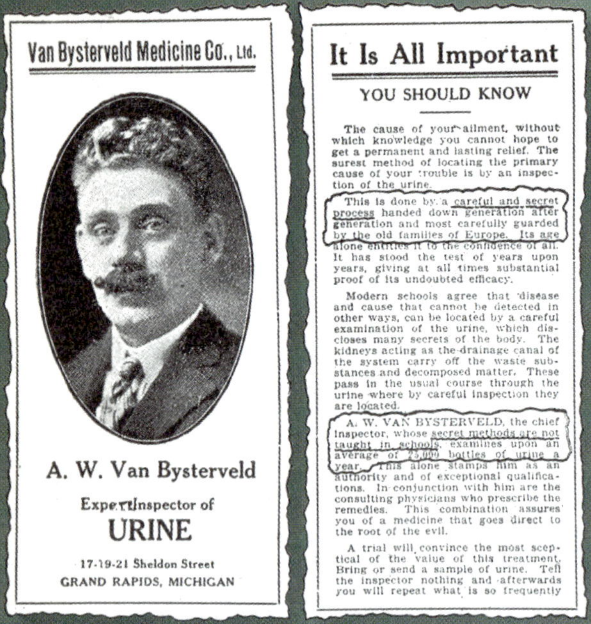

Van Bysterveld Medicine Co., Ltd.

A. W. Van Bysterveld

Expert Inspector of

URINE

17-19-21 Sheldon Street
GRAND RAPIDS, MICHIGAN

It Is All Important

YOU SHOULD KNOW

The cause of your ailment, without which knowledge you cannot hope to get a permanent and lasting relief. The surest method of locating the primary cause of your trouble is by an inspection of the urine.

This is done by a careful and secret process handed down generation after generation and most carefully guarded by the old families of Europe. Its age alone entitles it to the confidence of all. It has stood the test of years upon years, giving at all times substantial proof of its undoubted efficacy.

Modern schools agree that disease and cause that cannot be detected in other ways, can be located by a careful examination of the urine, which discloses many secrets of the body. The kidneys acting as the drainage canal of the system carry off the waste substances and decomposed matter. These pass in the usual course through the urine where by careful inspection they are located.

A. W. VAN BYSTERVELD, the chief inspector, whose secret methods are not taught in schools, examines upon an average of 25,000 bottles of urine a year. This alone stamps him as an authority and of exceptional qualifications. In conjunction with him are the consulting physicians who prescribe the remedies. This combination assures you of a medicine that goes direct to the root of the evil.

A trial will convince the most sceptical of the value of this treatment. Bring or send a sample of urine. Tell the inspector nothing and afterwards you will repeat what is so frequently

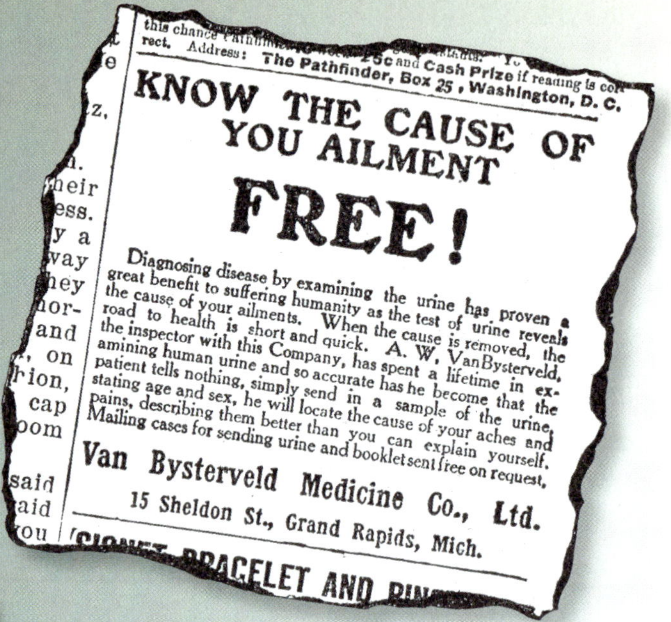

rect. Address: The Pathfinder, Box 25, Washington, D. C.

KNOW THE CAUSE OF YOU AILMENT

FREE!

Diagnosing disease by examining the urine has proven a great benefit to suffering humanity as the test of urine reveals the cause of your ailments. When the cause is removed, the road to health is short and quick. A. W. VanBysterveld, the inspector with this Company, has spent a lifetime in examining human urine and so accurate has he become that the patient tells nothing, simply send in a sample of the urine, stating age and sex, he will locate the cause of your aches and pains, describing them better than you can explain yourself. Mailing cases for sending urine and booklet sent free on request.

Van Bysterveld Medicine Co., Ltd.

15 Sheldon St., Grand Rapids, Mich.

# THE HUCKSTERS

"To delay for the sake of diagnosis is simply to waste valuable time. [Delay] is one of the errors of so-called scientific medicine, and should have nothing to do with the cure."

William Radam–1890
(Maker of Radam's Microbe Killer)

Chapter 13

# H.H. Warner- The Rise and Fall

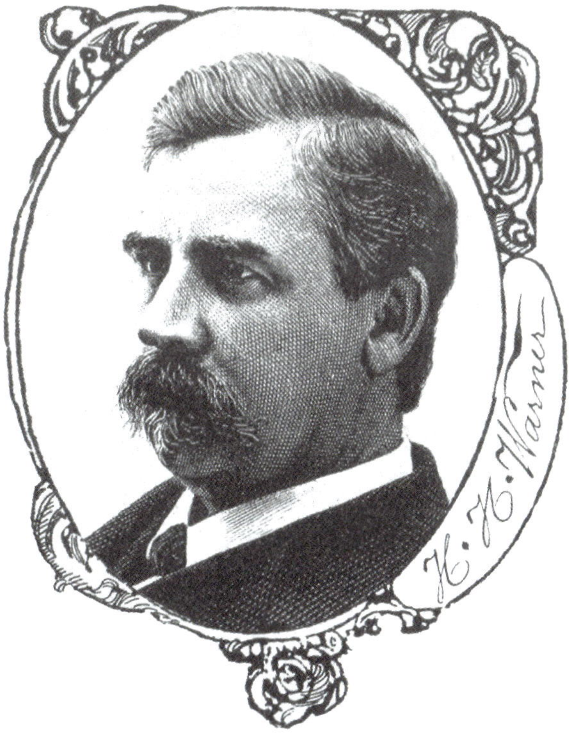


Hulbert Harrington Warner was one of the most charismatic and successful proprietary medicine manufacturers. He is remembered for the grand scale of his life style, philanthropy, and business success as well as his shady business practices, outrageous promotional claims, and questionable stock manipulation.[2]

In 1870 H.H. Warner began his career in Rochester, New York, selling fireproof safes. As business boomed, Warner, safe salesman extraordinaire soon became a millionaire. Warner's interest in the proprietary medicine business came from personal ill health allegedly thought to be Bright's disease. Uncertain as to its benefits, Warner tried Dr. Craig's Kidney Cure. Warner's dramatic improvement convinced him of the great possibilities in promoting such a miraculous medicine. He decided to sell the safe business and acquire Dr. Craig's patent medicine business. He felt inspired to "change the life of the hopeless suffering to the happiness of health." With promotional genius Warner soon enjoyed great success. Warner, no longer the safe salesman, now produced "safe" medicines with bottles that were embossed with the image of an iron safe.[1,3,4,5] Although he produced over 20 different "safe" medicines, by far his most successful nostrum was "Warner's Safe Kidney and Liver Cure." The formula or ingredients used to quicken and increase the efficiency of Kidney and Liver Cure were these:[4]

**TESTIMONIALS FOR WARNER'S SAFE CURE**

| Presidents: | Others: |
|---|---|
| J.A. Garfield | Longfellow |
| U.S. Grant | Oliver Wendell Holmes |
| R.B. Hayes | Whittier |
| C.A. Arthur | W.J. Bryan |
| W. McKinley | Thomas A. Edison |
| | Mark Twain |

| | |
|---|---|
| • Extract lycopus virginiana | 308 grains |
| • Extract liverwort | 322 grains |
| • Extract wintergreen | 7.5 grains |
| • Potassium Nitrate | 39 grains |
| • Alcohol (90 percent) | 2.5 ounces |
| • Glycerin | 10 drams |
| • Water sufficient to make | 1 pint |

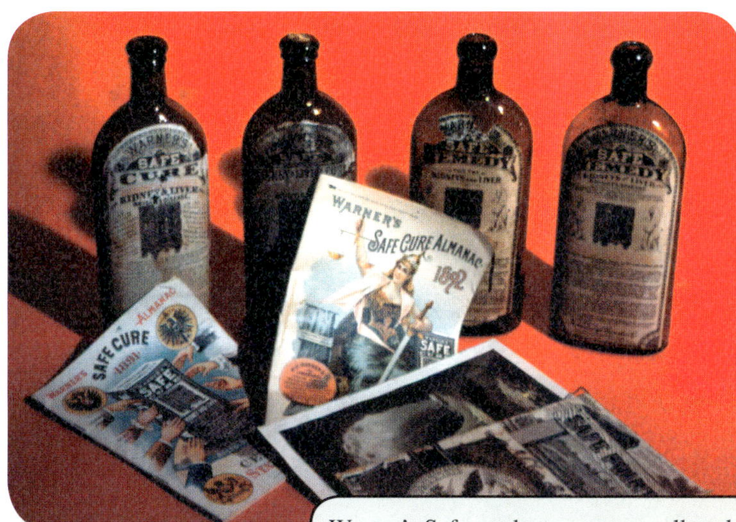

Warner's Safe products are very collectable.

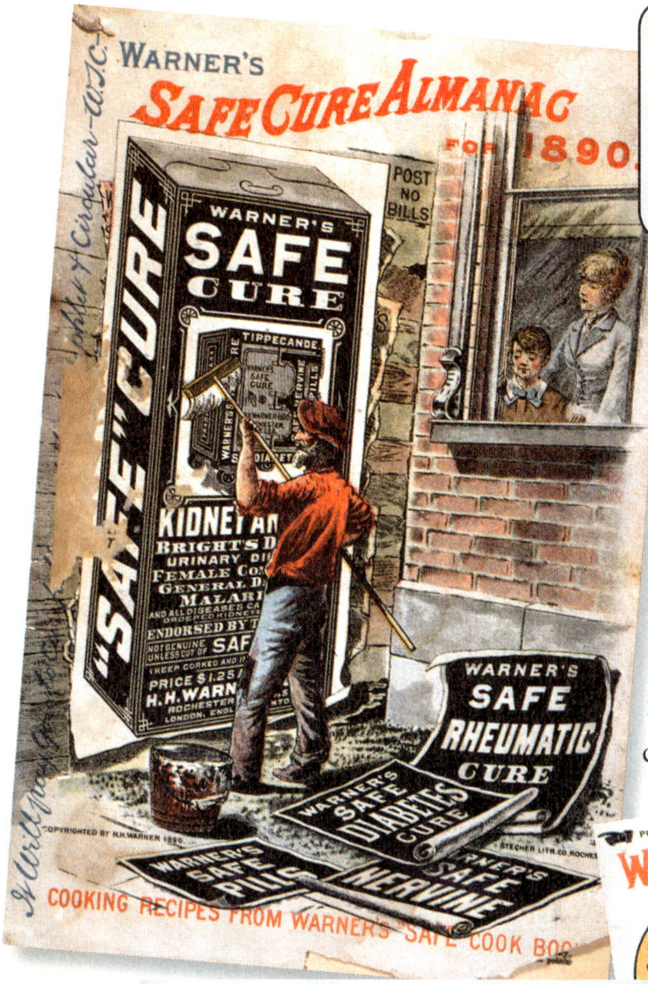


**Almanac 1890**
In the free and easy days, before the public was protected by the Food and Drug Act, Warner's Safe Cure was advertised extensively - and fraudulently. Efforts were made to advertise that "most aches and pains are due to diseased kidneys, - that a pain in the back is a sure sign of Bright's Disease, - the only sure cure is the Warner's nostrum." Also purported was a sure and simple test for kidney disease. "Put some urine in a glass or bottle; let it stand for twenty-four hours. If it is cloudy etc. your kidneys are diseased. This is the supreme moment when you should begin to take Warner's Safe Cure."
*Nostrums and Quackery. Vol.II, p.208, 1921.*

Warner embarked on a campaign of flamboyant philanthropy, entrepreneurial schemes, and sustained promotions that lasted almost a decade. In the process, he brought himself and Rochester international fame. His factory had the capacity of producing 7000 gallons of medicine daily, or 56,000 pint bottles, each of which sold for $1.25. His profits were estimated to be a half million dollars annually. From the Rochester based company branches were opened internationally first in London, England and Toronto, Canada. Further company expansion in Australia, Germany, Austria–Hungary, Switzerland, and New Zealand made it the world's leader for the manufacture of proprietary medicines.[1,5]

The signs and symptoms of various maladies were described in almanacs and packaged literature. Self-diagnosis and treatment were grandly promoted and guaranteed. Fervent followers, who had imbibed and benefitted from Warner's concoctions, issued testimonials. Warner continually offered a $5,000 reward to anyone who could prove that one of the testimonials he supplied was not authentic. Each year Warner repeated that the reward had not been collected. Of significance were the testimonials of presidents J.A. Garfield, U.S. Grant, R.B. Hayes, C.A. Arthur, W. McKinley, as well as such notables as Henry Wadsworth Longfellow, Oliver Wendell Holmes,

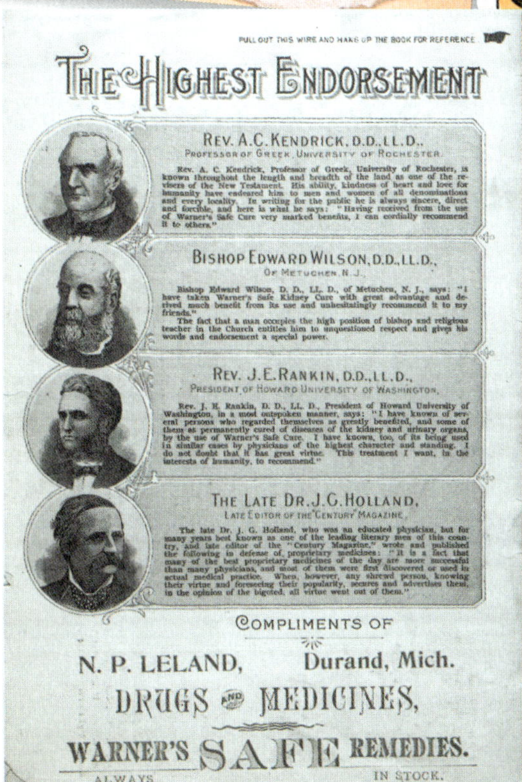


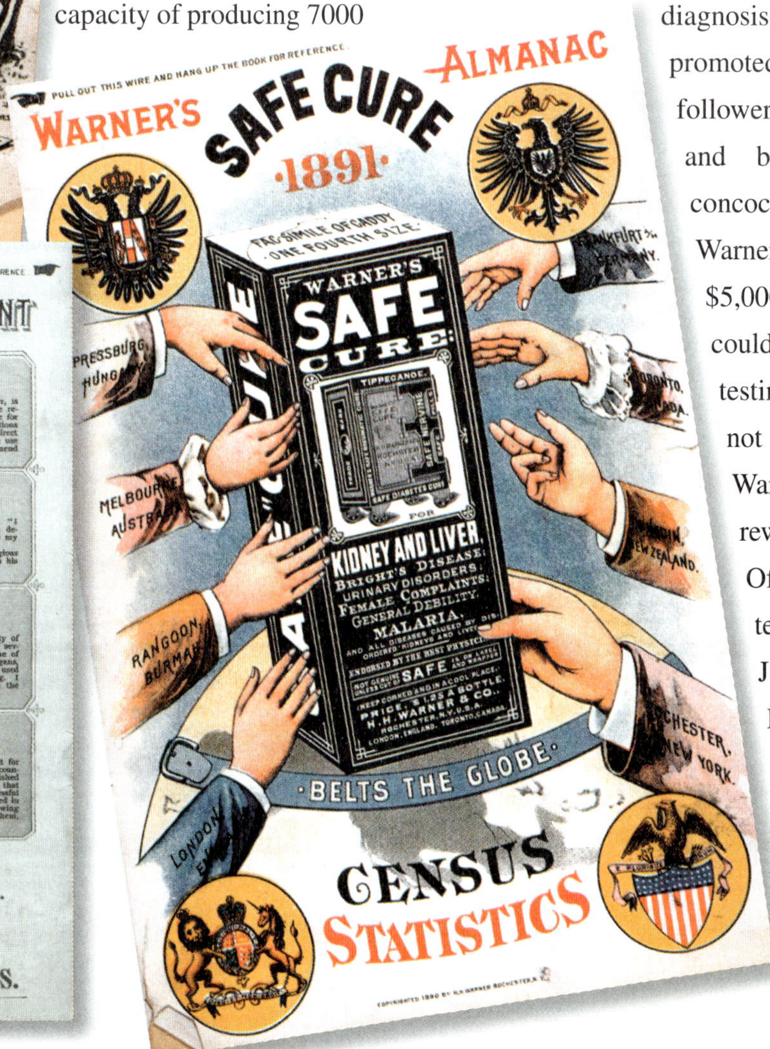

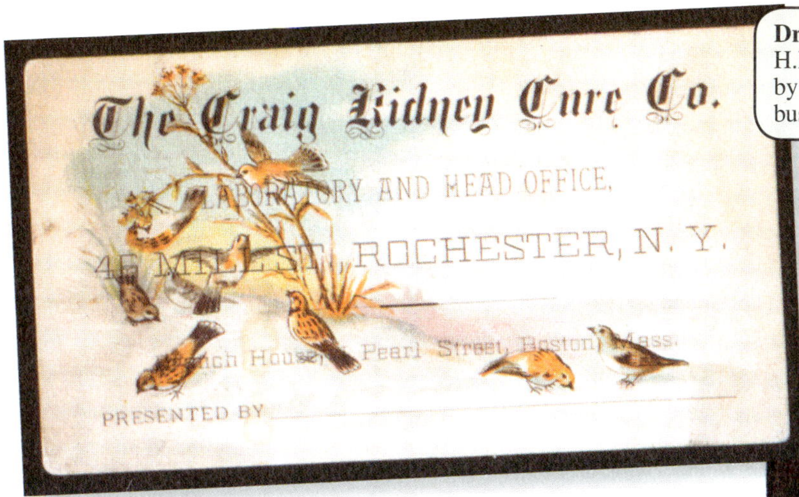


**Dr. Craig's Kidney Cure Co.**
H.H. Warner's apparent cure of his Bright's Disease by Dr. Craig's medicine, prompted him to sell his safe business and become the foremost patent medicine maker.

John Greenleaf Whittier, William Jennings Bryan, Thomas A. Edison, and Mark Twain.[1,5,6]

In keeping with his flamboyant style Warner built next to his luxurious Victorian mansion the largest private observatory in the nation into which was installed the nation's fourth largest telescope. Warner helped organize the Rochester Chamber of Commerce and became its first president. Later he was chosen Man of the Year over George Eastman of Eastman Kodak.[1,5]

Due to his high-flying style and penchant for a high stakes gamble, Warner's empire soon began to totter. He eventually sold his medicine company to an English syndicate in 1892 for $3.4 million, quite a sum in those days. But because of the recession in England in 1893, payment could not be made to Warner. Warner's financial plight worsened until his creditors forced him into bankruptcy. Warner lived for 30 years after his fortunes came crashing down. Every one of his last years was marked by loneliness, struggle, and poverty. "His fall," wrote Blake McKelvey, a Rochester city historian, "was . . . more spectacular than his rise."[1,3,5]

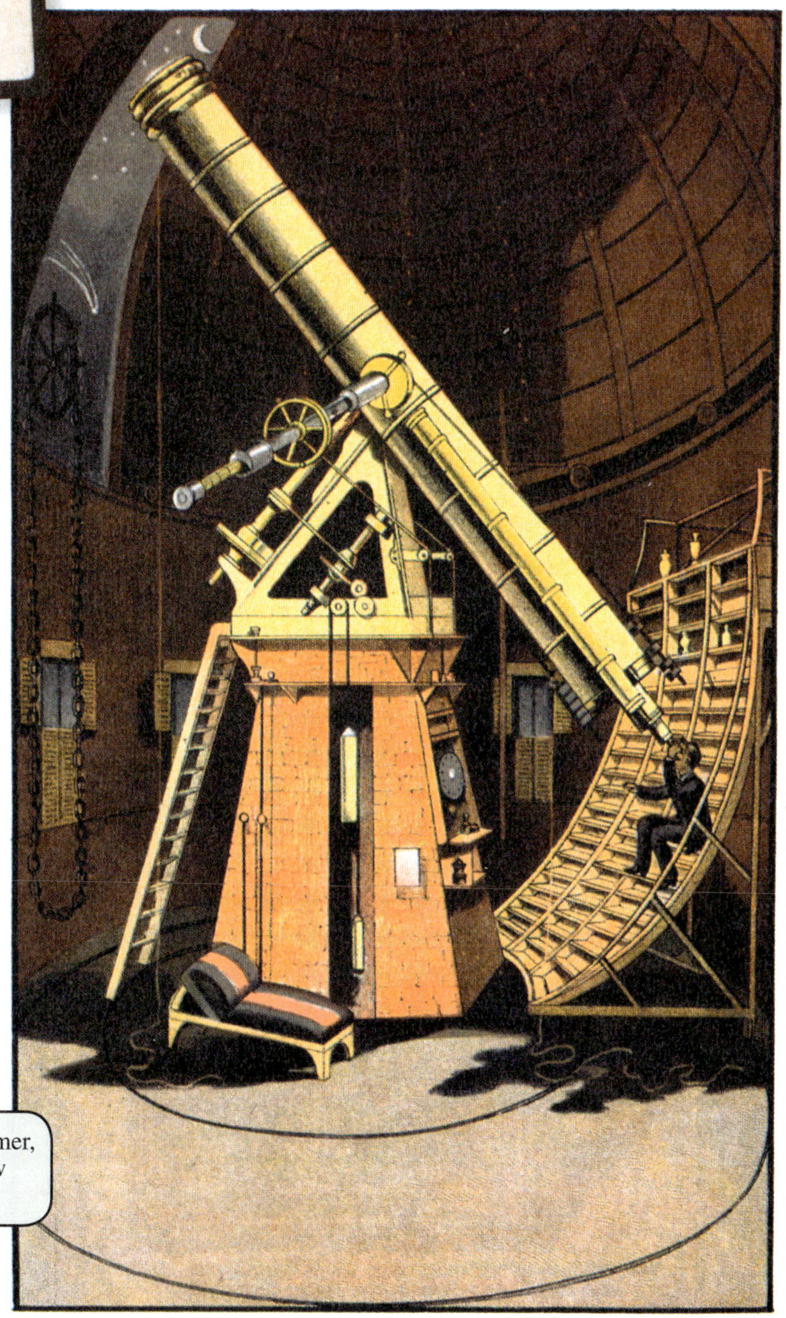

H.H. Warner's private observatory was managed by an amateur astronomer, "Doctor" Lewis Swift. In ten years Swift was credited in finding six new comets and 900 nebulae.

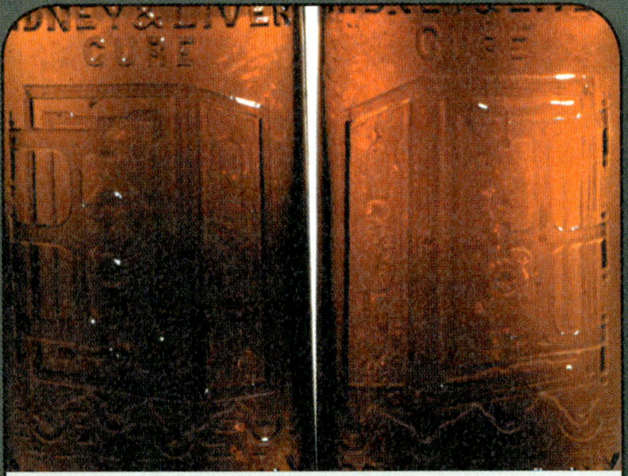


Warner's Kidney and Liver Cure bottle was a 10.25 inch amber glass bottle. It had a full label on one side and bold embossing on the other. In the center of the embossing was the Warner trademark, a banker's safe. The safe was at times reversed.

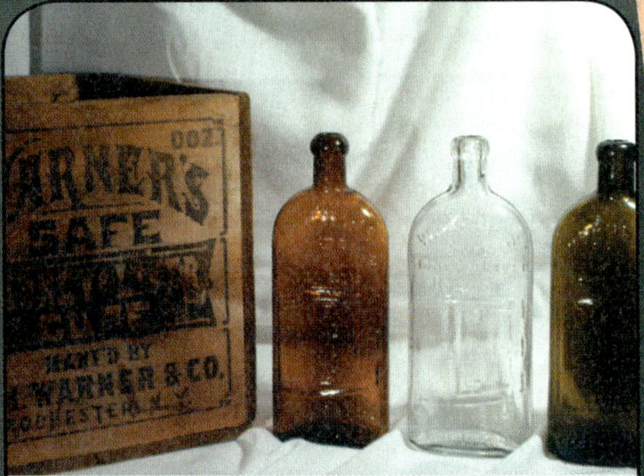


Warner's Kidney and Liver Remedy Bottles in amber, clear and green glass are very desirable. After 1906 medicine like Warner's Safe Cure was renamed Warner's Safe Remedy and dropped entirely all alcohol by adding more glycerin.

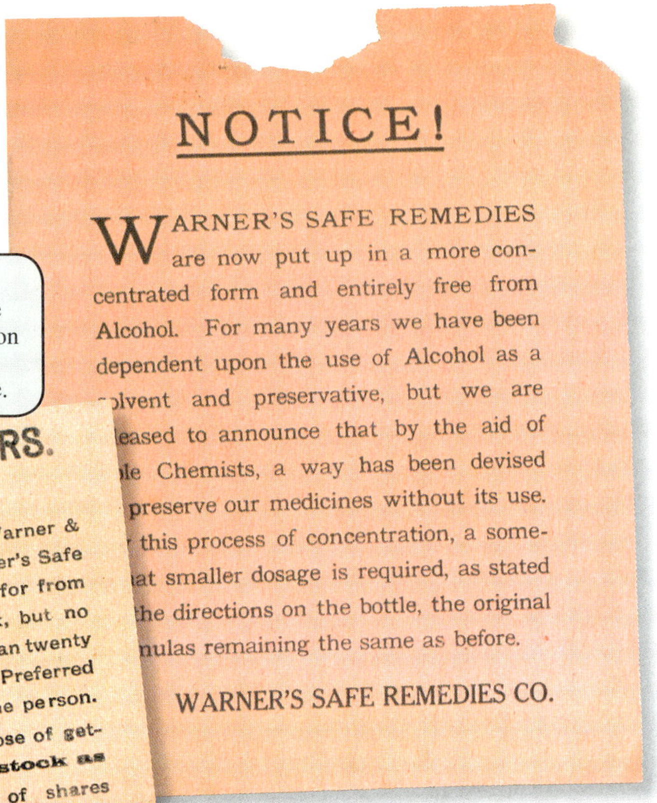

NOTICE!

WARNER'S SAFE REMEDIES are now put up in a more concentrated form and entirely free from Alcohol. For many years we have been dependent upon the use of Alcohol as a ...olvent and preservative, but we are ...leased to announce that by the aid of ...le Chemists, a way has been devised ... preserve our medicines without its use. ... this process of concentration, a some...at smaller dosage is required, as stated ... the directions on the bottle, the original ...nulas remaining the same as before.

WARNER'S SAFE REMEDIES CO.

A notice to subscribers that they were limited to no more then twenty shares of common stock to achieve the widest distribution of stock possible.

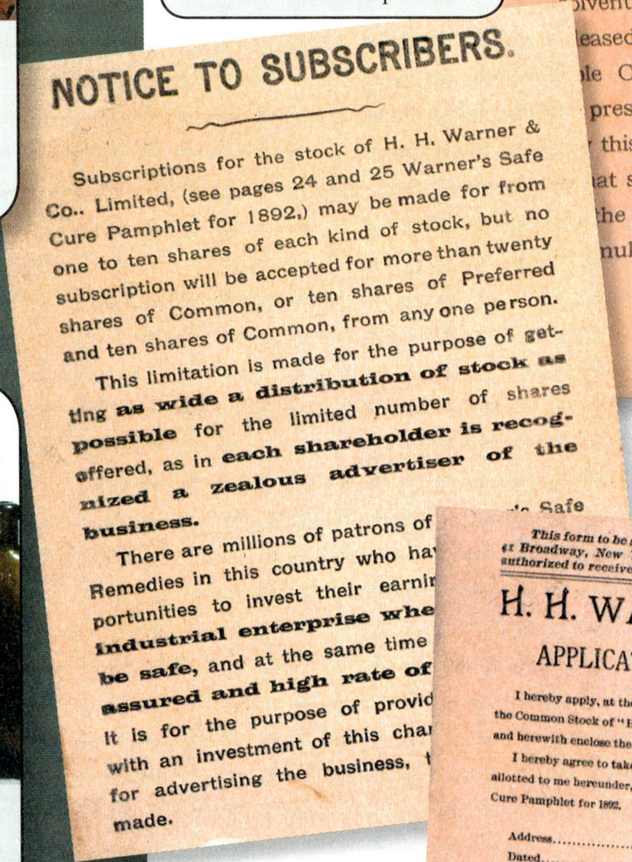

NOTICE TO SUBSCRIBERS.

Subscriptions for the stock of H. H. Warner & Co.. Limited, (see pages 24 and 25 Warner's Safe Cure Pamphlet for 1892,) may be made for from one to ten shares of each kind of stock, but no subscription will be accepted for more than twenty shares of Common, or ten shares of Preferred and ten shares of Common, from any one person.

This limitation is made for the purpose of getting **as wide a distribution of stock as possible** for the limited number of shares offered, as in **each shareholder is recognized a zealous advertiser of the business.**

There are millions of patrons of ...'s Safe Remedies in this country who ha... portunities to invest their earni... **industrial enterprise whe... be safe,** and at the same time ... **assured and high rate of** ... It is for the purpose of provid... with an investment of this cha... for advertising the business, ... made.

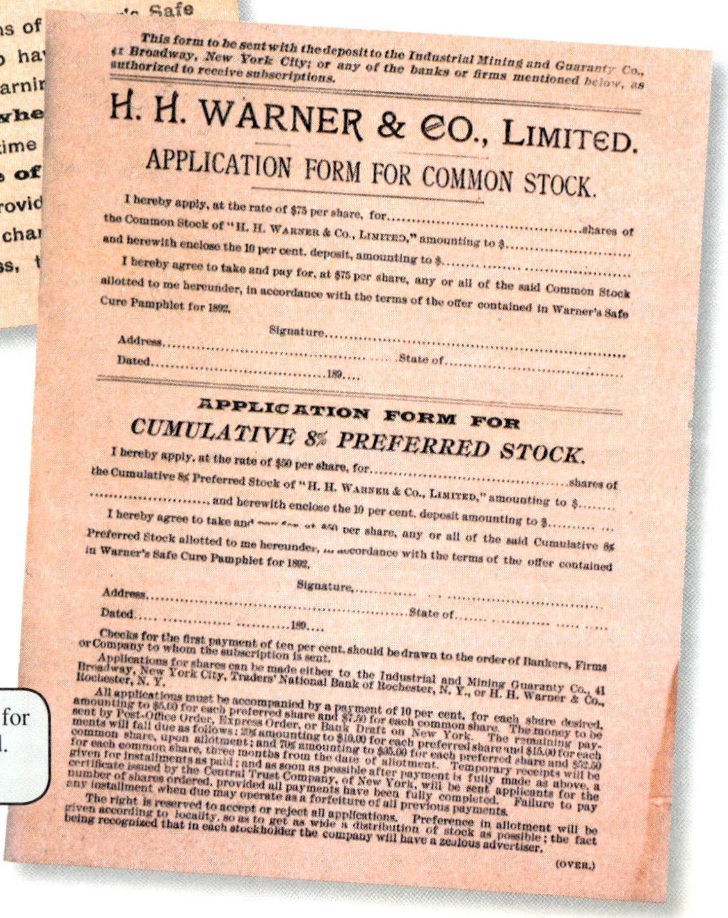

*This form to be sent with the deposit to the Industrial Mining and Guaranty Co., 41 Broadway, New York City; or any of the banks or firms mentioned below, as authorized to receive subscriptions.*

H. H. WARNER & CO., LIMITED.

APPLICATION FORM FOR COMMON STOCK.

I hereby apply, at the rate of $75 per share, for.................................shares of the Common Stock of "H. H. Warner & Co., Limited," amounting to $........................ and herewith enclose the 10 per cent. deposit, amounting to $........................

I hereby agree to take and pay for, at $75 per share, any or all of the said Common Stock allotted to me hereunder, in accordance with the terms of the offer contained in Warner's Safe Cure Pamphlet for 1892.

Signature........................................

Address.................................State of..............................

Dated..................................189....

APPLICATION FORM FOR

CUMULATIVE 8% PREFERRED STOCK.

I hereby apply, at the rate of $50 per share, for.................................shares of the Cumulative 8% Preferred Stock of "H. H. Warner & Co., Limited," amounting to $....... ........................, and herewith enclose the 10 per cent. deposit amounting to $..........

I hereby agree to take an... per share, any or all of the said Cumulative 8% Preferred Stock allotted to me hereunder, ... accordance with the terms of the offer contained in Warner's Safe Cure Pamphlet for 1892.

Signature,........................................

Address.................................State of..............................

Dated..................................189....

Checks for the first payment of ten per cent. should be drawn to the order of Bankers, Firms or Company to whom the subscription is sent.

Applications for shares can be made either to the Industrial and Mining Guaranty Co., 41 Broadway, New York City, Traders' National Bank of Rochester, N. Y., or H. H. Warner & Co., Rochester, N. Y.

All applications must be accompanied by a payment of 10 per cent. for each share desired, amounting to $5.00 for each preferred share and $7.50 for each common share. The money to be sent by Post-Office Order, Express Order, or Bank Draft on New York. The remaining payments will fall due as follows: 20% amounting to $10.00 for each preferred share and $15.00 for each common share, upon allotment; and 70% amounting to $35.00 for each preferred share and $52.50 for each common share, three months from the date of allotment. Temporary receipts will be given for installments as paid; and as soon as possible after payment is fully made as above, a certificate issued by the Central Trust Company, of New York, will be sent applicants for the number of shares ordered, provided all payments have been fully completed. Failure to pay any installment when due may operate as a forfeiture of all previous payments.

The right is reserved to accept or reject all applications. Preference in allotment will be given according to locality, so as to get as wide a distribution of stock as possible; the fact being recognized that in each stockholder the company will have a zealous advertiser.

(OVER.)

An application form for the H.H. Warner, Ltd. stock offering.

Chapter 14

# Swamproot
# The Kidney Cure

S. Andral Kilmer, M.D. of Binghamton, New York was the concocter of "Swamproot, the Great Kidney, Liver and Bladder Specific."[1,6] He received from several medical colleges including Jefferson in Philadelphia, Bellevue in New York, Albany in Albany and Bennett in Chicago three scholastic degrees including the doctorate of medicine. Beginning with the general practice of medicine Dr. Kilmer soon branched out to establish hygienic or sanitary institutions. Ten miles east of Binghamton he built a sanatorium at Sanatoria Springs. In the mid 1870s he established a "Can-certorium."

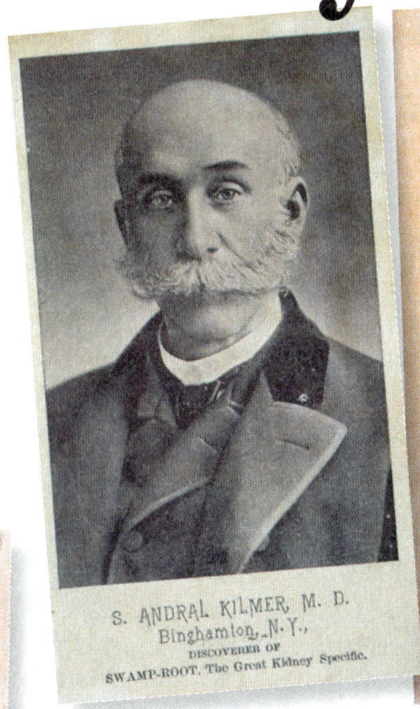

S. ANDRAL KILMER, M. D.
Binghamton, N. Y.,
DISCOVERER OF
SWAMP-ROOT, The Great Kidney Specific.


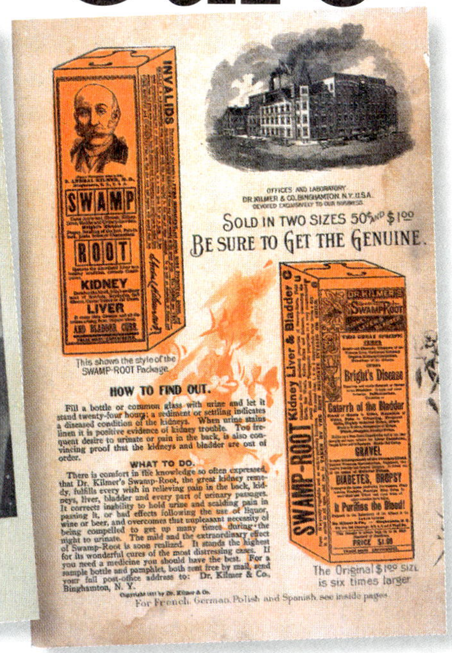


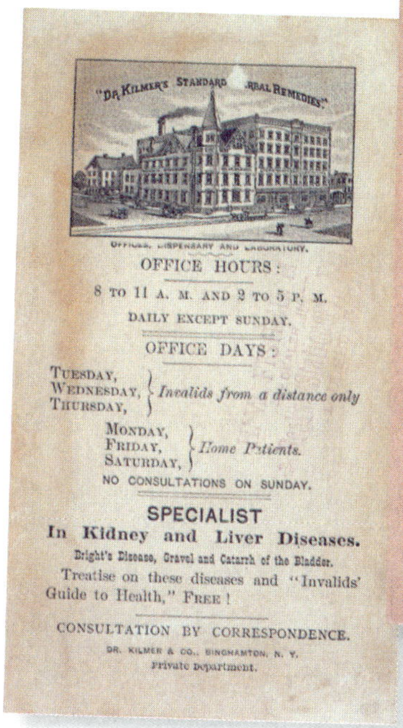


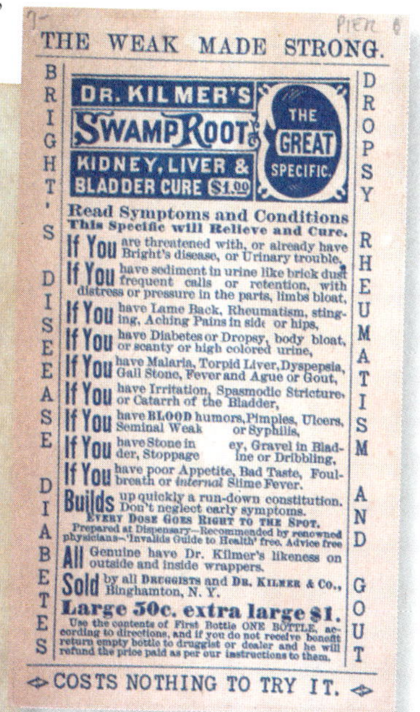


Dr. Kilmer would apply ointments of secret ingredients as a non-operative treatment for cancer. The tumor would reportedly "just fall off." He was also a promoter of a line of pills, ointments, and home medicines for every ailment.[2,4,5]

Five years younger, Jonas M. Kilmer joined his doctor brother, Andral, in 1878 and became a full partner in the nostrum business in 1881. They produced medicines that included "Indian Cough Cure," "Autumn Leaf Extract," "Ocean Weed Heart Remedy," "Prompt Parilla Pills," and of course "Swamp Root." In 1882 the brothers built a five story building that included a machine that could fill 2000 bottles per hour. A conveyer belt operation facilitated corking, waxing, labeling and packaging of the bottles. Unfortunately conflict developed between Andral and Jonas which resulted in Jonas becoming sole owner in 1893. Andral disappeared medically, but he did leave behind his face, his whiskers, and his MD degree, which were used as the trademark for "Dr. Kilmer's Standard Herbal Remedies."[3,4]

*Reprinted with permission of The New York Public Library.*

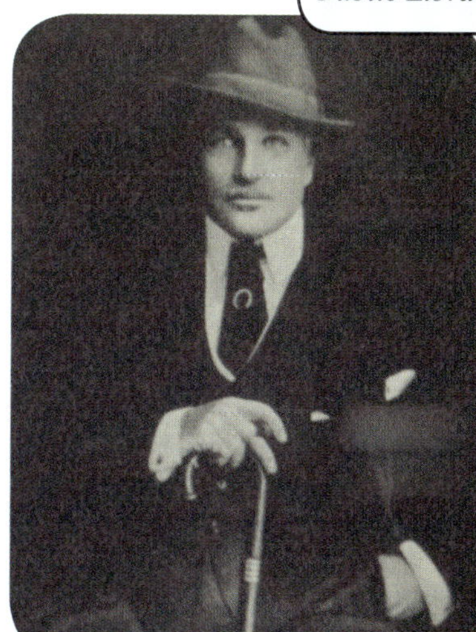

Willis Sharpe Kilmer

The Swamproot ads said that "Dr. Kilmer" wanted folks to write to him about their kidney troubles. Since Andral was no longer with the

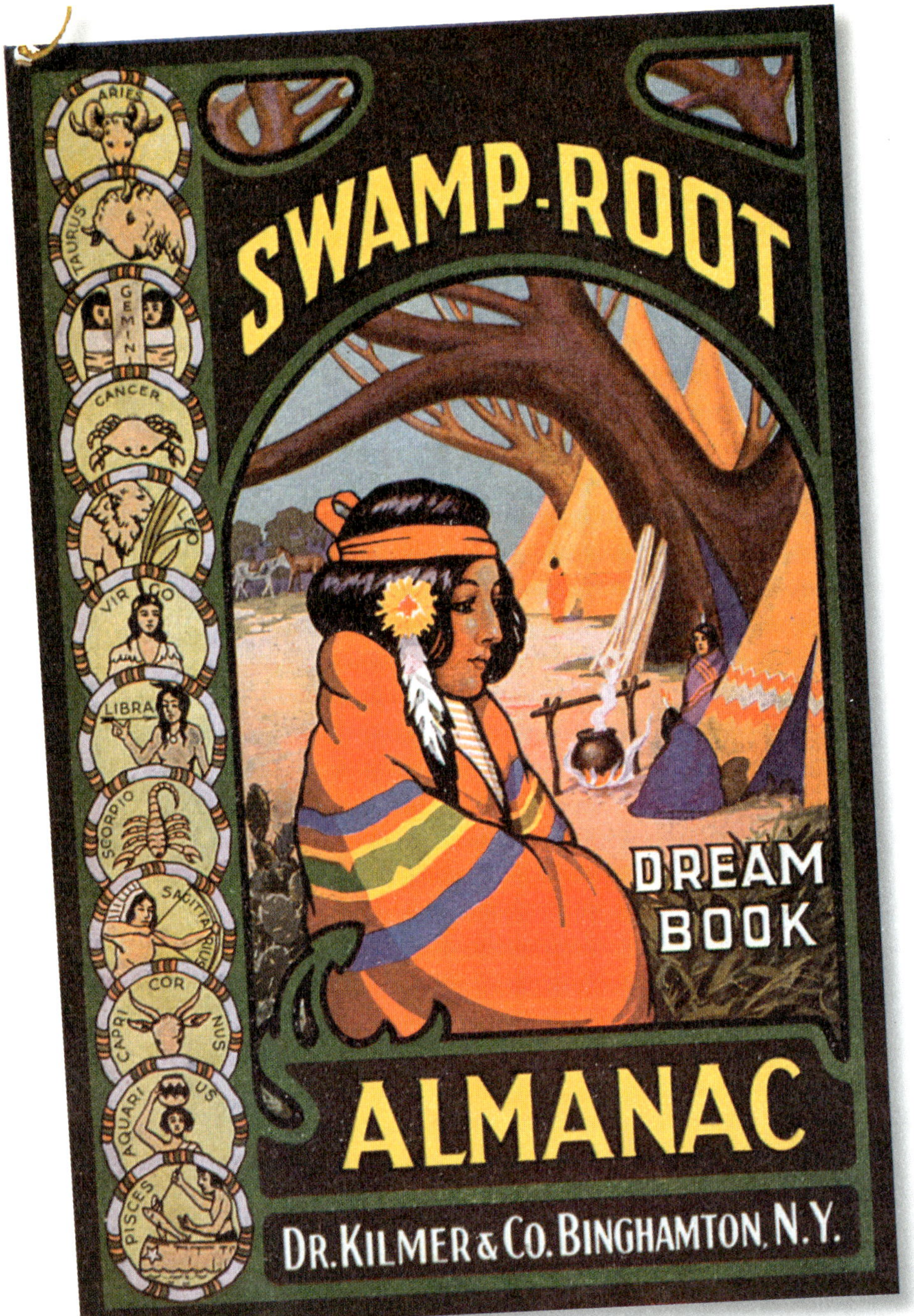


**Dr. Kilmer's Swamp Root Almanac**
The loyalty of the people who medicined themselves, with their raw courage, are as astonishing as their capacity to take the medicine. As the Kilmers pointed out, thousands have kidney trouble and don't know it, but much more important is the reverse. There are thousands who "knew" they had kidney trouble but in reality were well. Thus, the truism is "A cured patient pays no fee. Keep 'um sick!"

company, he complained bitterly and brought legal proceedings against Jonas. Although Jonas could handle his doctor brother, Andral, he was not able to effectively reap the profits of the nostrum trade.

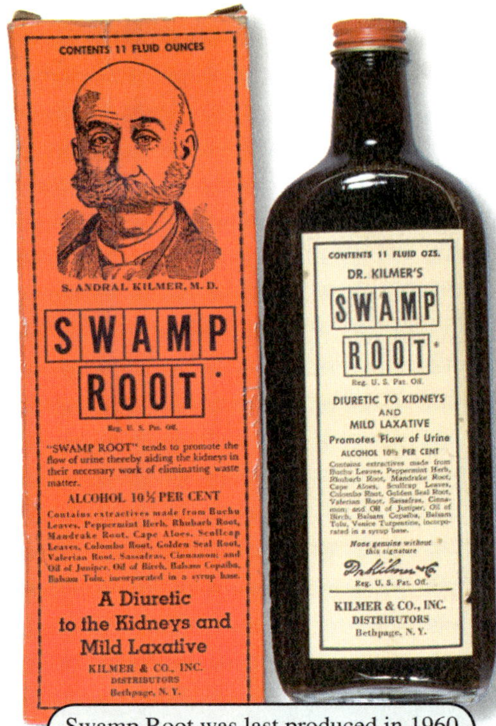


Swamp Root was last produced in 1960 in a screw topped bottle, with simple labeling, in a bright red box.

But the real story of Swamproot begins with Willis Sharpe Kilmer, nephew of Andral and son of Jonas. Willis, having just returned from Cornell University, was a dashing, good-looking son, who was full of derring-do. His willful and imaginative style combined to give the flamboyant promotion that Swamproot needed. "Swamproot, the Great Kidney Specific," was very profitable and it became the bellwether of the Kilmer Herbal Remedies. Country folks living in remote Southern hamlets could identify the bewhiskered Dr. Kilmer, but could not recall the name of the President of the United States.[2,3,4,5]

Willis became the company president in 1912. From the Binghamton based company branches were opened in Rio de Janeiro, Brazil; Kingston, Jamaica; and London, England. Advertising and almanacs were still being produced as late as 1933–1940. Swamproot was still being distributed when zip codes came out in 1960.[3,4]

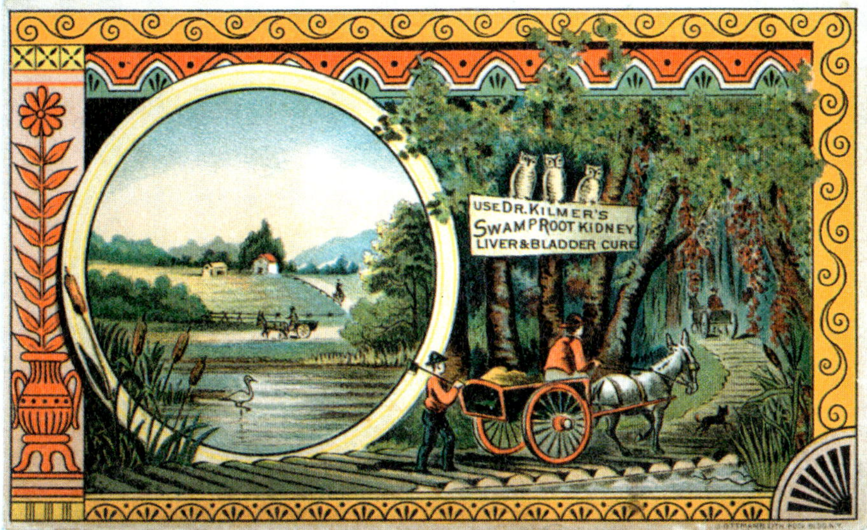


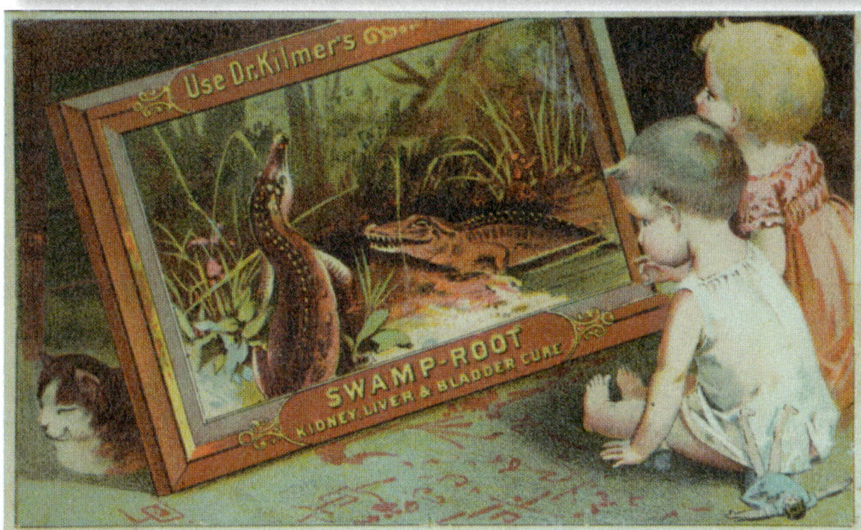


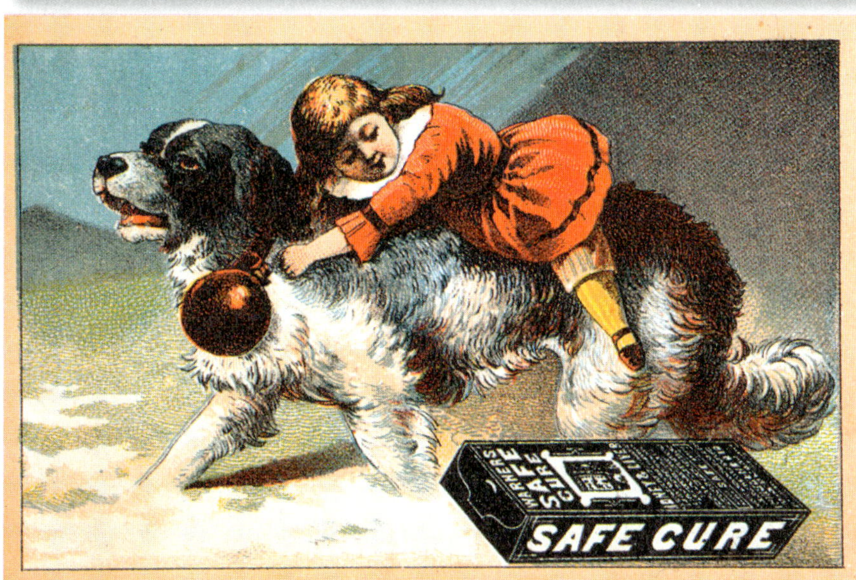


**Dr. Kilmer's Swamp-Root Kidney, Liver and Bladder Cure**

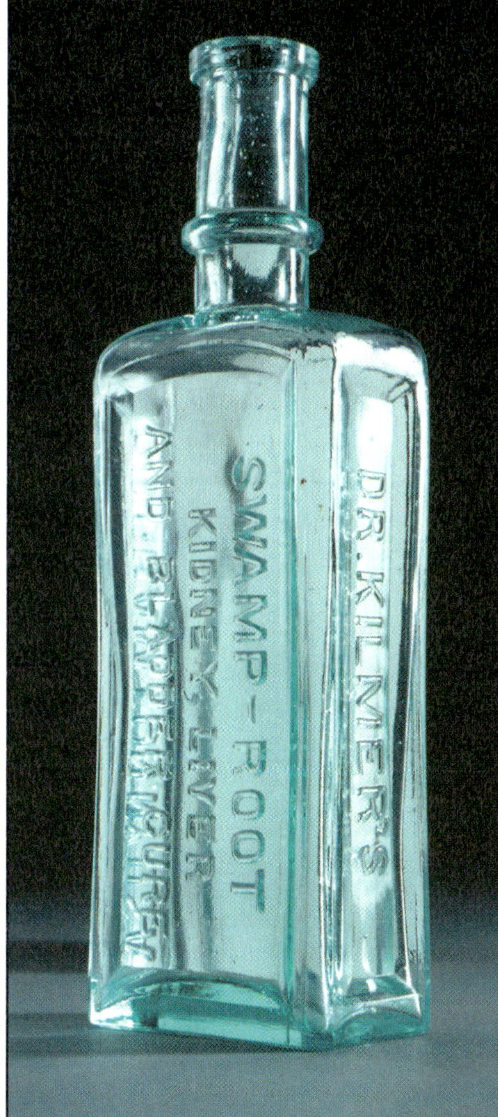


This rare Kilmer Cure bottle has a double ring or collar.

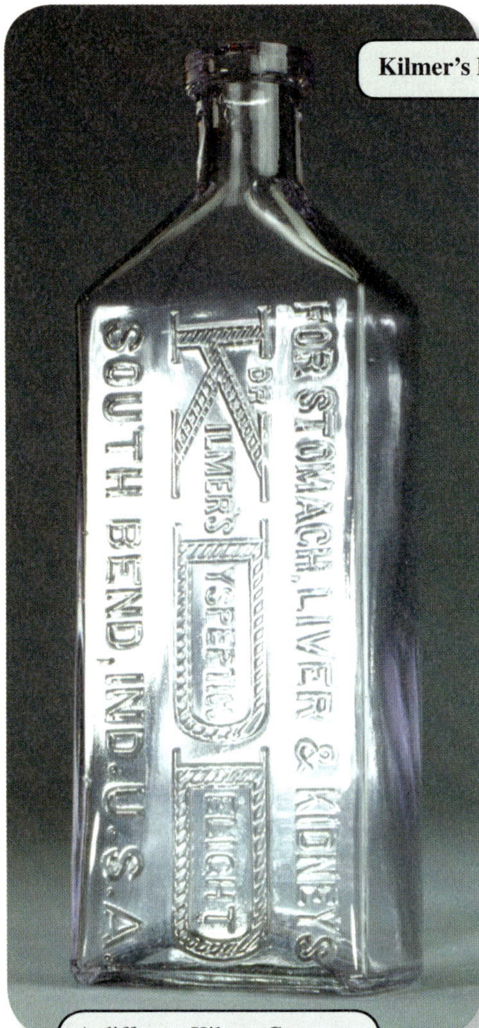


Kilmer's Dyspeptik Delight For Stomach, Liver and Kidneys

The Home of the "other" Kilmer Company from South Bend, Indiana.

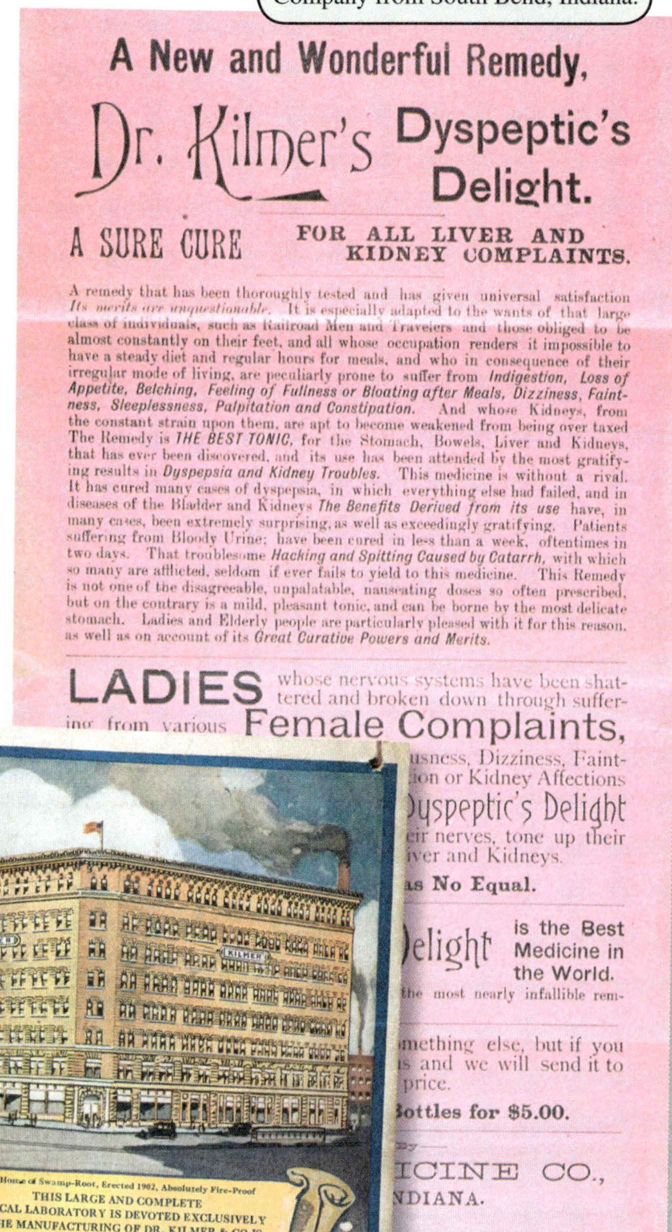


Living life on a grand scale, flamboyant Willis turned his energies to dogs, horses, travel, and to founding a newspaper, thereby keeping Binghamton on the edge of its seat. He exhibited jumpers at Madison Square Garden and had the joy of winning the Kentucky Derby. Bloodlines of his horses can be traced to the great Triple Crown winner Secretariat. Willis became a patron of the arts. His first automobile was a Gasmobile. He had an oceangoing yacht and an estate in Virginia both known as Remlik, which is Kilmer spelled backward.

A different Kilmer Company from South Bend, Indiana advertising a sure cure and attempting to benefit from name recognition.

The fast life and good times ended for Willis in 1940. He left his widow an estate valued between ten and fifteen million dollars. At his funeral at the North Presbyterian Church of Binghamton there were lengthy and glowing eulogies. However, mourners were surprised that there was not one mention of Swamproot.[3]

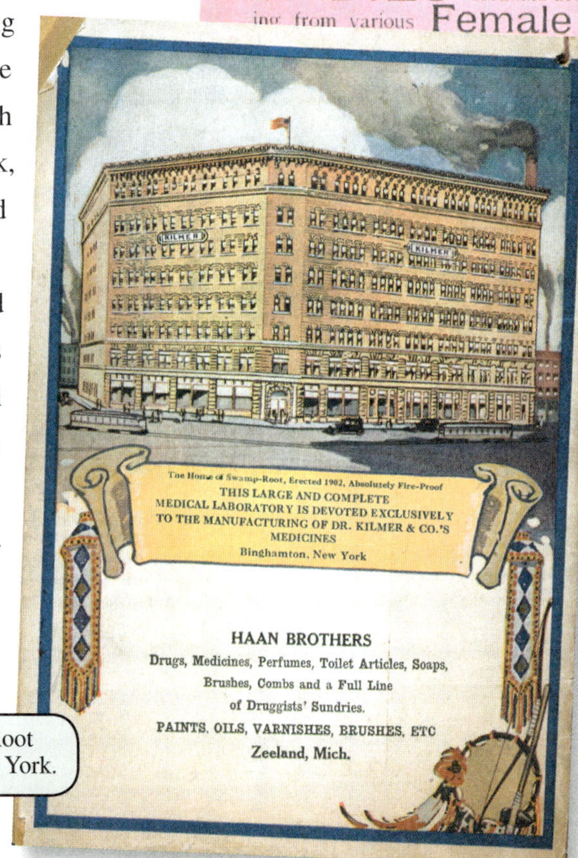


The Home of Dr. Kilmer's-Swamp Root erected in 1902 in Binghamton, New York.

Chapter 15

# Dr. Chase & His Recipe Book

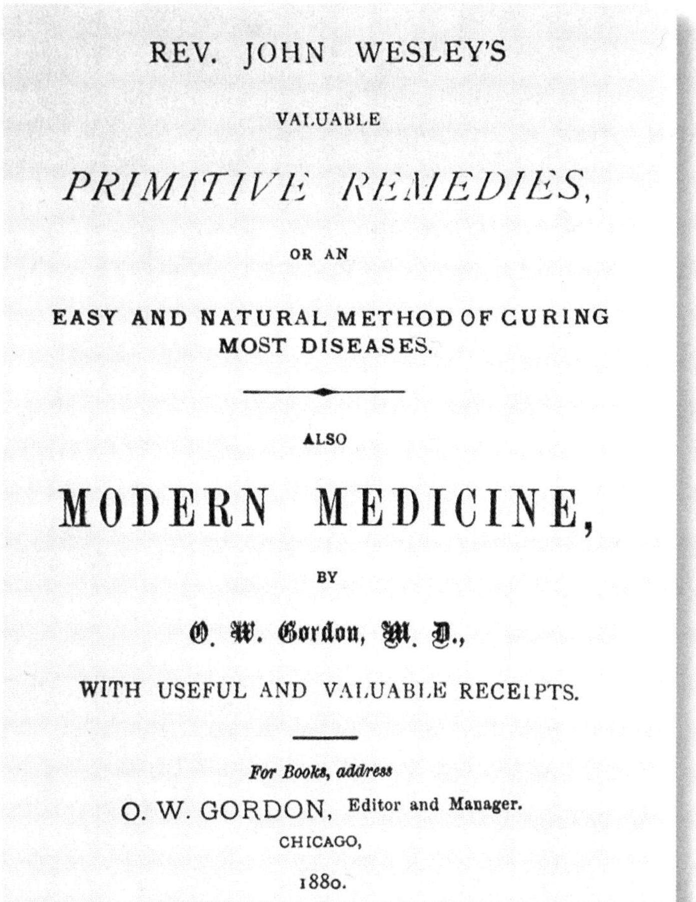

REV. JOHN WESLEY'S

VALUABLE

*PRIMITIVE REMEDIES,*

OR AN

EASY AND NATURAL METHOD OF CURING MOST DISEASES.

ALSO

MODERN MEDICINE,

BY

O. W. Gordon, M. D.,

WITH USEFUL AND VALUABLE RECEIPTS.

*For Books, address*

O. W. GORDON, Editor and Manager.

CHICAGO,

1880.

Rev. John Wesley's *Primitive Remedies* was combined with *Modern Medicine* in 1880. Since the original Wesley book was unchanged by Dr. Gordon, all the original quaintness is there.(1)

In the days before 1900 much medical treatment was domestic and primitive. It was not easy nor at times helpful to secure the services of the one physician in the area. Every family had its own home medical books and supply of medicines, usually herbs, and other nostrums listed in the books. Caring for the sick involved homemade science, empiricism, and superstition. Herb recipes were passed along from person to person, copied down in odd places, recorded in household remedy books, and published in almanacs and newspapers. Eventually enterprising authors and publishers put the recipes into book form for general use. These "Cook Books" described medications that could be concocted at home, but also had sections that dealt with general health and marriage as well as the weather.

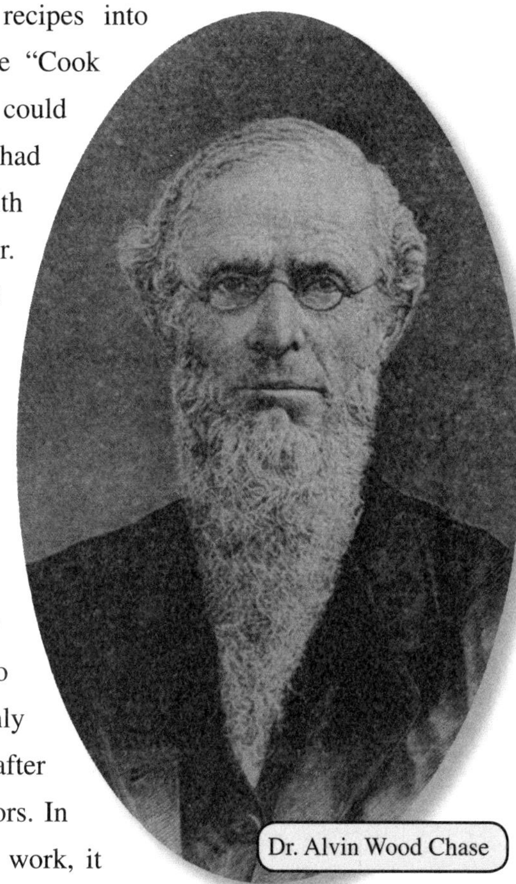

Dr. Alvin Wood Chase

In the preface to the *Household Physician*, one can find the following: "Hippocrates said, 'All men ought to be acquainted with the medical art. We believe that knowledge of medicine is the sister and companion of wisdom.' Such knowledge would shield many from the impositions of quackery. No one who reads this book thoroughly will be often imposed upon thereafter by quack nostrums, or quack doctors. In accordance with the design of the work, it has been written in plain, simple English, and brought within the comprehension of all who have medium powers of mind."[1]

Most books included a set of diagrams showing the various parts of the body so the subscriber would know what area the author was referring to. Using the diagram the "home doctor" determined the "nature of the ailment" by isolating the symptoms. Once the reader made a diagnosis, he could go on to a list of remedies. One of the first such books was *Primitive Physic* published in 1747 by Rev. John Wesley. During the 19th century there were many

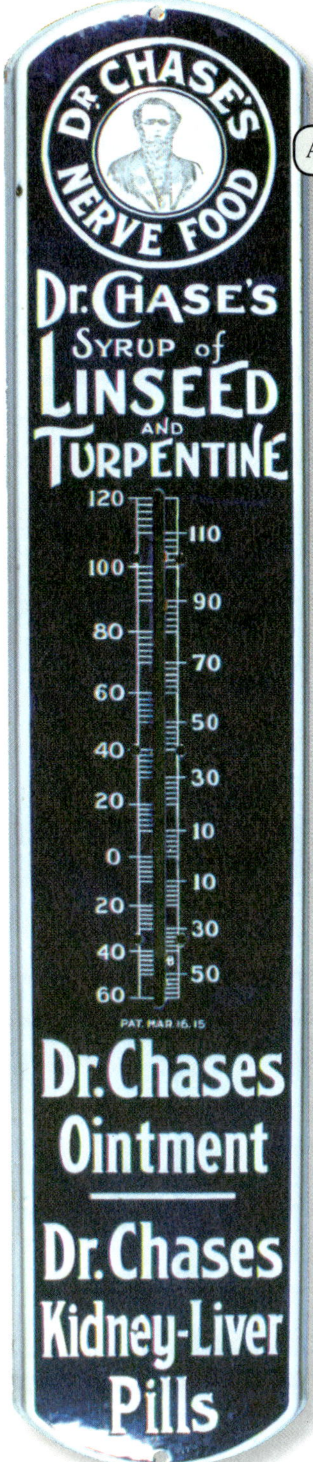


Advertising Thermometer

such books published. One of the most famous was *Dr. Chase's Recipes or Information for Everybody.*[1]

Dr. Alvin Wood Chase was born in the county of Cayuga, N.Y., in 1817. After receiving his early education in a log cabin school in the Buffalo vicinity, he took to the road at age 17 as an itinerant peddler. While Chase was centering his operations in Michigan and Northern Ohio, he was also collecting recipes of nostrums for whatever ailed man or beast.[2]

After a while Chase decided that his true calling was that of a physician. He settled in Ann Arbor in 1856 and began taking medical classes at the University of Michigan. But he could not graduate, because he lacked a background in Latin and natural history. He then enrolled in the Eclectic Medical Institute of Cincinnati in 1858. With hard work

The slogan that Dr. Chase used on the title page of his recipe book was "We learn to live, by living to learn."

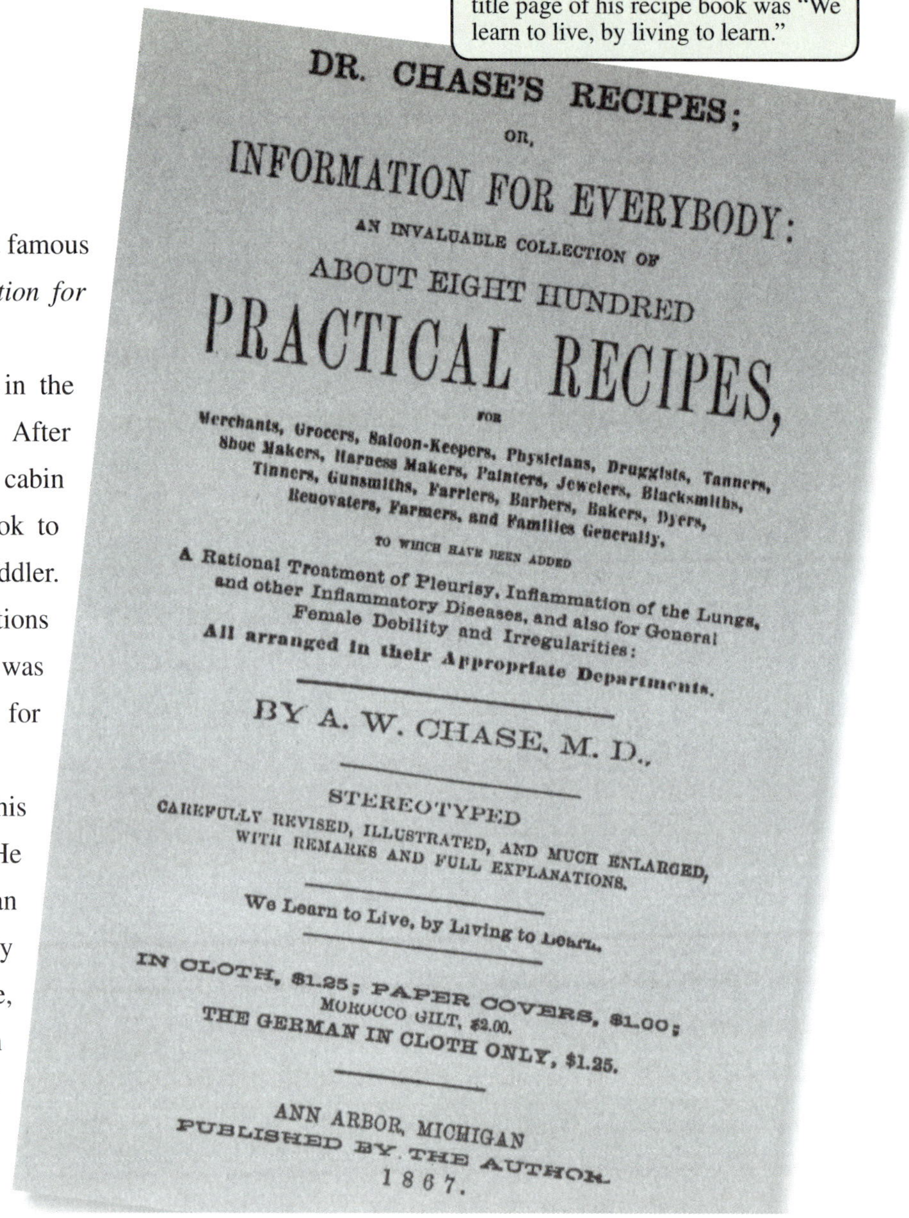

DR. CHASE'S RECIPES;

OR,

INFORMATION FOR EVERYBODY:

AN INVALUABLE COLLECTION OF

ABOUT EIGHT HUNDRED

PRACTICAL RECIPES,

FOR

Merchants, Grocers, Saloon-Keepers, Physicians, Druggists, Tanners, Shoe Makers, Harness Makers, Painters, Jewelers, Blacksmiths, Tinners, Gunsmiths, Farriers, Barbers, Bakers, Dyers, Renovaters, Farmers, and Families Generally,

TO WHICH HAVE BEEN ADDED

A Rational Treatment of Pleurisy, Inflammation of the Lungs, and other Inflammatory Diseases, and also for General Female Debility and Irregularities:

All arranged in their Appropriate Departments.

BY A. W. CHASE, M. D.,

STEREOTYPED

CAREFULLY REVISED, ILLUSTRATED, AND MUCH ENLARGED, WITH REMARKS AND FULL EXPLANATIONS.

We Learn to Live, by Living to Learn.

IN CLOTH, $1.25; PAPER COVERS, $1.00;
MOROCCO GILT, $2.00.
THE GERMAN IN CLOTH ONLY, $1.25.

ANN ARBOR, MICHIGAN
PUBLISHED BY THE AUTHOR.
1867.

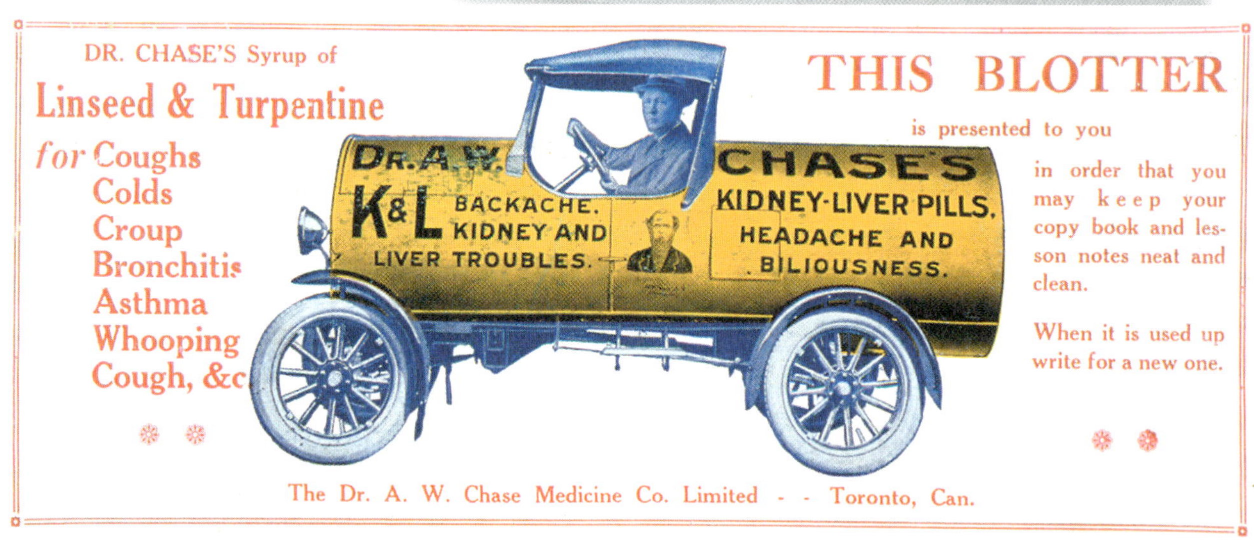

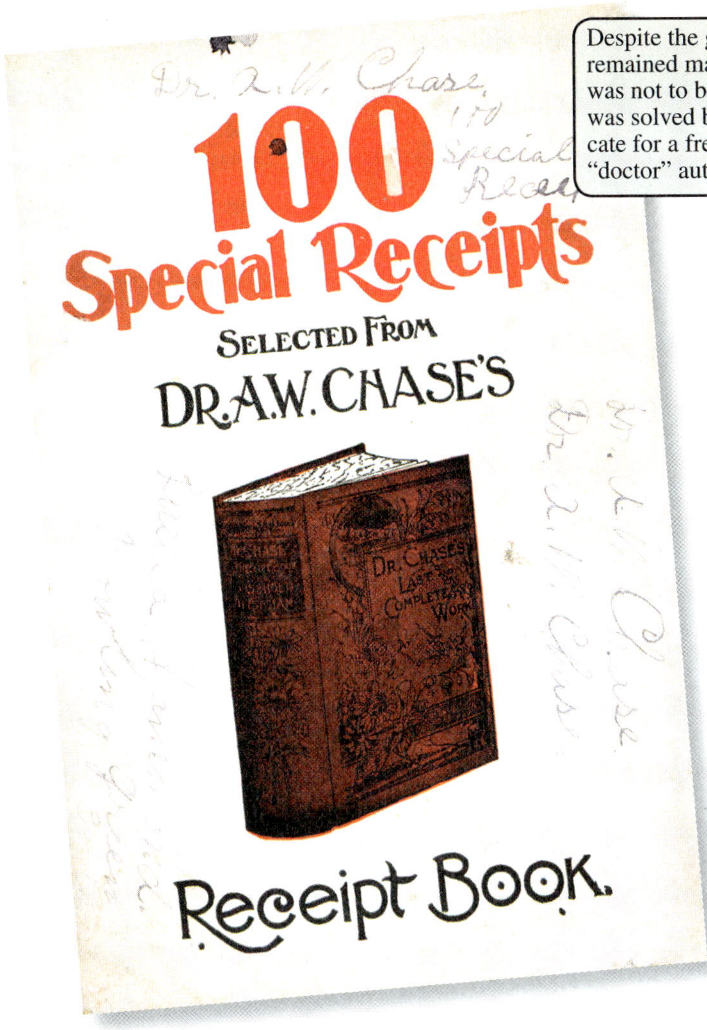


Despite the growing volume of books, there remained many ailments the cure for which was not to be found in a book. This problem was solved by offering the purchaser a certificate for a free consultation by mail with the "doctor" author of the book. (1)

and studying 16 hours a day he earned his medical diploma in four months graduating as class valedictorian.[3]

The practitioners of eclectic medicine chose freely from the myriad of remedies that were currently advocated by the diverse theories of medical practice. Frequently the patient or the next of kin had to choose one of the many treatments offered.

Following graduation Dr. Chase returned to Ann Arbor and hung out his shingle as a general practitioner. To augment his income he peddled his own recipe book. Each succeeding edition became more comprehensive and successful. By 1860 the eighth edition contained 600 recipes. Three years later he had added 200 more recipes to the 10th, until then the most popular edition.[2,3]

Undoubtedly there was some good in the old fashioned folk wisdom contained in the pages of the recipes. Peculiar by today's standards was the offering of multiple cures for a single aliment like ague, as malaria was called. Steeping

*Cure for Bright's Disease of the Kidneys and Dropsy.*—Drink of an infusion of the dry pods of the common white soup bean or corn bean. When the latter cannot be readily obtained the pods of the "snap short" bean will answer, and even the Lima bean, though the latter is of inferior strength. Take a double handful of the pods to three quarts of water; boil slowly for three hours until it is reduced to three pints. Use no drink of any kind but this, the patient drinking as much as he conveniently can; it may be taken either hot or cold. In every case in which it has been tried, it is claimed, a cure has been effected.

one tablespoon of soot scraped from the chimney into a pint of hot water made the remedy, soot coffee. Another ague cure was to have come from the spirit world via a clairvoyant. Several herbs were dissolved in a gallon of rye whiskey. The dosage of five or six well-filled wine glasses per day must at least have brightened up the sickroom.[1,3]

A no-fail remedy for the croup was kindly supplied by

Cure of Cancer.—The extract of wood sorrel, used as a plaster through the day, and slippery elm bark at night, will cure any cancer that has ulcerated or that has not live skin over it; the skin should be broken in some way. To burn a piece of punk on the place, is a good method, then apply the salve, as before directed. The extract is obtained simply by pounding the common sorrel in a mortar, or other vessel, and pressing out the juice, then put it in a pewter dish or basin, and place it in the sun, until it dries to the consistence of tar, when it is fit for use.

an old Dutch woman as her favorite. It was a teaspoon of urine and goose grease taken every 15 minutes until one got well. Equally awful was Chase's remedy for sprains—toad ointment. Boiling four large toads until soft and adding the resulting liquid to butter produced the ointment.

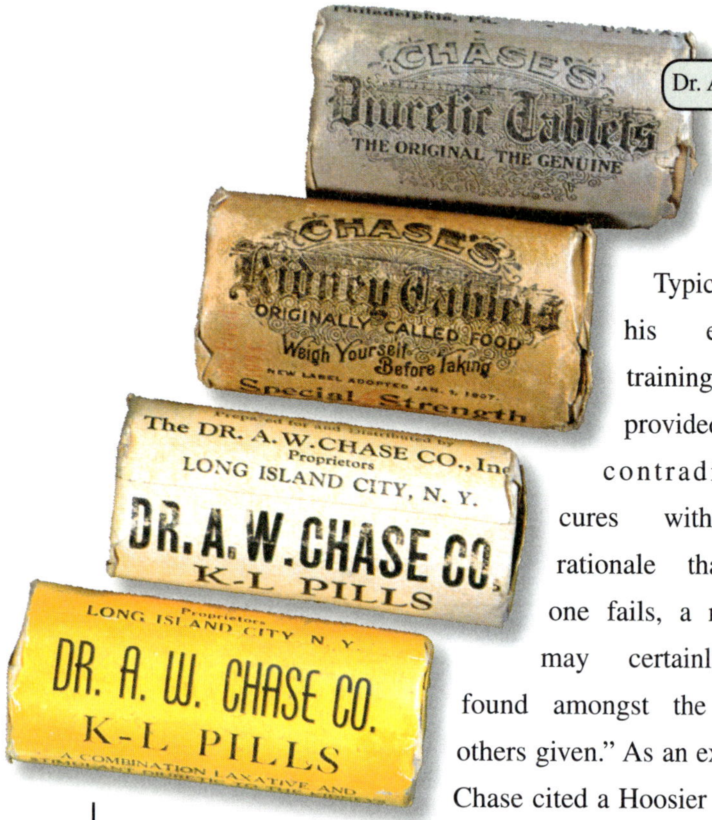


Dr. A.W. Chase Kidney and Liver Pills

Typical of his eclectic training, Chase provided many contradictory cures with the rationale that "If one fails, a remedy may certainly be found amongst the many others given." As an example Chase cited a Hoosier couple who were troubled with piles. The wife cured herself by sitting in warm water while her mate enjoyed the same success with cold water. One may wonder as to the effectiveness of the various medical recipes that Chase collected and offered his ailing readers. Just remember that Chase's wife and five children, whom he often used as guinea pigs for his remedies, all preceded him in death.[3]

In addition to his cookbook, Chase also distributed his own medicines. He marketed a line of family medicines that included "Dr. Chase's Kidney and Liver Pills." Well into the 20th century these medicines were manufactured and distributed from offices in Buffalo, Toronto, and London.

> **Pills**
> All ye that are of Venus' race
> Apply yourself to Dr. Chase
> Who with a box or two of pills
> Will soon remove your painful ills.

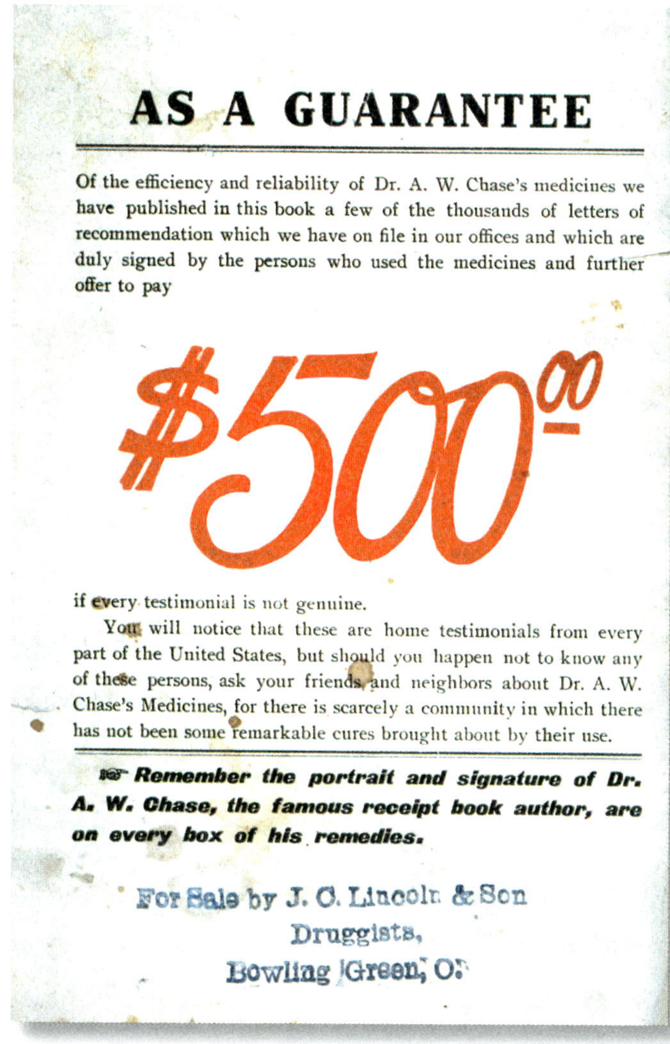

**AS A GUARANTEE**

Of the efficiency and reliability of Dr. A. W. Chase's medicines we have published in this book a few of the thousands of letters of recommendation which we have on file in our offices and which are duly signed by the persons who used the medicines and further offer to pay

**$500.00**

if every testimonial is not genuine.

You will notice that these are home testimonials from every part of the United States, but should you happen not to know any of these persons, ask your friends and neighbors about Dr. A. W. Chase's Medicines, for there is scarcely a community in which there has not been some remarkable cures brought about by their use.

***Remember the portrait and signature of Dr. A. W. Chase, the famous receipt book author, are on every box of his remedies.***

For Sale by J. C. Lincoln & Son
Druggists,
Bowling Green, O.

To enlarge the business, Chase began construction in 1864 of his own printing establishment. Four years later, because of booming sales of *"Dr. Chase's Recipe or Information for Everybody,"* he tripled the size of the building and added 50 typesetters, pressmen, and binders to produce his books. By 1869 Chase had sold approximately 500,000 copies of his book. However, he sold out to Rice A. Beal signing a contract never to return to the recipe business in Michigan. He then moved to Sauk Rapids, Minnesota, in an effort to regain his failing health.

After three years the rejuvenated Dr. Chase returned to Ann Arbor and attempted to publish another book of recipes. The result was a lawsuit that forced Chase to move to Toledo, Ohio, and eventually to lose all his money. Although Chase's books continued to sell very well, the author received none of the proceeds.[3]

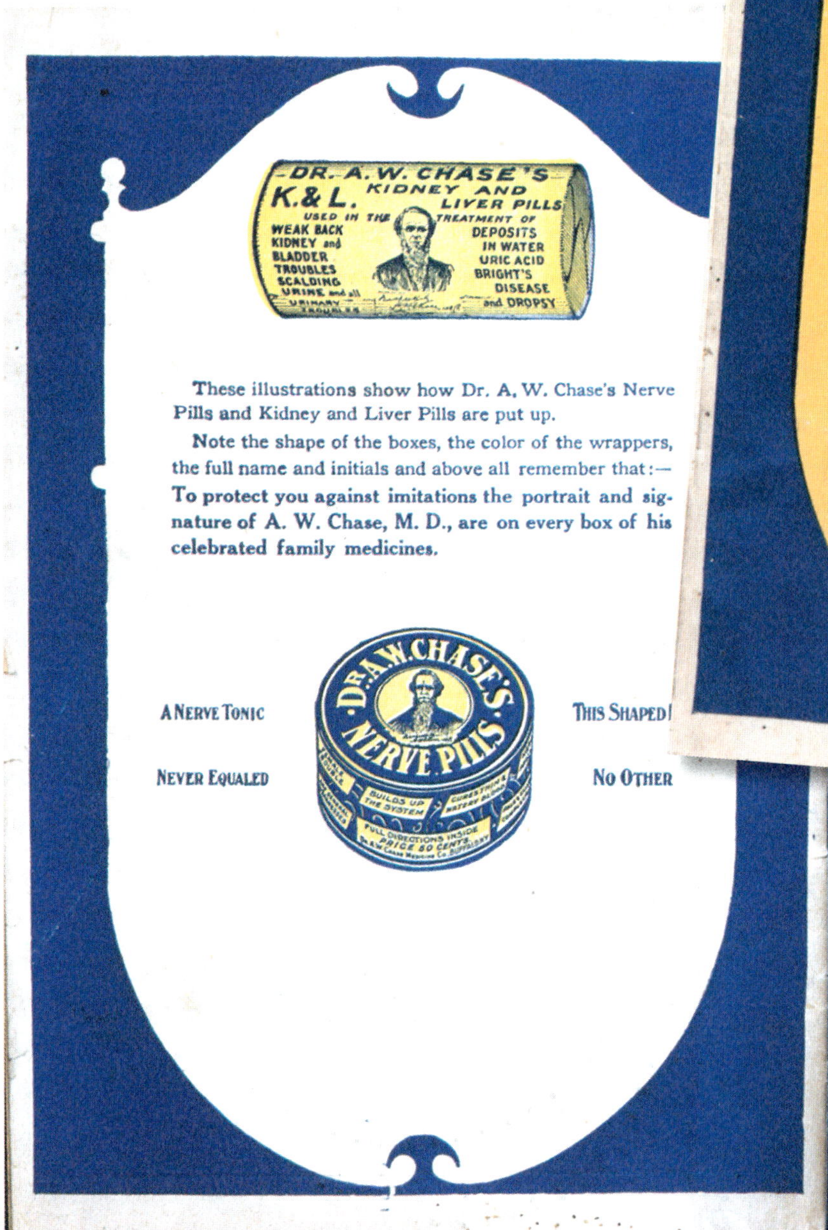


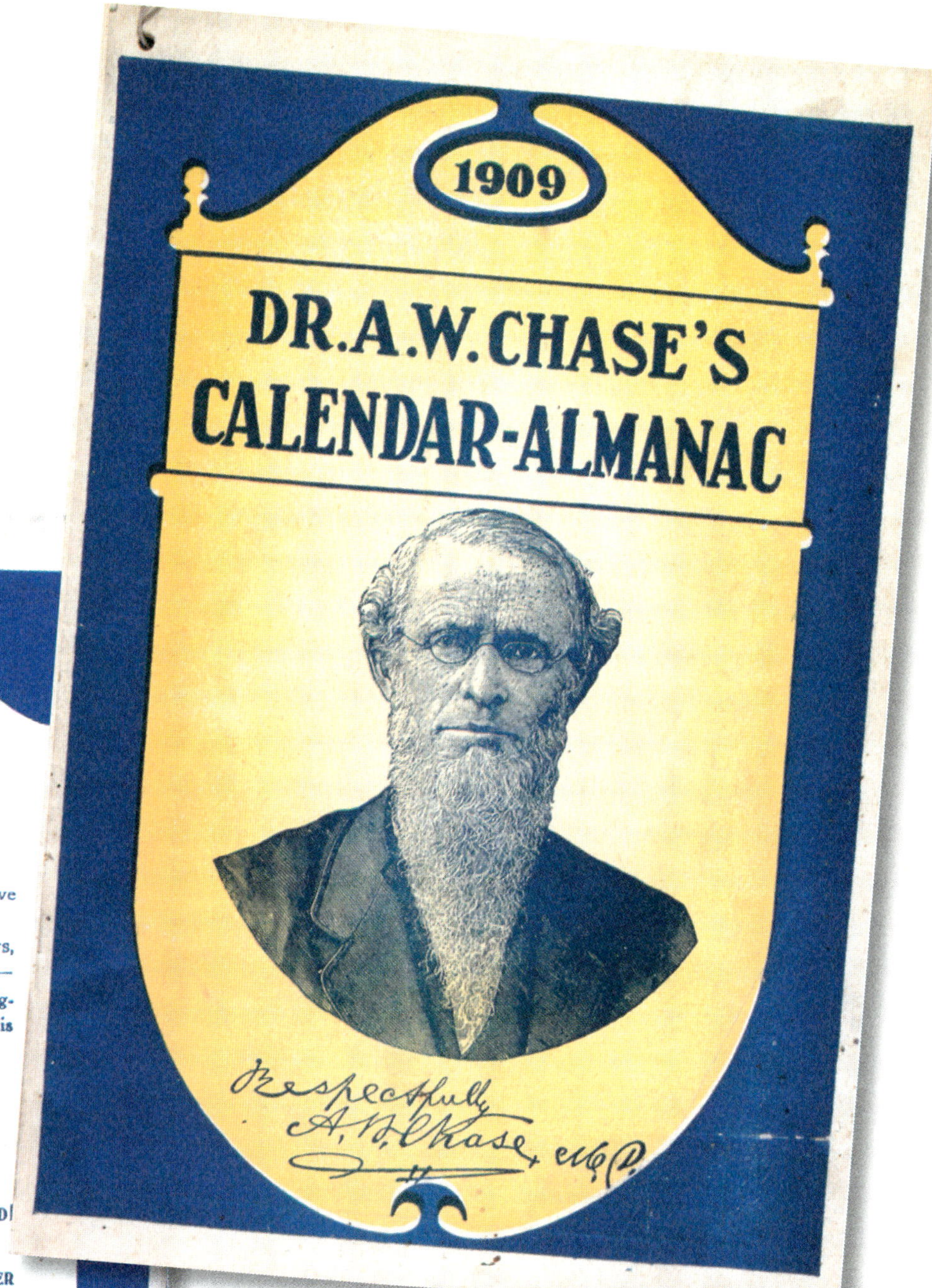


"If each inhabitant of America could have an experienced doctor constantly at his elbow to advise him in all the medical and sanitary emergencies of life, these pages would never be needed."

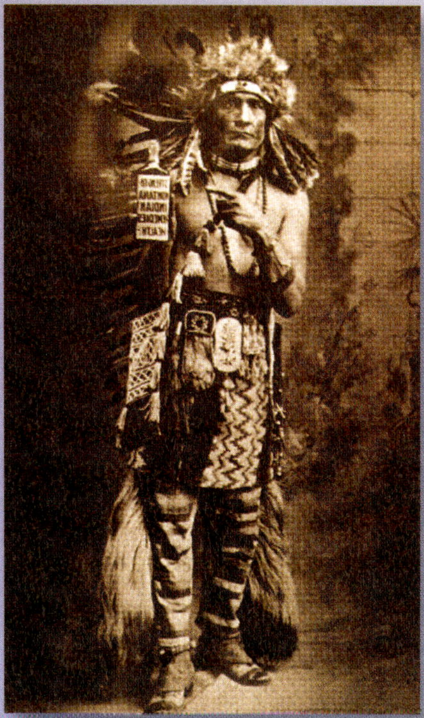

# MARKETING

"The advertising quack...is the black wolf, aye, the Bengal Tiger of the profession...He is full of shrewdness and cunning, and knows poor, weak human nature like a book."

Dr. Willis P. King, 1882

Chapter 16

# Trade Cards

Advertising in the nostrum trade assumed different marketing forms, but no form was more vivid and artistic than the advertising trade card. Its success was phenomenal and its history was unique. During the last two decades of the nineteenth century trade cards were produced in vast quantities since they were an effective marketing medium during this period of active consumerism.[1]

Victorian trade cards or advertising trade cards, as they are often called today, date mostly from 1876 to 1900. Although dimension varies considerably, they were usually 3 x 5 inches in size. Exactly when the first trade card was issued is a matter of debate. The onset may be associated with early eighteenth century tradesmen who used their black and white business cards as an advertising handout. The evolution of the trade card followed the progress of the Industrial Revolution. The technical advances in printing and the increase in the production of cards went hand in hand with the cultural changes taking place in our country.[2,3,5]

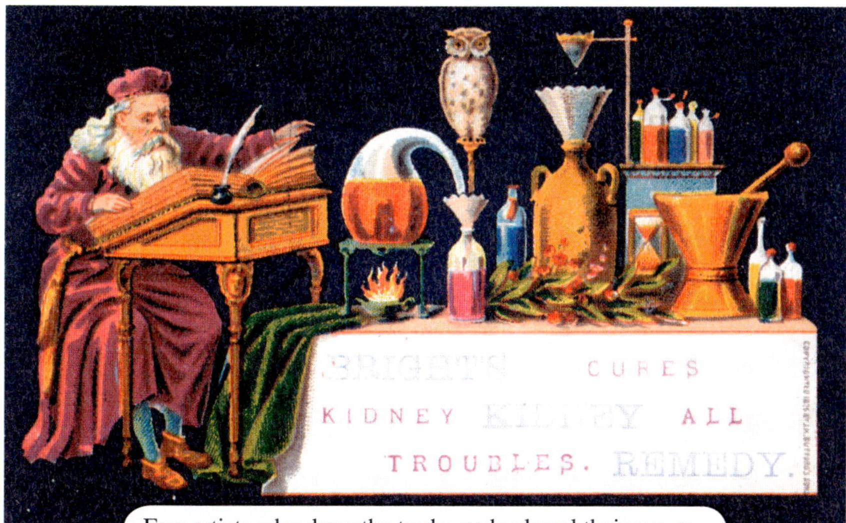


Few artists who drew the trade cards placed their names on the cards for identification.

Initially trade cards were produced by the established method of printing with etched or engraved metal copper plates. The steel or copper engravings could produce very fine line drawings and designs, but their method was slow, labor intensive, and required frequent recutting of the worn out plates. Further innovations introduced lithography, which provided a means for mass producing printed material. With lithography (literally, "stone writers") a limestone block is substituted for the metal plate on which the design is placed. Beautiful color prints (chromo-lithography) were achieved by overprinting with a different stone for each color. Another advance in lithography occurred in the form of steam presses. Once the steam press was perfected, lithography firms could crank out volumes of trade cards and advertising material at a rate of thousands per day.[2,3]

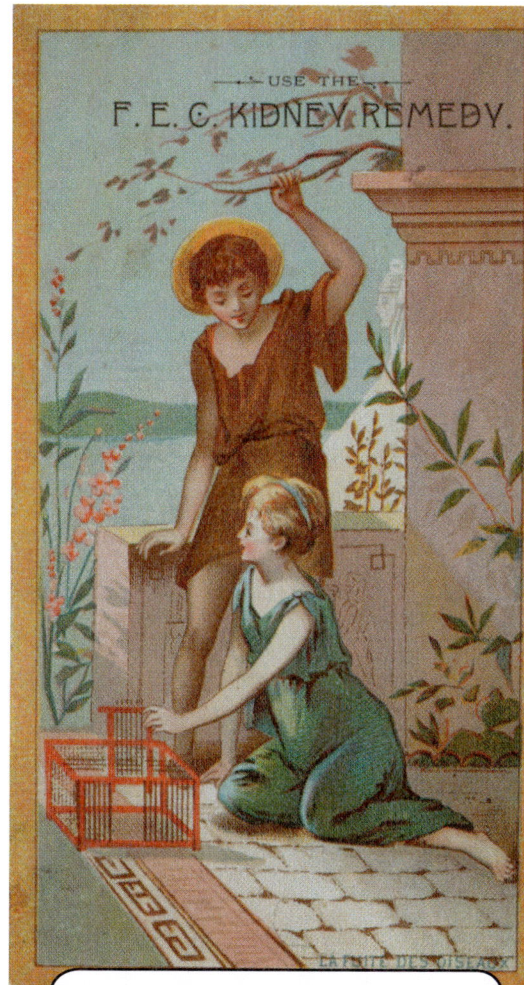


When one sees the number of cards that were produced, one wonders whether the trading cards were issued to advertise the product - or did one buy the product to get the cards?

The name of the printer or lithographer was occasionally found along the bottom margin of the trade card. Currier

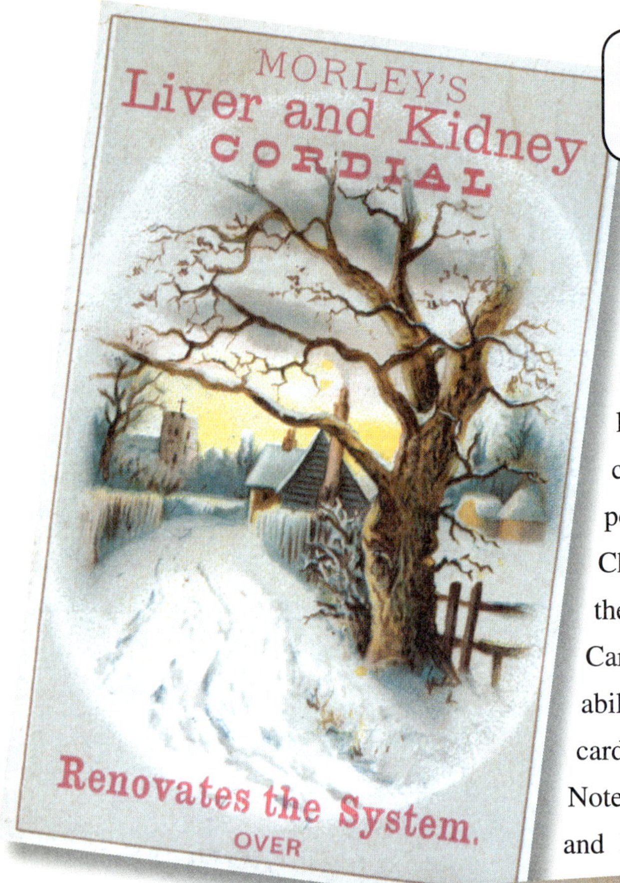


**Morley's Liver and Kidney Cordial**
The labeling of some of the nostrums made a clear reference to the alcohol contained in the concoction. Kidney gins, cordials, wines were sold as medicinals.

and Ives and Louis Prang & Co. are the best known of the early American lithographers. Prang is credited today with the popularization of the Christmas card and is called the "Father of the Christmas Card." Considerable artistic ability is reflected on the trade card, but rarely is credit given. Noted illustrators Palmer Cox and Kate Greenaway as well as artist Winslow Homer were identified. Also making a timely contribution were the papermakers who produced a wood pulp product of light cardboard.[2,3]

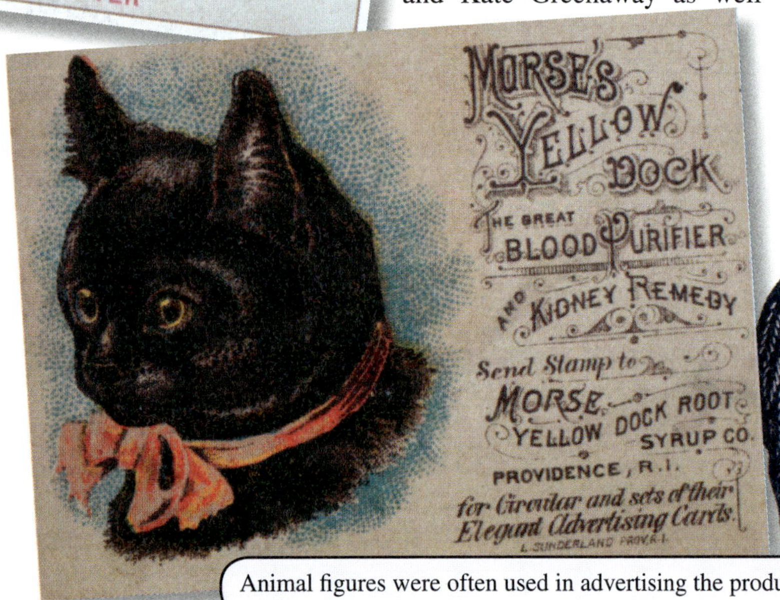


Animal figures were often used in advertising the product.

Color advertising trade cards were seldom produced prior to the International Centennial Exposition of 1876 held in Philadelphia. It was there that the trade card received instant and widespread prominence as an advertising medium when Louis Prang & Co. gave away thousands of cards. Within a short time nearly all-serious advertisers began ordering the chromolithographed cards. Trade cards became so popular and cheap that some firms began distributing them by the tens of thousands. The rapidly expanding economy created a compelling need for the attractive and easily distributed advertising. Trade cards were also produced in Europe but the volume was comparatively small. Trade card advertising by the patent medicine industry was a uniquely American phenomenon.[5,6] Nostrum manufacturers utilizing the medium were "Morse's Yellow Dock—The Great Liver and Kidney Remedy," "Dr. Kermott's Mandrake Pills—Cure for Liver and Kidney Disease," "Morley's Liver and Kidney Cordial," "The Great Sierra Kidney and Liver Cure," and many more.

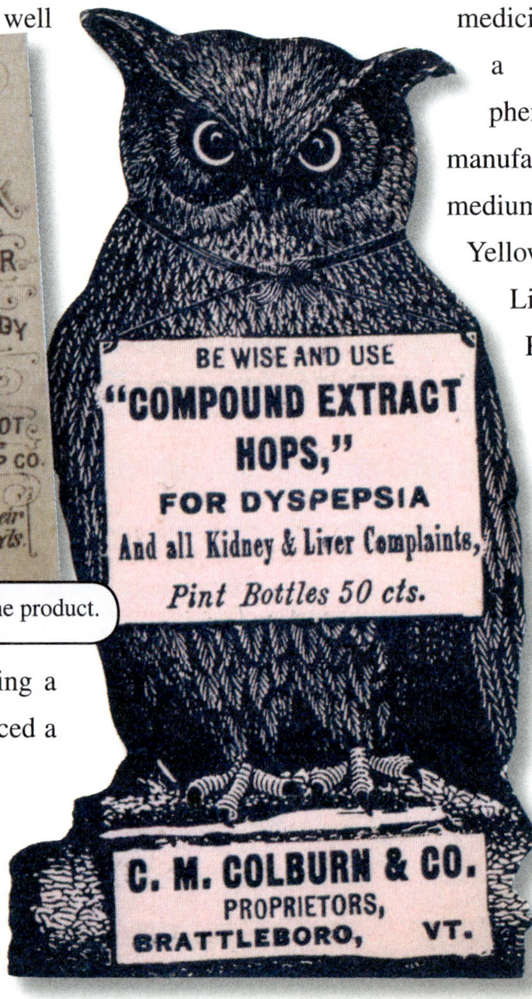

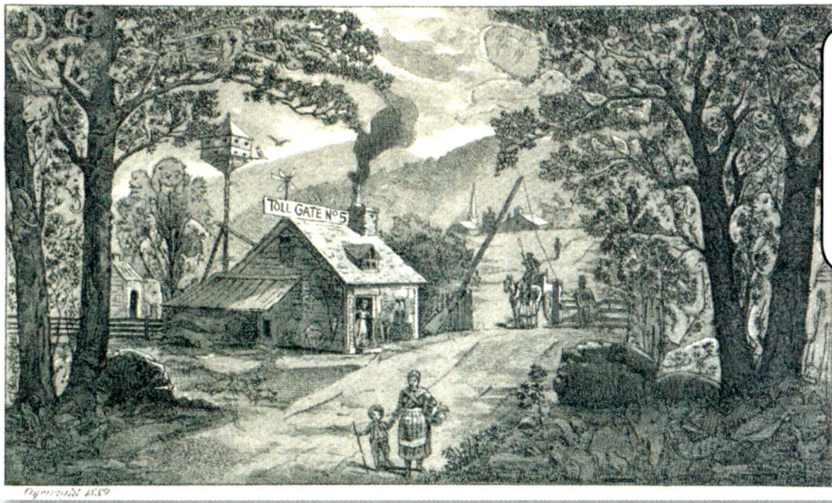


**Toll Gate No. 5 - Puzzle Card**
The most numerous category of the specialty cards was the puzzle card. It was a simple line drawn picture often in black and white or monochromes in red or blue. The most common contained a number of "hidden" figures, usually animals that could be found upon viewing the card from different angles. The card entitled "Toll Gate No. 5" contained 160 hidden figures. This card is one of a series of cards used to advertise a book by E.C. Abbey, M.D. entitled *"The Sexual System and It's Derangements"*, which sold 3 for 25¢ - postpaid.

Eventually untold millions of trade cards were issued, exchanged and collected—creating the Victorian card-collecting craze. Cards were collected and pasted in albums, which at times were presented as gifts. Trade cards came in a variety of forms: the metamorphic or changing cards, mechanical cards, hold-to-light cards, book mark cards, perfumed cards, toy cards, chemically impregnated cards, puzzle cards—all collectibles. In time, card collecting, in common with many leisurely forms of home-oriented recreation, was displaced by competition from other pastimes.[4]

The novelty of the trade card decreased, not only because of the glut of cards at the peak of their popularity, but also because of the wide spread presence of colored pictures in magazines and even newspapers. Once advertising and marketing reached a national scale, other forms of visual persuasion became more efficient. By 1900 the advertising trade card was considered "old fashioned" and the issuance of the card had declined markedly.[2,4]

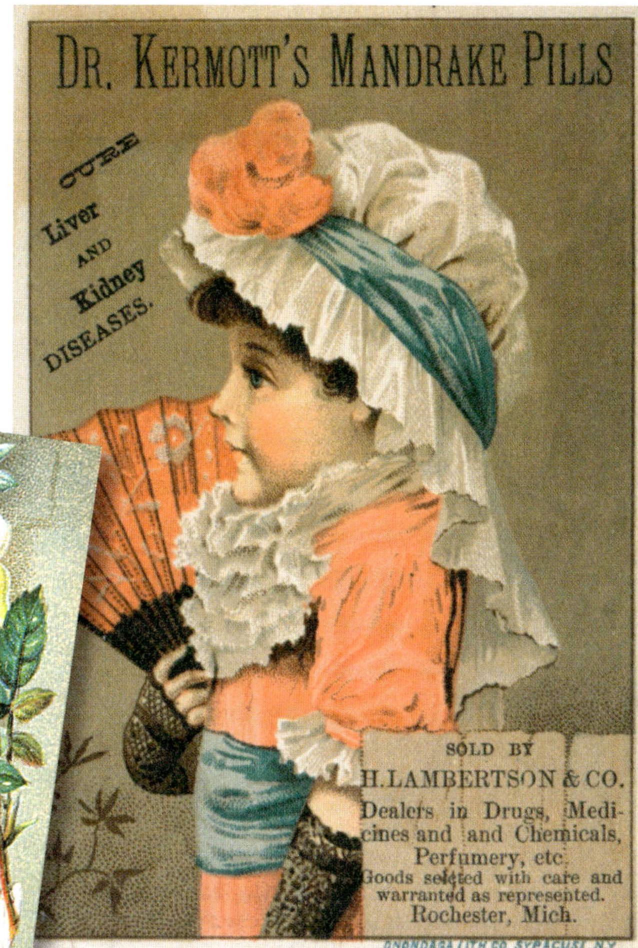


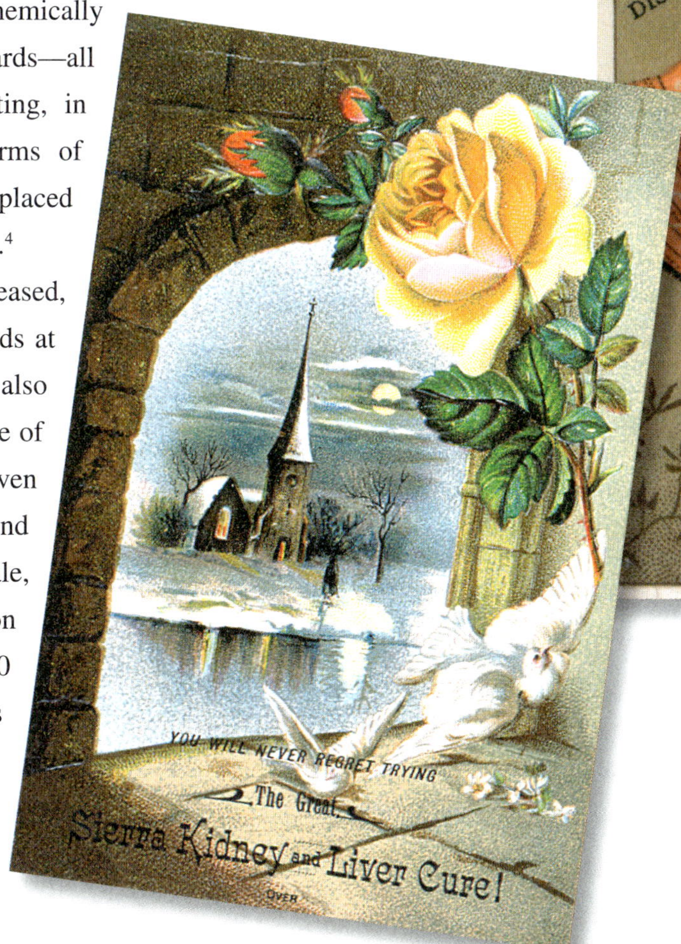

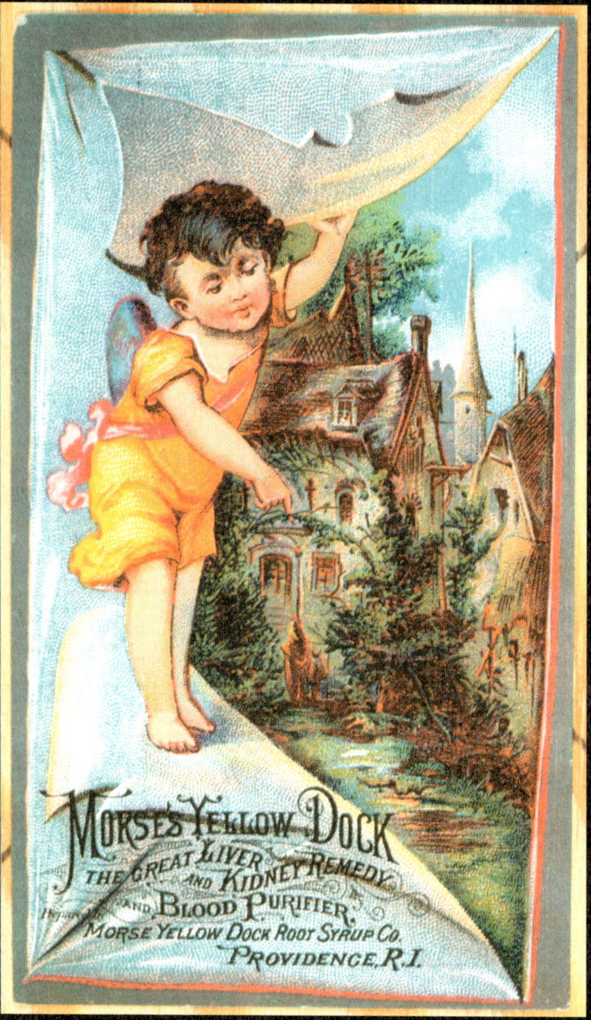
MORSE'S YELLOW DOCK
THE GREAT LIVER AND KIDNEY REMEDY
AND BLOOD PURIFIER.
Prepared by MORSE YELLOW DOCK ROOT SYRUP CO.
PROVIDENCE, R.I.

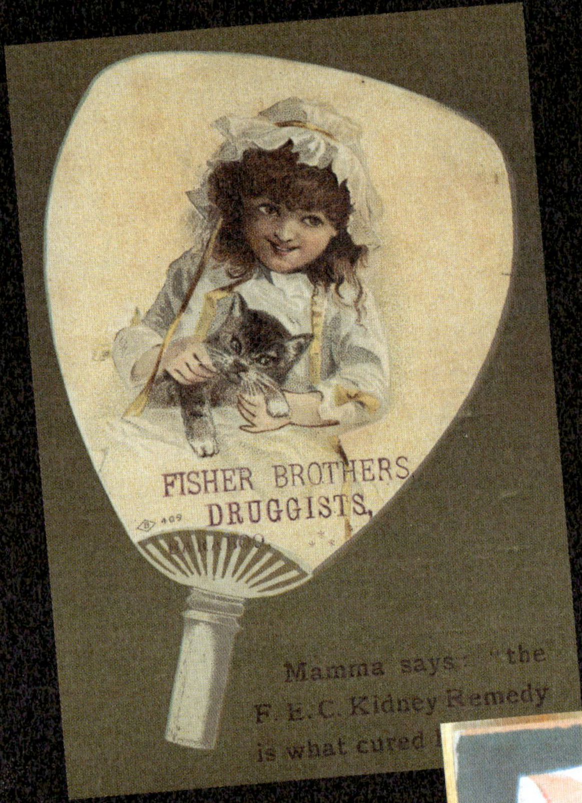
FISHER BROTHERS
DRUGGISTS.
Mamma says: "the
F. E. C. Kidney Remedy
is what cured

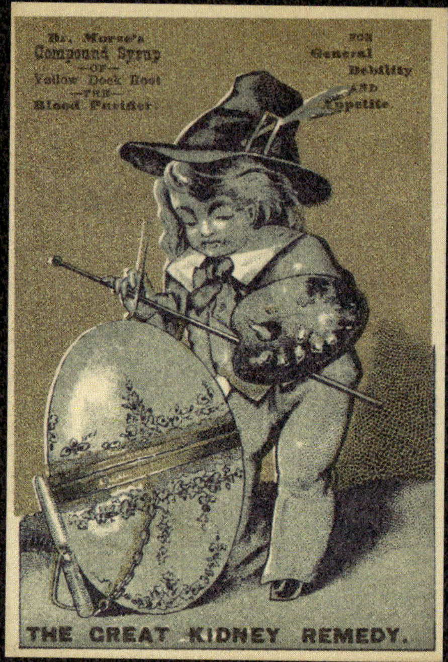
Dr. Morse's
Compound Syrup
—OF—
Yellow Dock Root
—THE—
Blood Purifier.
FOR
General
Debility
AND
Appetite.
THE GREAT KIDNEY REMEDY.

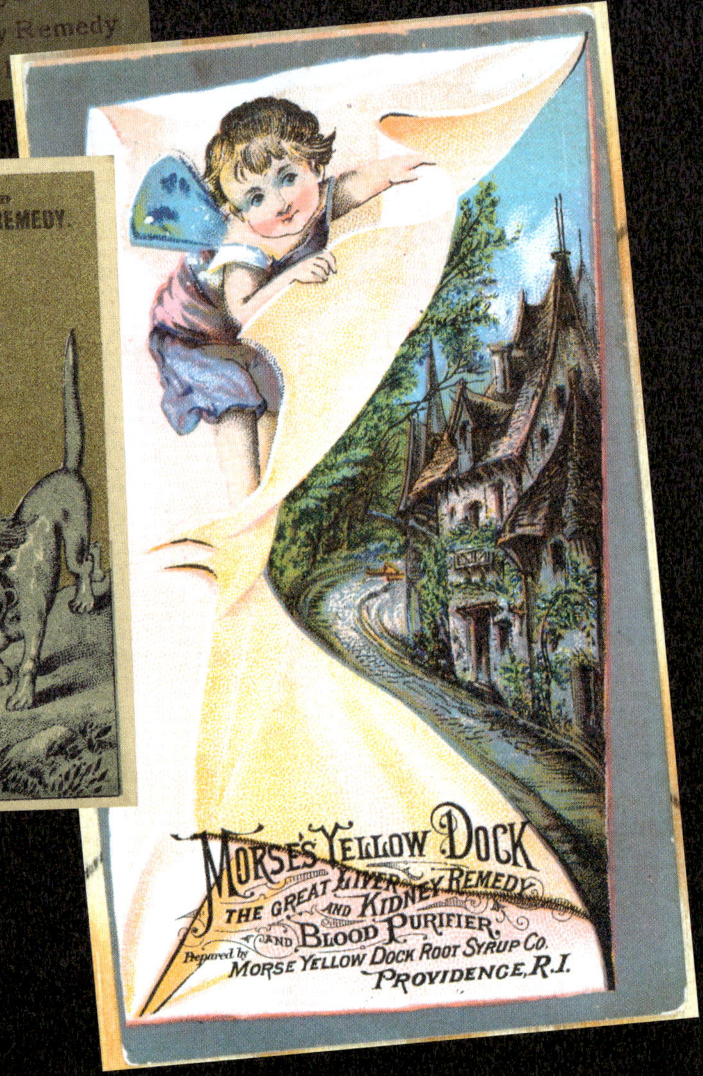
MORSE'S YELLOW DOCK
THE GREAT LIVER AND KIDNEY REMEDY
AND BLOOD PURIFIER.
Prepared by MORSE YELLOW DOCK ROOT SYRUP CO.
PROVIDENCE, R.I.

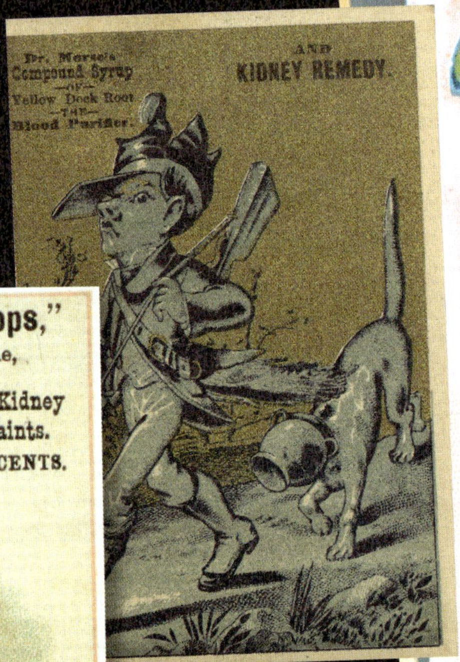
Dr. Morse's
Compound Syrup
—OF—
Yellow Dock Root
—THE—
Blood Purifier.
AND
KIDNEY REMEDY.

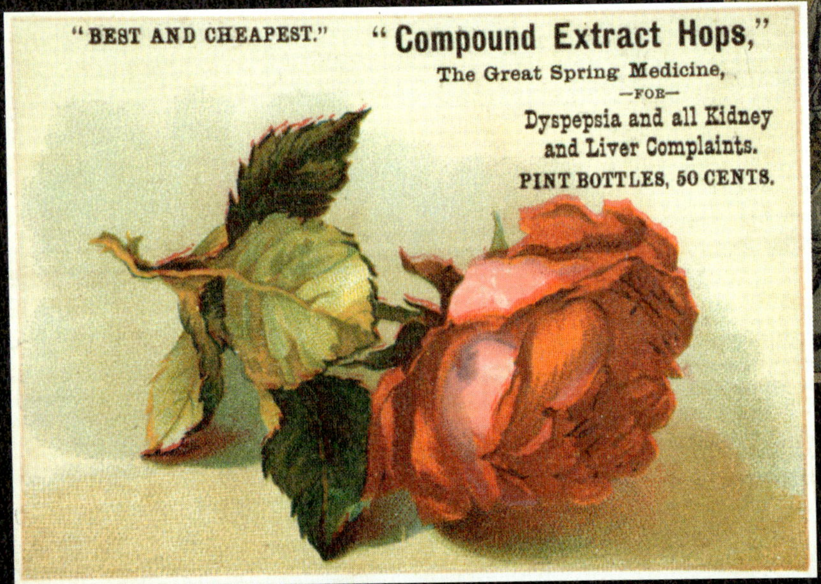
"BEST AND CHEAPEST."
"Compound Extract Hops,"
The Great Spring Medicine,
—FOR—
Dyspepsia and all Kidney
and Liver Complaints.
PINT BOTTLES, 50 CENTS.

# Almanacs

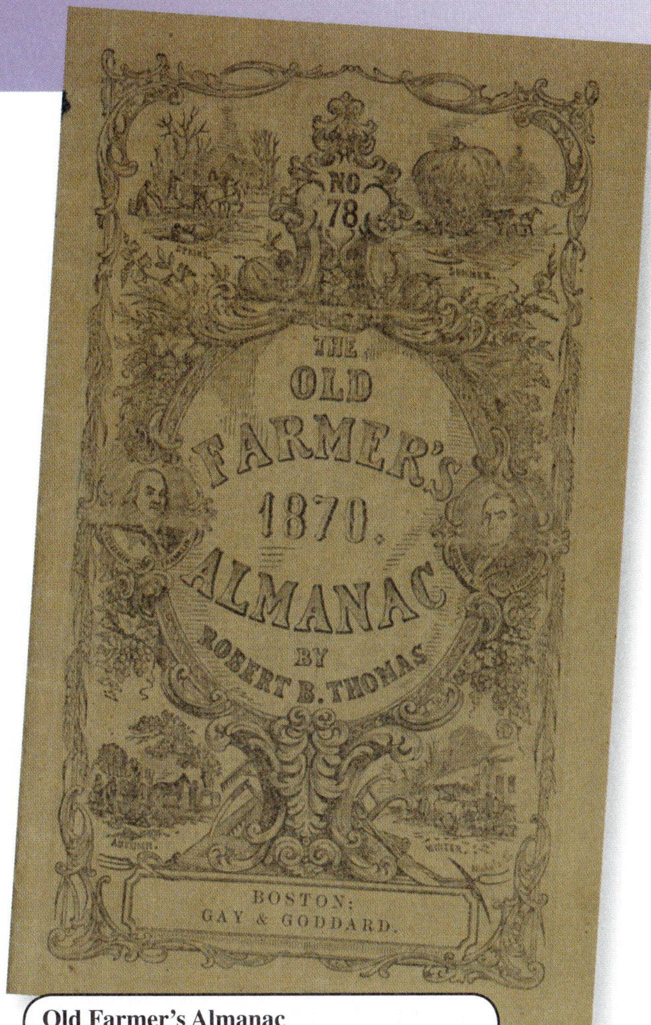


**Old Farmer's Almanac**
The ever popular and enduring Old Farmer's Almanac is still published today.

During the middle of the eighteenth century the almanac became a part of the early American cultural scene. Those Americans who could read were enjoying the wit and wisdom of Benjamin Franklin's *Poor Richard's Almanack*. Proverbs were plentiful within its pages as well as gems of advice on how to live successfully. Franklin wrote "some are weather wise, some are otherwise" and "at twenty years of age the will reigns; at thirty, the wit; at forty, the judgement." [1,2,3,5]

While Ben Franklin was our best known author of almanacs, he was not alone. The nineteenth century saw a boom in the publication of almanacs. Adding to the proliferation was the use of colorful cover pages that captured the imagination of readers by displaying natural world wonders, dramatic Indian scenes, and famous historical events. The contents of earlier almanacs were mostly astronomical and weather information interspersed with proverbs, anecdotes, and scraps of poetry and items of history. However, by mid-century the purpose of the almanac was not always the edification of the general public, nor the dispensing of wisdom and advice for the general good. The

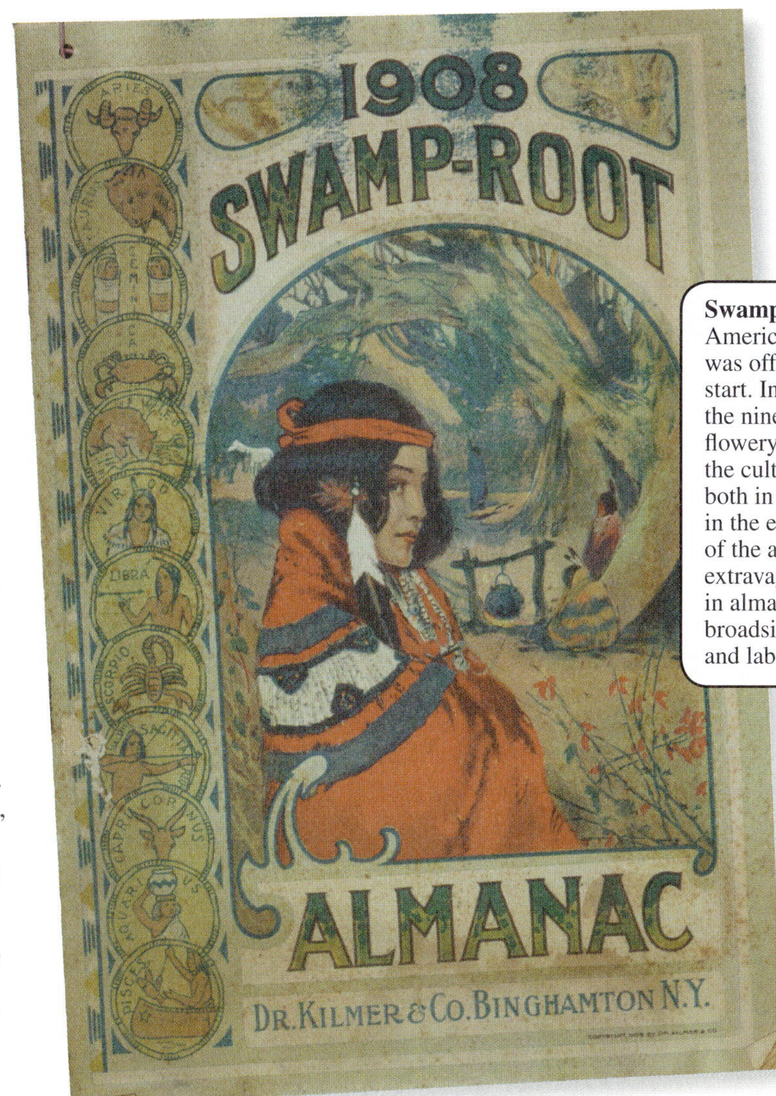


**Swamp Root Almanac**
American advertising was off to an impressive start. In the latter part of the nineteenth century the flowery extravagance of the culture was displayed both in the language and in the elaborate artwork of the advertising. This extravagance was visible in almanacs, trade cards, broadsides, newspapers and labels.

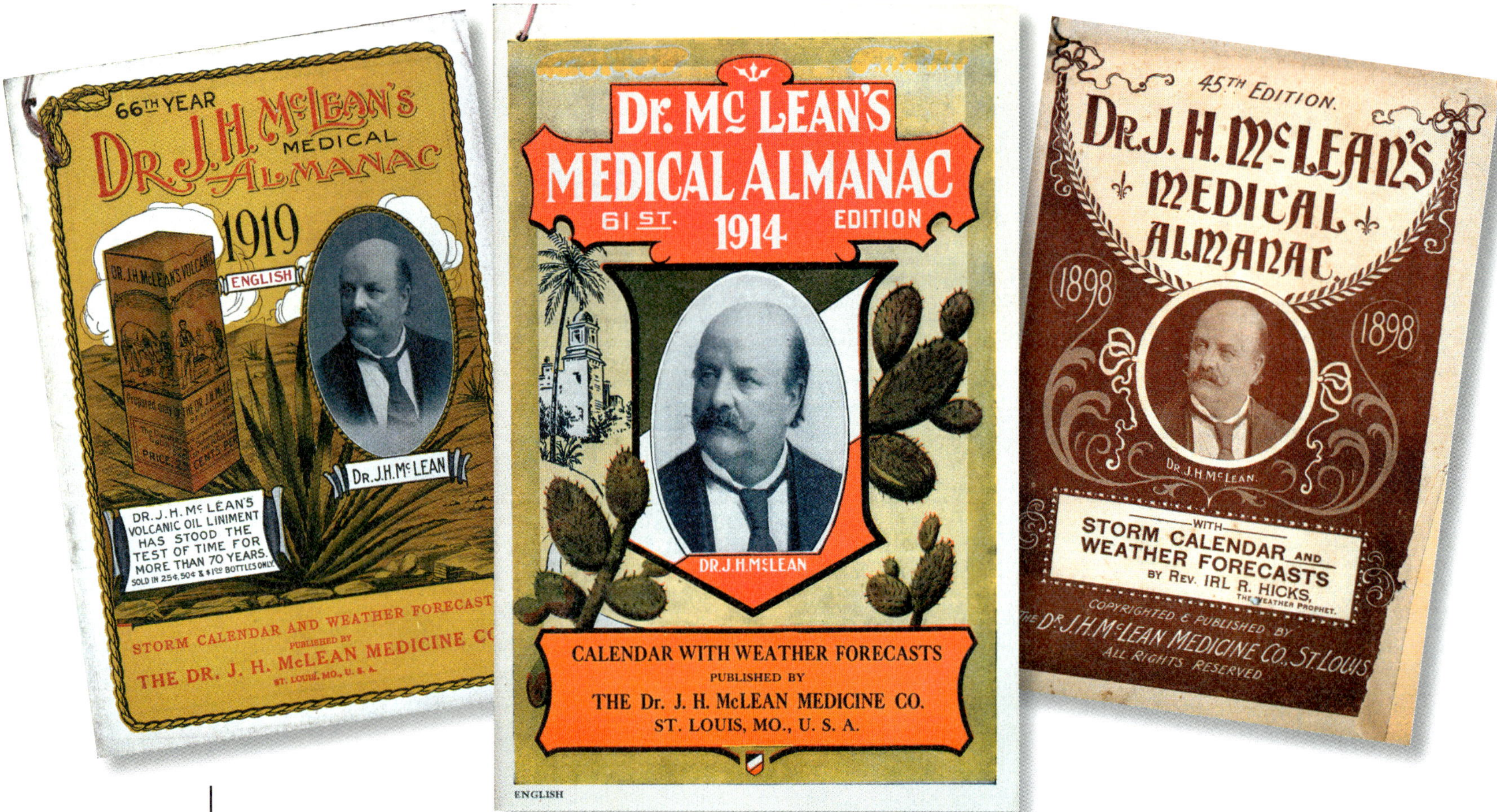


makers of proprietary medicines published a number of the almanacs. According to Robb Sagendorph's *America and Her Almanacs*, the first "health" almanac appeared in 1817.[4] By the late nineteenth century, such almanacs were printed by the millions and distributed by dozens of medicine makers. The quantity issued by the largest proprietors grew to enormous proportions. The makers of "Ayer's Cherry Pectoral" boasted that their almanac was second only to *The Bible* in circulation. An average year for the J.C. Ayer Company was about sixteen million almanacs but in 1889 they distributed more than twenty-five million, written in twenty-one languages.[1]

As was typical of any almanac, the Dr. J.H. McLean Medicine Company almanac in 1896 contained monthly calendars and a list of important holidays along with the weather forecasts. Included were tips in the management of everything from consumption to corns. It was soon evident that advertising was most important. The booklet was crammed with ads and claims for such products as "McLean's Liver and Kidney Balm," "McLean's Strengthening Cordial and Blood Purifier," "McLean's Tar and Lung Balm," "McLean's Volcanic Oil Liniment," and "McLean's Liquid Vermifuge." The ad for "Dr. McLean's Liver and Kidney Pillets" claimed a certain cure for neuralgia, biliousness, costiveness, bad taste in the mouth, and mental depression. There was no mention of liver or kidney disease.

Almanac manufacturers soon made no pretense of copying the monthly calendar format and instead were filling the pages with many testimonials along with a few ads. From cover to cover testimonials and line drawings of the grateful customers filled the pages with descriptions of their dramatic and even miraculous cures.

In due time, as the public became increasingly saturated with hard-sell health material, the alert merchandiser wooed his customer's attention with booklets on many unrelated subjects of general interest, which contained an occasional advertisement. Such medicinal booklets were produced in a number of categories. There were the fortune-telling variety, "dream books," "fate books," and horoscopes. There were

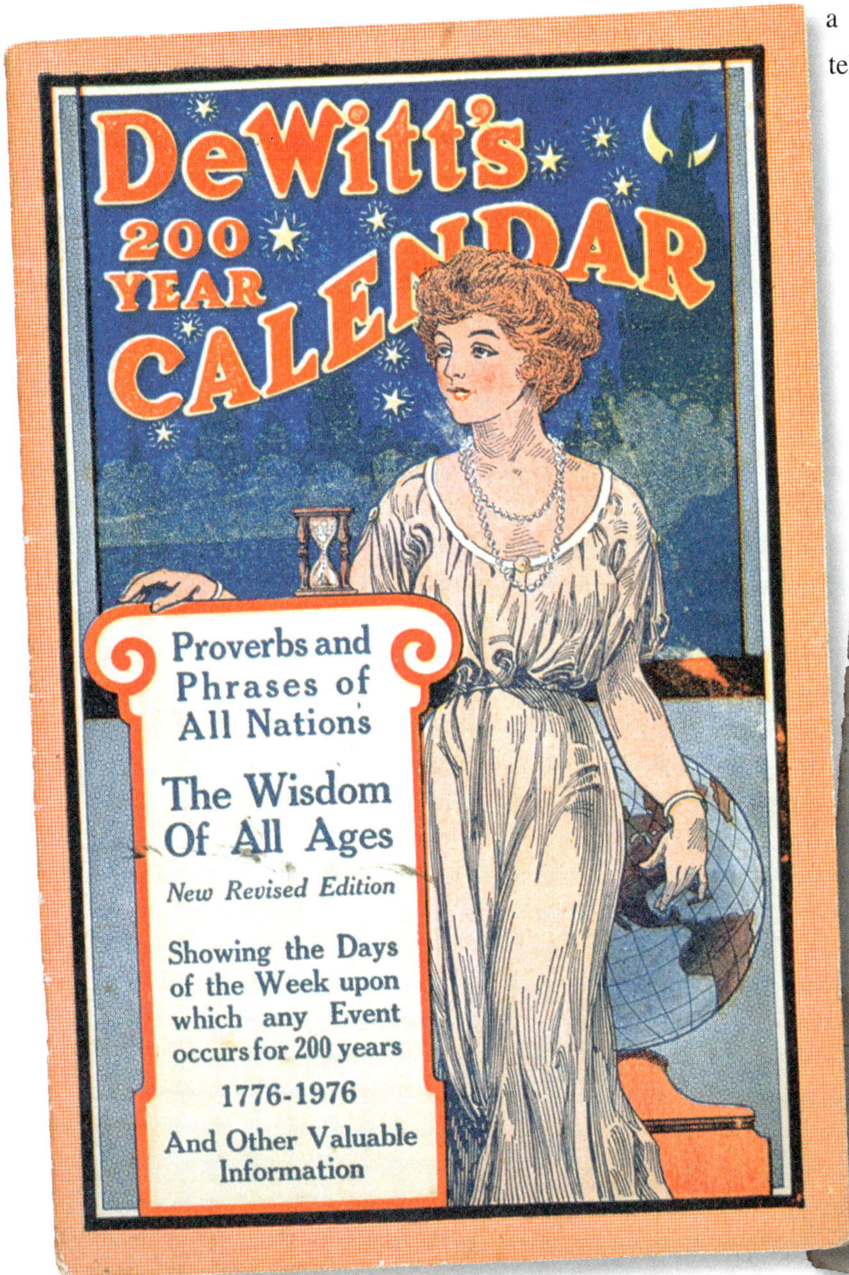


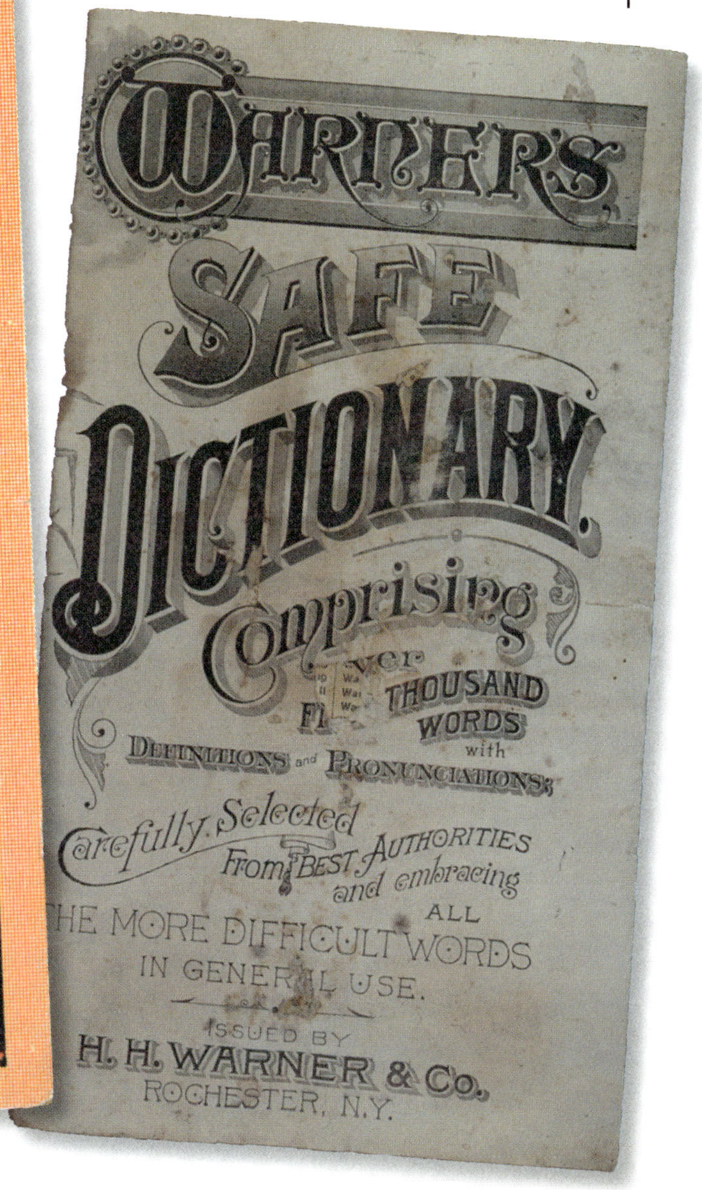

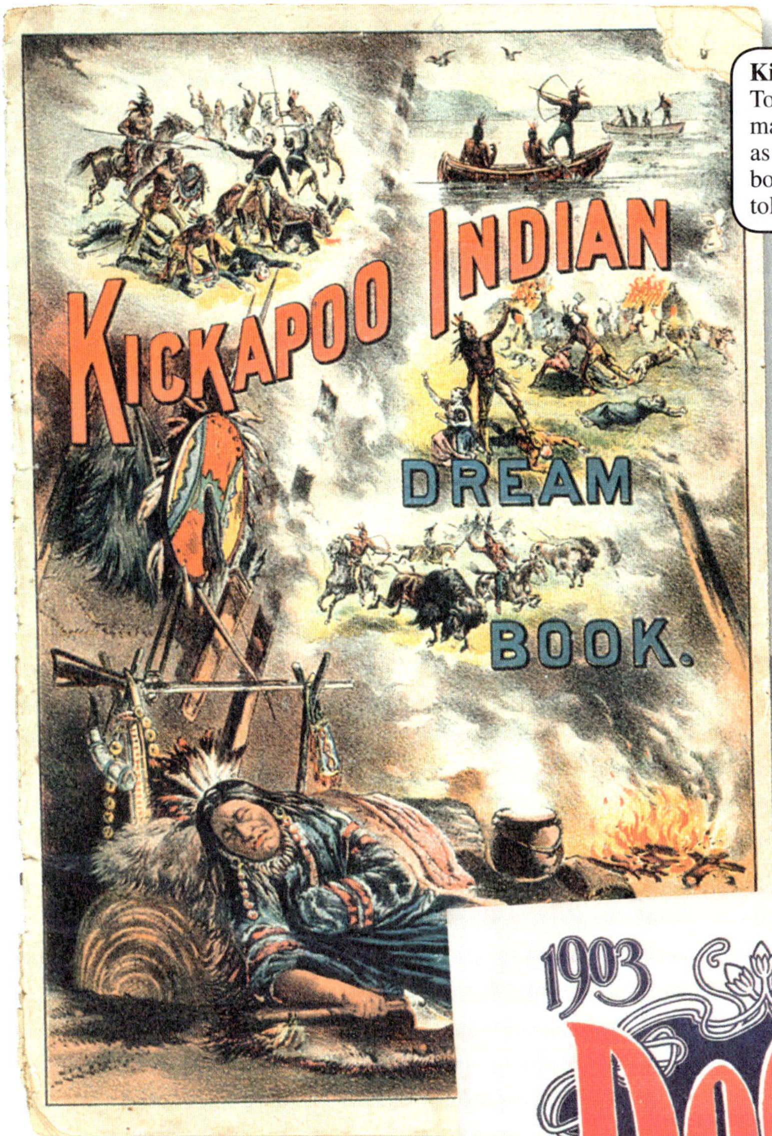


**Kickapoo Indian Dream Book**
To offer wisdom and timely advice, the almanac makers engaged in forecasting such imponderables as weather, as well as producing prognosticating books that explained dreams, predicted the future or told fortunes.

the recipe booklets coupled with culinary axioms. Included were song booklets, memorandum booklets, joke booklets, and for the children color and paint booklets.[1,3,4]

Though they may not measure up to the almanacs of Ben Franklin, the patent medicine almanacs of the nineteenth century are worth a closer look. Since they reveal to us how American people once believed and behaved, they are an important link to a past century.

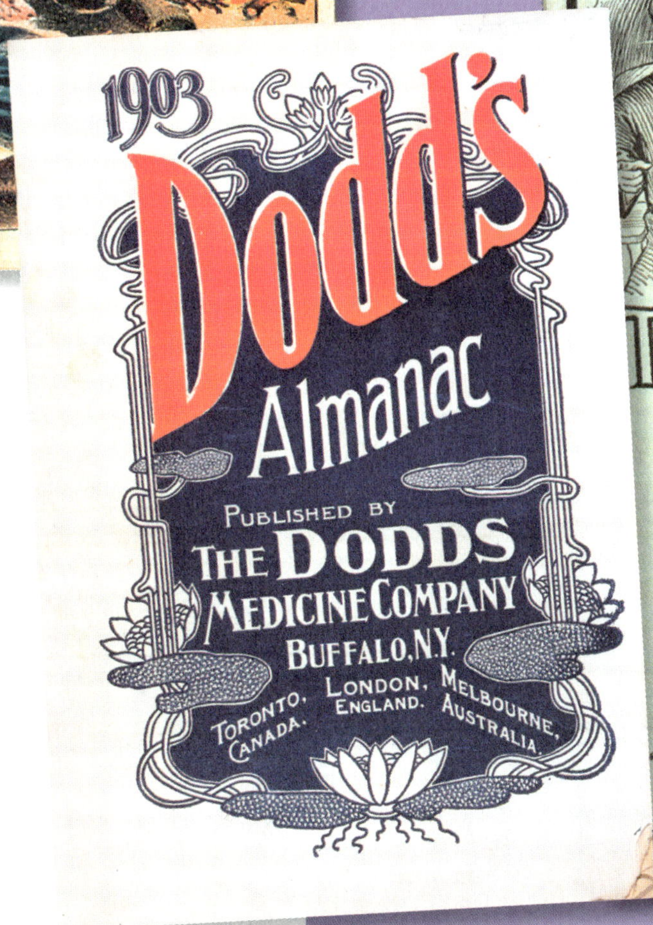


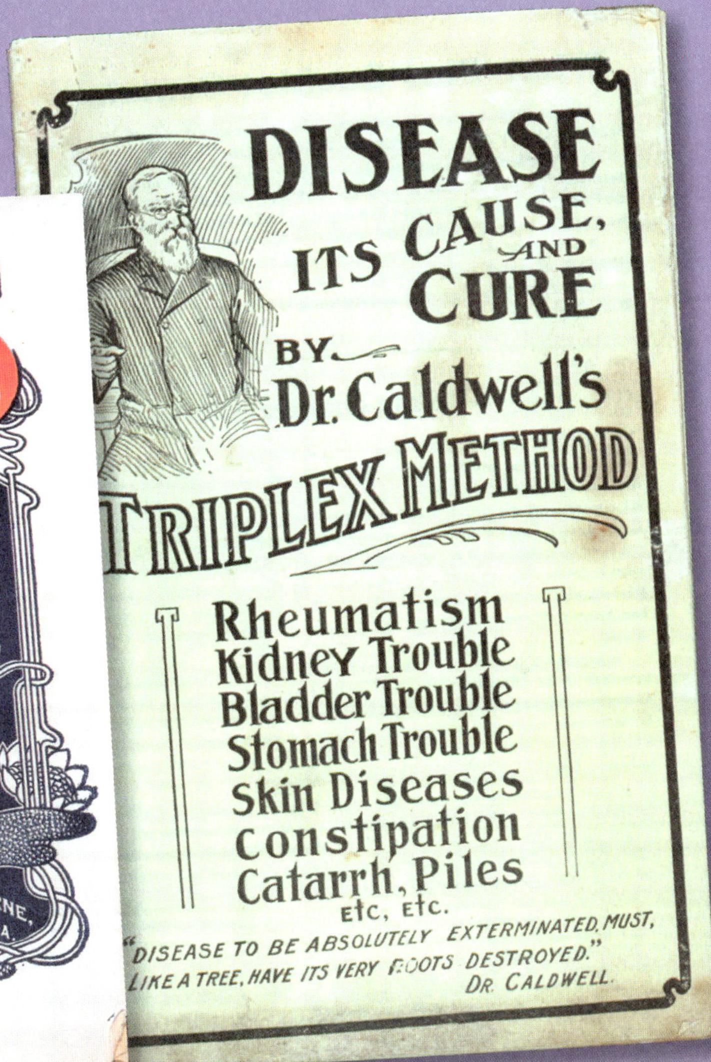

Chapter 18

# Medicine Shows

Conning people—cheating them and making them like it---was the skill of the itinerant medicine showman. For nearly a century, traveling medicine shows were a curious part of American life, with their fast-talking pitchman, their flamboyantly named remedies, and their entertainers who attracted the crowds. The medicine-selling troupes moved from town to town, first in wagons, much later in trucks, all of the vehicles gaudily painted to catch the eye. The territory traveled was mainly rural America with audiences of folks from the farms and villages. They came to towns and hamlets at such times as fairs, when outsiders swelled the native population. It was neither a circus nor a carnival, but a show with entertainment put on for the purpose of selling "medicine."[1,2,5]

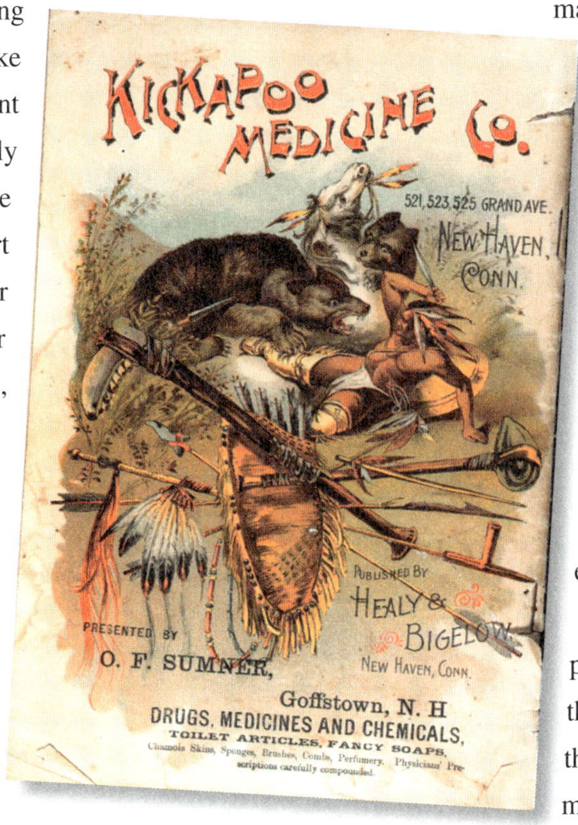


Traveling medicine shows, common to virtually all cultures, have been part of the minstrel tradition that provided rural entertainment. Medicine shows usually started with the same format. First came the ballyhoo or the come-on. It could be a noon parade or a street corner concert—whatever it took to attract attention. For a description of the colorful scene, Nevada Ned, a big-time showman, summed it up well: "Here full evenings of drama, vaudeville, musical comedy, Wild West shows, minstrels, magic, burlesque, dog and pony circuses, pantomime, movies, menageries, bands, parades and pie eating contests, have been thrown in with Ho-Ang-Nan, the great Chinese herb remedy. Medicine shows have played in opera houses, halls, storerooms, ballparks, show boats, and tents, large and small, as well as doorways, street corners, and fairs."[5] Music was always an integral part of any medicine show and perhaps the biggest draw of the evening's entertainment.

Hucksters would augment their presentations by using Native Americans that appealed to the popular notion of the supposedly primitive. The Indian medicine show was particularly popular and was a format adopted by many of the touring companies. The purveyors could count upon the Easterner's awed curiosity about a bronze-skinned people. While massacres of these Native Americans were still

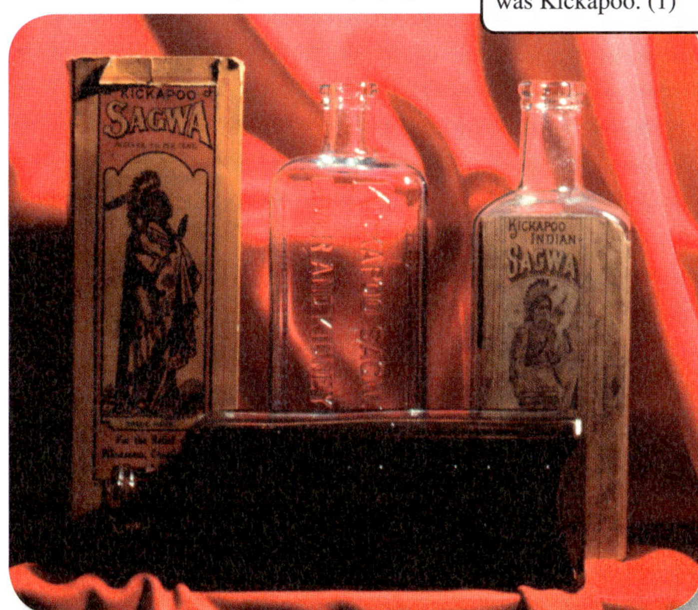


**Kickapoo Medicine Company**
The Kickapoo were a minor branch of the Algonquin tribe that helped the British capture Detroit in the French and Indian War. At the peak of business more than a thousand Indians were hired from the U.S. Government Indian Agents at $30 per head a month plus upkeep. Not one was Kickapoo. (1)

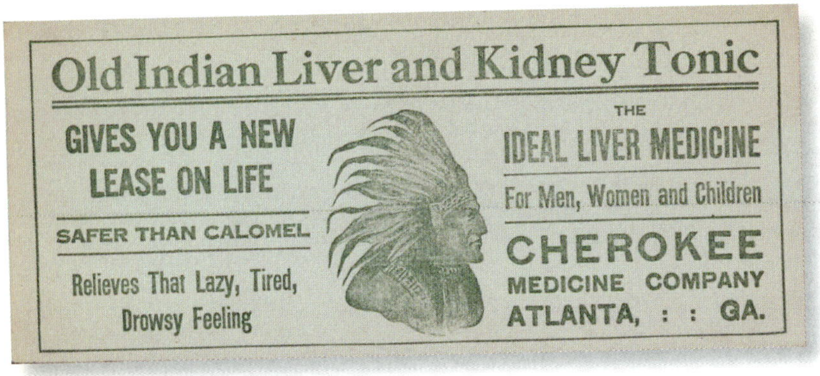


taking place in the West, travelling medicine shows with Indians in full regalia vouching for "Indian Compounds" crisscrossed the East. The razzle-dazzle of the show included war whoops, full Indian dress of feathers and buckskins and a display of Indian curiosities. The beating of drums and the blaring of horns produced frenzied accompaniment for the pitchman's continual harangue. In such a noisy atmosphere, medicine and money changed hands.[2,4,5]

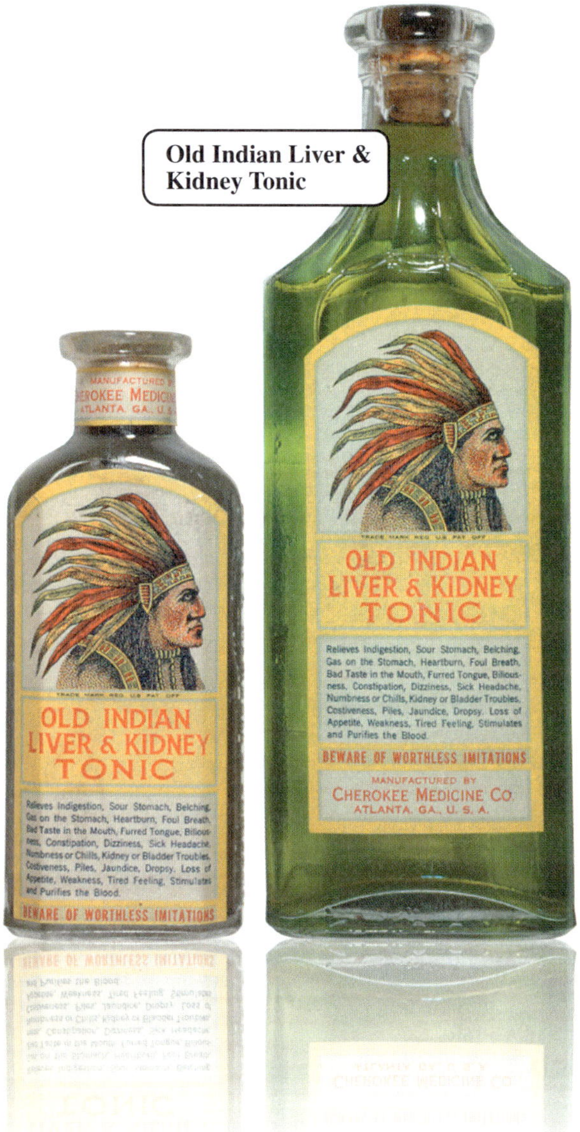


**Old Indian Liver & Kidney Tonic**

The medicine show began with music and laughter to warm up the crowd. When the audience was full of good cheer and enjoyment, the medicine showman or show doctor took the stage to deliver his "pitch." The show doctor's art was in understanding human nature. In his sales pitch he appealed to the basic human reactions: anxiety about health, greed, curiosity, mob psychology—and always credulity, a readiness to believe out of lack of understanding. If a few shills could be hired to start the action, the crowd would become affected by the excitement of buying the miracle cure. The show doctor also seemed to work a bit of hypnotism. It was talk with a purpose and the medicine showman delighted in the skillful way he worked his con. They were talkers and they prided themselves on their gift of oratory by polishing it, exploiting it, and glorying in it. Nothing made the show doctor happier than to hold-in-sway an audience with his voice, playing out his spiel, corralling a crowd, and bringing them in with finesse like a bunch of sheep.[2,4]

The medicine show business started to flourish widely in the 1880s. Two giants, the Kickapoo Indian Medicine Company and Hamlin's Wizard Oil Company, maintained their medicine

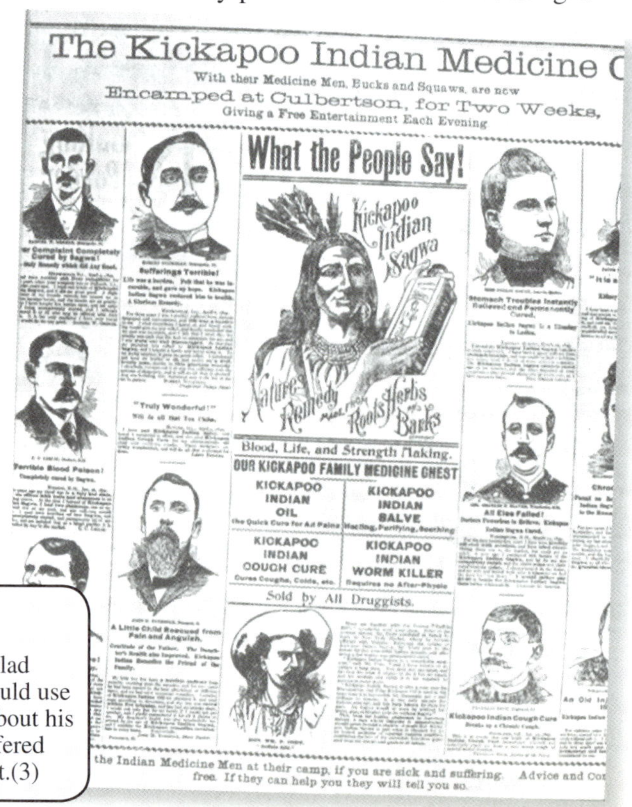
The Kickapoo Indian Medicine C
With their Medicine Men, Bucks and Squaws, are now
Encamped at Culbertson, for Two Weeks,
Giving a Free Entertainment Each Evening

What the People Say!

Kickapoo Indian Sagwa
Nature's Remedy Made from Roots, Herbs and Barks
Blood, Life, and Strength Making.

OUR KICKAPOO FAMILY MEDICINE CHEST
KICKAPOO INDIAN OIL
KICKAPOO INDIAN SALVE
KICKAPOO INDIAN COUGH CURE
KICKAPOO INDIAN WORM KILLER
Sold by All Druggists.

the Indian Medicine Men at their camp, if you are sick and suffering. Advice and Con
free. If they can help you they will tell you so.

**Kickapoo Testimonials**
Sometimes the show doctor put away the buckskins and Indian regalia and would clad himself in gorgeous eastern robes. He would use Oriental banter to tell an absorbing tale about his precious medicinal root that had been pilfered from the long-lived lama of faraway Tibet.(3)

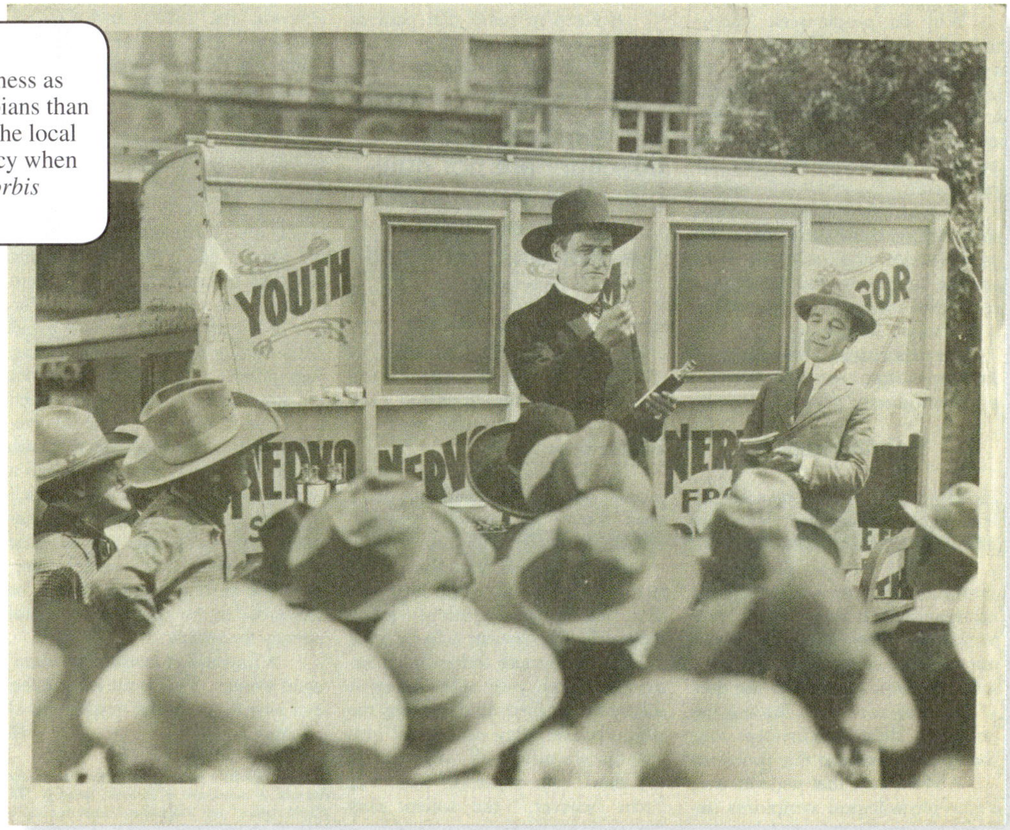


**Picture of Show Doctor**
Some nostrum hucksters were known in medicine show business as "Quacker Doctors." These merry gentlemen were more thespians than doctors. They "thee'd" and "thou'd" on the stage and called the local knave "Friend." The Quacker gimmick caught the public fancy when wigwam medicine was becoming ho-hum.(3) *Courtesy of Corbis Archives.*

factories in the East and sent out show troops to hawk their product along with hundreds of other companies with touring shows. Medicine show business was truly big business.[2,3,4]

The headquarters of the Kickapoo Indian Medicine Company in Hartford, Connecticut was known as the Big Wigwam. At any given time they had as many as seventy-five Kickapoo shows on the road. The shows featured American Indians who were hired by the hundreds—but not one was Kickapoo.

Hamlin's Wizard Oil Company was the other titan of medicine show business. In sharp contrast, it differed from the hoopla of the Indian shows. The Hamlin image was that of dignity, performing refined music, wearing stylish attire, and offering a distinguished doctor. The parlor organ built on each handsome six-horse drawn wagon would accompany the impeccably dressed musicians and male-quartet. The troupe would visit a town for two to six weeks to promote goodwill by performing many free concerts and creating a demand for Wizard Oil medicines among the spectators. Local merchants also began ordering and stocking these nostrums.[2,3,4]

Why did the medicine man become the con artist? First of all, for the money. Also, life on the road offered adventurous living, traveling to new places, and meeting new people. As a showman he would always be center stage, persuading audiences with his compelling voice and skillful oratory. But—alas, medicine men lived high with expensive habits, generous tips, costly clothes, and fancy women. From 1880 to 1910 was the golden age, the most prosperous time for the hucksters in the medicine show business.[2,4]

Hucksters, purveyors, swindlers, show doctors—what characterized these artists of con? It was their con—as concealer, conspirator, contentious, contrary, and controversial—without a conscience toward the objects of their guile.

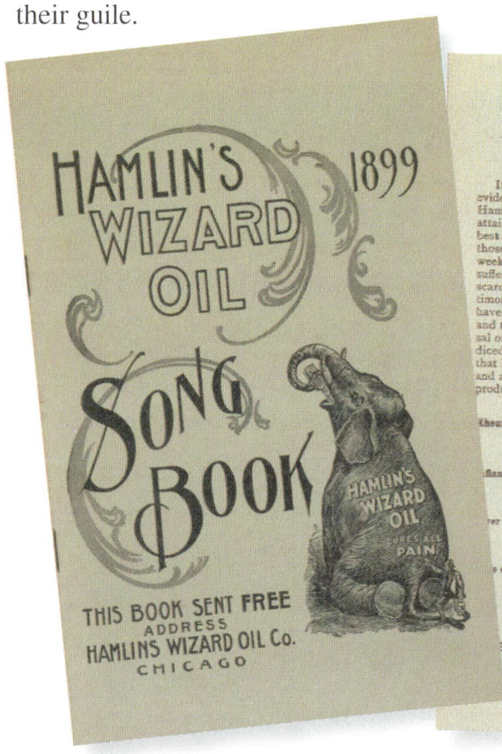


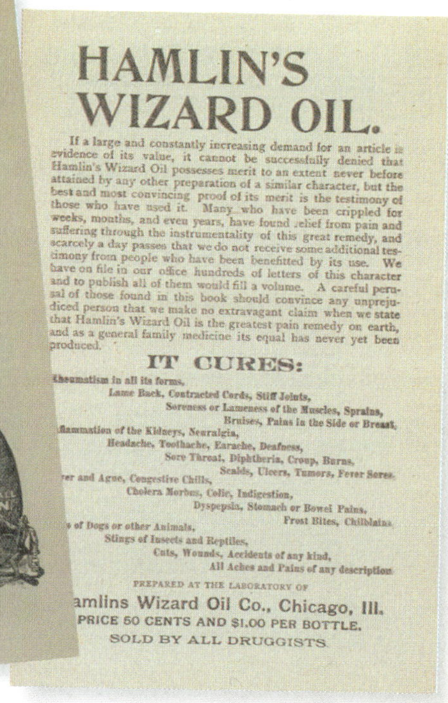

HAMLIN'S
WIZARD OIL.

If a large and constantly increasing demand for an article is evidence of its value, it cannot be successfully denied that Hamlin's Wizard Oil possesses merit to an extent never before attained by any other preparation of a similar character, but the best and most convincing proof of its merit is the testimony of those who have used it. Many who have been crippled for weeks, months, and even years, have found relief from pain and suffering through the instrumentality of this great remedy, and scarcely a day passes that we do not receive some additional testimony from people who have been benefitted by its use. We have on file in our office hundreds of letters of this character and to publish all of them would fill a volume. A careful perusal of those found in this book should convince any unprejudiced person that we make no extravagant claim when we state that Hamlin's Wizard Oil is the greatest pain remedy on earth, and as a general family medicine its equal has never yet been produced.

IT CURES:

heumatism in all its forms,
Lame Back, Contracted Cords, Stiff Joints,
Soreness or Lameness of the Muscles, Sprains,
Bruises, Pains in the Side or Breast,
flammation of the Kidneys, Neuralgia,
Headache, Toothache, Earache, Deafness,
Sore Throat, Diphtheria, Croup, Burns,
Scalds, Ulcers, Tumors, Fever Sores,
er and Ague, Congestive Chills,
Cholera Morbus, Colic, Indigestion,
Dyspepsia, Stomach or Bowel Pains,
Frost Bites, Chilblains,
of Dogs or other Animals,
Stings of Insects and Reptiles,
Cuts, Wounds, Accidents of any kind,
All Aches and Pains of any description

PREPARED AT THE LABORATORY OF
amlins Wizard Oil Co., Chicago, Ill.
PRICE 50 CENTS AND $1.00 PER BOTTLE.
SOLD BY ALL DRUGGISTS

# CHINESE MEDICINE

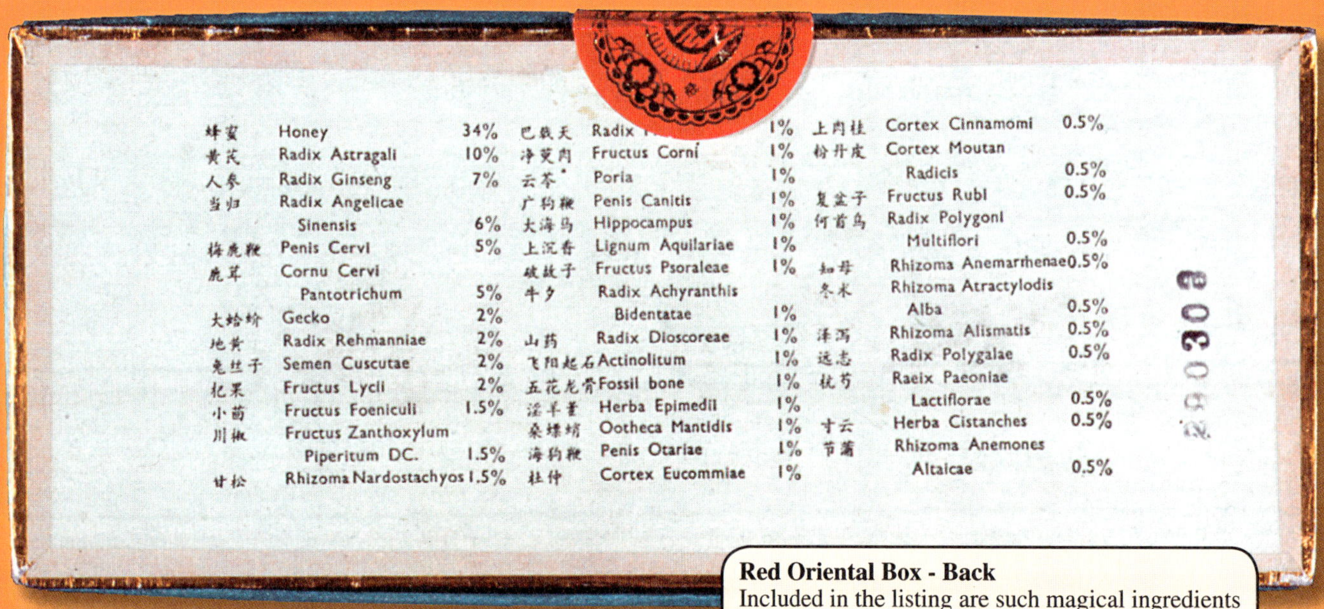

蜂蜜 Honey 34%
黄芪 Radix Astragali 10%
人参 Radix Ginseng 7%
当归 Radix Angelicae Sinensis 6%
梅鹿鞭 Penis Cervi 5%
鹿茸 Cornu Cervi Pantotrichum 5%
大蛤蚧 Gecko 2%
地黄 Radix Rehmanniae 2%
菟丝子 Semen Cuscutae 2%
杞果 Fructus Lycii 2%
小茴 Fructus Foeniculi 1.5%
川椒 Fructus Zanthoxylum Piperitum DC. 1.5%
甘松 Rhizoma Nardostachyos 1.5%
巴戟天 Radix 1%
净萸肉 Fructus Corni 1%
云苓 Poria 1%
广狗鞭 Penis Canitis 1%
大海马 Hippocampus 1%
上沉香 Lignum Aquilariae 1%
破故子 Fructus Psoraleae 1%
牛夕 Radix Achyranthis Bidentatae 1%
山药 Radix Dioscoreae 1%
飞阳起石 Actinolitum 1%
五花龙骨 Fossil bone 1%
淫羊藿 Herba Epimedii 1%
桑螵蛸 Ootheca Mantidis 1%
海狗鞭 Penis Otariae 1%
杜仲 Cortex Eucommiae 1%
上肉桂 Cortex Cinnamomi 0.5%
粉丹皮 Cortex Moutan Radicis 0.5%
覆盆子 Fructus Rubi 0.5%
何首乌 Radix Polygoni Multiflori 0.5%
知母 Rhizoma Anemarrhenae 0.5%
冬术 Rhizoma Atractylodis Alba 0.5%
泽泻 Rhizoma Alismatis 0.5%
远志 Radix Polygalae 0.5%
杭芍 Raeix Paeoniae Lactiflorae 0.5%
寸云 Herba Cistanches 0.5%
节菖 Rhizoma Anemones Altaicae 0.5%


**Red Oriental Box - Back**
Included in the listing are such magical ingredients as Penis Cervi, Gecko, Fossil bone.

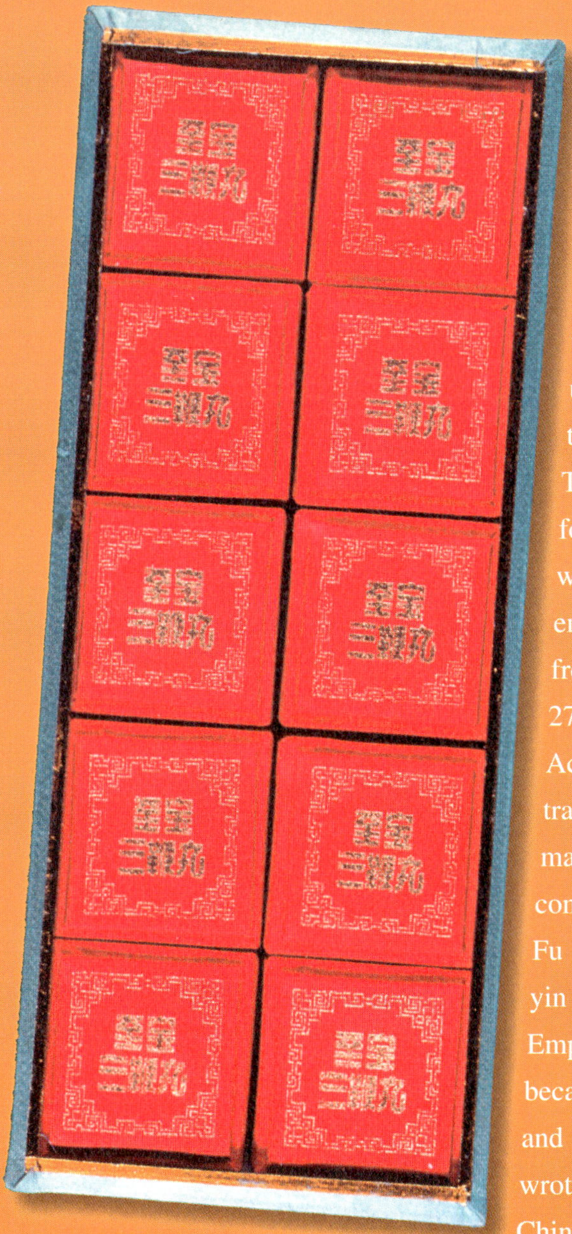


Chinese medicine traces its history to unwritten legends thousands of years old. The true foundations for Chinese medicine were laid by three emperors who reigned from the 29th to the 27th centuries B.C. According to oral tradition each emperor made a significant contribution. Emperor Fu Hsi authored the yin and yang doctrine, Emperor Shen Hung became the first herbalist, and Emperor Huang Ti wrote the earliest book on Chinese medicine.[1,4,5]

These emperors taught that the health of all creation and especially humanity was dependent on harmony of the yin and the yang. Within the human body the polar elements of the yin and yang exist such as cold and hot, wet and dry, body and mind. In acupuncture, the aim was to restore the balance and harmony between these attributes.[1,4,5]

The ancient Chinese considered a dead body to be sacrosanct. Their doctors were not allowed to dissect any human corpses, and thus learned nothing about human anatomy.[2] Principles of bodily function included the Ch'I, as the energy or animating force, coursing along pathways called meridians. It was believed that the body, as in all nature, consisted of five elements: water, fire, earth, metal and wood. Each element was associated and in harmony with an organ system of the body.

Legend says that Emperor Shen Nung, the father of Chinese medicinal herbs, classified these plants and provided details on preparation and dosage. The complex combinations of herbs along with the use of animal parts, metals, minerals, insects, shells, rocks eventually resulted in today's form of medicinal treatment called traditional medicine.[3] Currently herbal medicines continue to play an important role in the prevention as well as the treatment of disease in China. However, the emphasis of Chinese medicine is prevention. When illness does occur, the treatment can include acupuncture, massage, dietary changes, as well as medicinal herbs.[3] Most 21st century Chinese physicians practice some form of traditional medicine along with the practice of Western medicine.

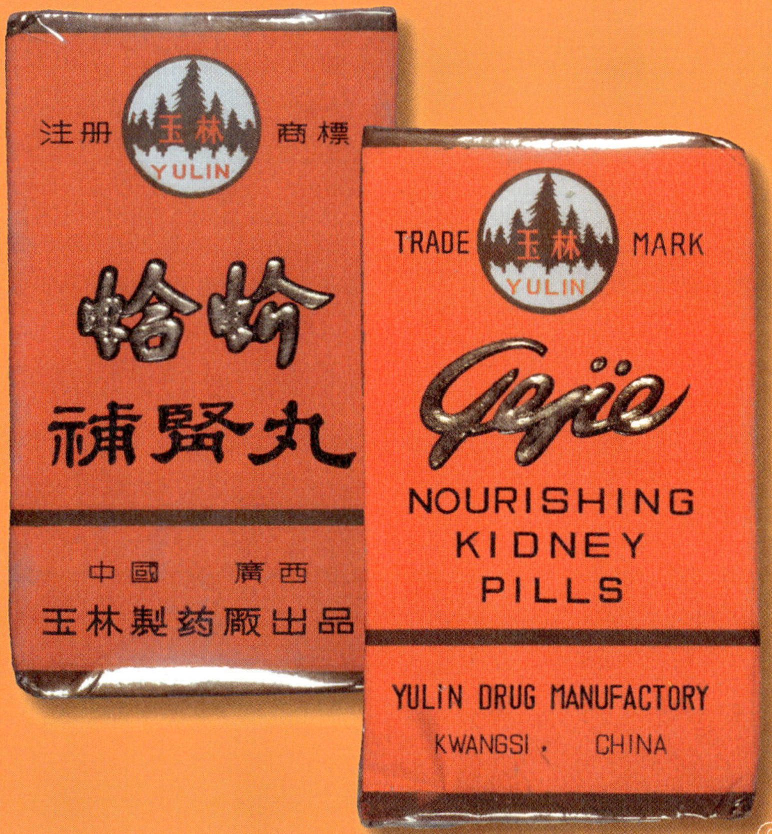

PART TWO

# TODAY, THE GREAT DECEPTION CONTINUES

"I know it is common to speak of the 'good old days' of snake oil and soothing syrups as though they were gone forever. The amazing fact is that to a very great extent those good old days, so-called, are still with us."

- Commissioner George P. Larrick, Food and Drug Administration, 1955

After returning from his worldwide search for the best cures on earth, Dr. David Williams declares...

# "These AMAZING NEW CURES Could Make Disease Extinct!"

"As you read this, brilliant medical researchers are curing (yes, curing) high blood pressure (p. 7 *inside*), heart disease (p. 6), cancer (p. 10), diabetes (p. 6), osteoporosis (p. 19), prostate problems (p. 10), alzheimers (p. 4), allergies (p. 21), asthma (p. 21), and ulcers (p. 9)—without resorting to a pill or scalpel. Ten years from now, these almost miraculous cures will be commonplace.

"**But you can't wait.** You or someone you love may be in pain now. Or facing life-threatening surgery. Or taking toxic drugs. I'm 'going public' with these cures *now*."

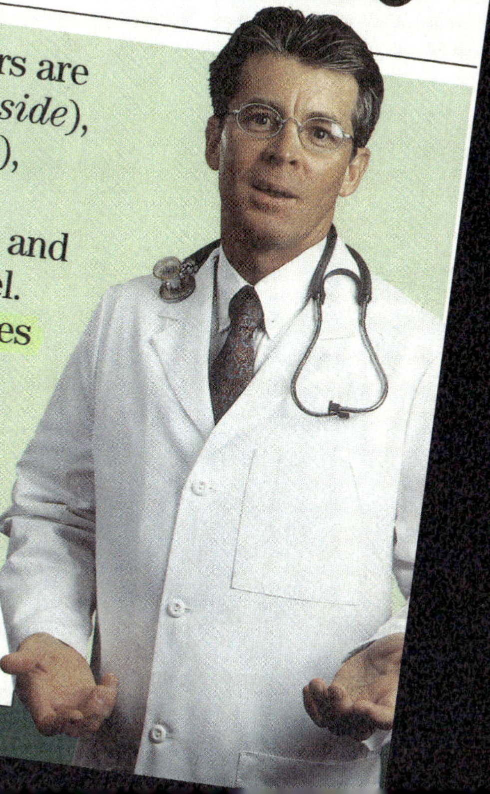

Dr. David Williams: The doctor trusted by over a hundred thousand Americans because he brings them tomorrow's cures *today*.

# MOVING FORWARD

"While the physician seeks to help his patient if he can, he must sometimes confess that he cannot. The quack need make no such confession, for honesty is not contained in his code of ethics. This gives the charlatan great advantage in competing with the physician."

- James Harvey Young, P.H.D., Professor of History, Emory University, 1967

# What About Alternative Medicine?

For thousands of years of human history, plants have been the chief source of medicinal remedies. From the doctor-philosopher of classical antiquity to the shamans of yesterday's rain forests, healers have prescribed a variety of herbs culled from the flora around them. Scant documentation resulted in a limited recording of remedies used in the era. Traditional societies accumulated knowledge about medicinal plants, but passed it on orally from one generation to the next. The village healers considered the knowledge of plants and their healing properties as a gift from the gods. Their information was guarded to protect their livelihood and position of power.

Before the advent of modern science, in rural America, women maintained herb gardens and served as village healers. In time they concocted more than 14,000 herbal remedies for problems associated with fertility, childbirth, and menstruation. During his childhood in Missouri, Mark Twain noted that "every old woman was a doctor, and gathered her own medicines . . . ."[10]

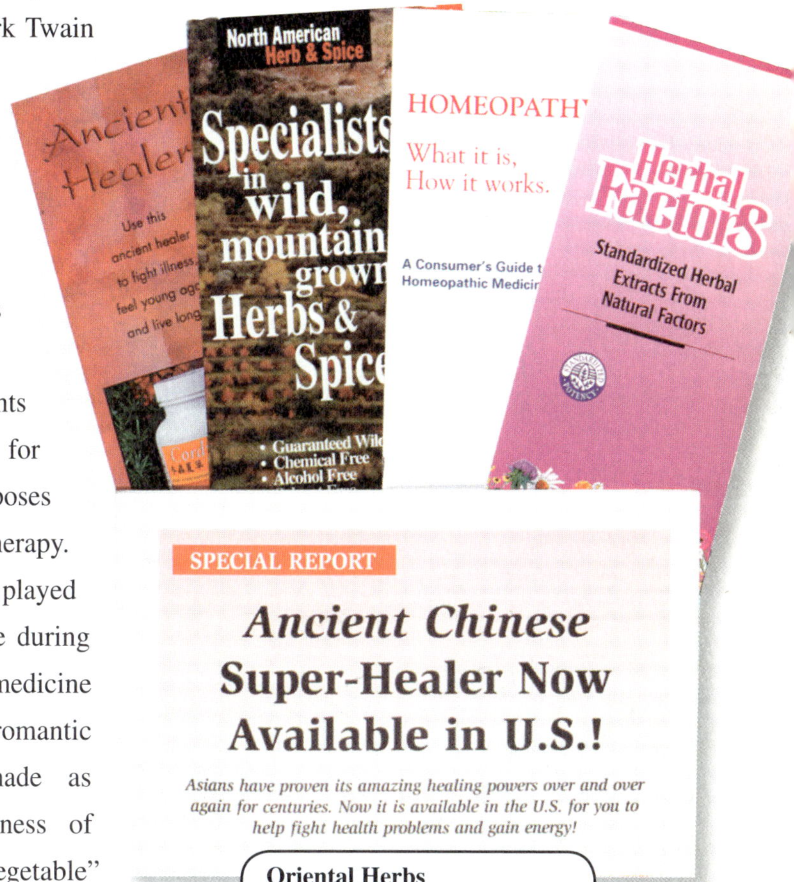


**Oriental Herbs**
The lure of mystical healing and magical herbal medicine is enhanced with ads that suggest ancient and oriental origins.

The use of plants or plant extracts for medicinal purposes is called phytotherapy. Phytotherapy played an important role during the patent medicine era. Bold and romantic claims were made as to the effectiveness of the "purely vegetable" ingredients. Herbal combinations were marketed as remedies, alternatives, tonics, cures, and teas. But today in the 21st century "it's déjà vu all over again" (as Yogi Berra said) since the use of plants and plant extracts enjoy wide acceptance as medicinals. Also, there is the assumption that if it is advertised, some federal agency must have approved it.

One of the most profound trends affecting physicians today is the growing

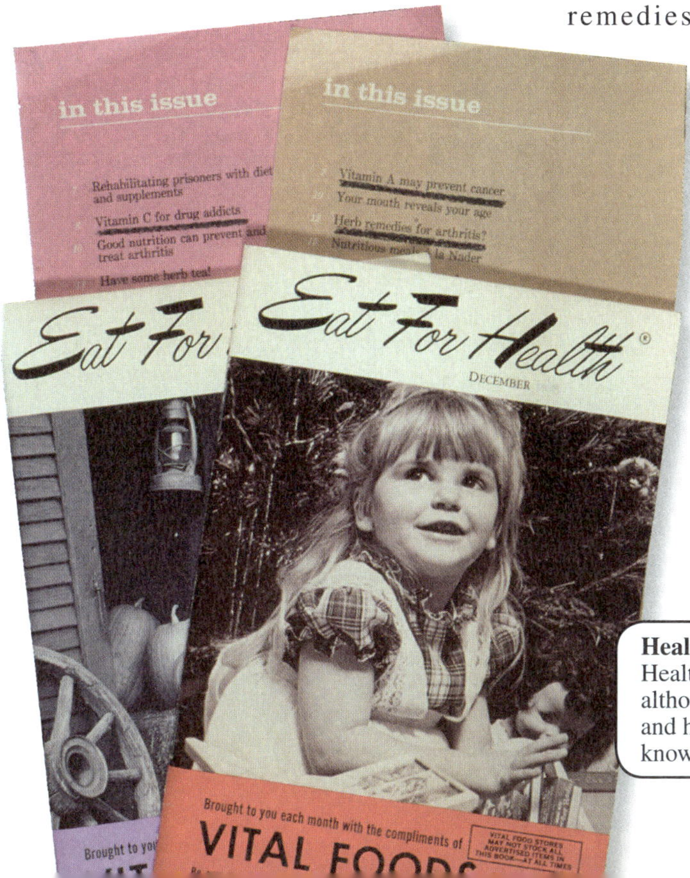


**Health Food Stores**
Health Food Stores are not pharmacies, although they promote food supplements and herbal medicines as remedies for all known illnesses.

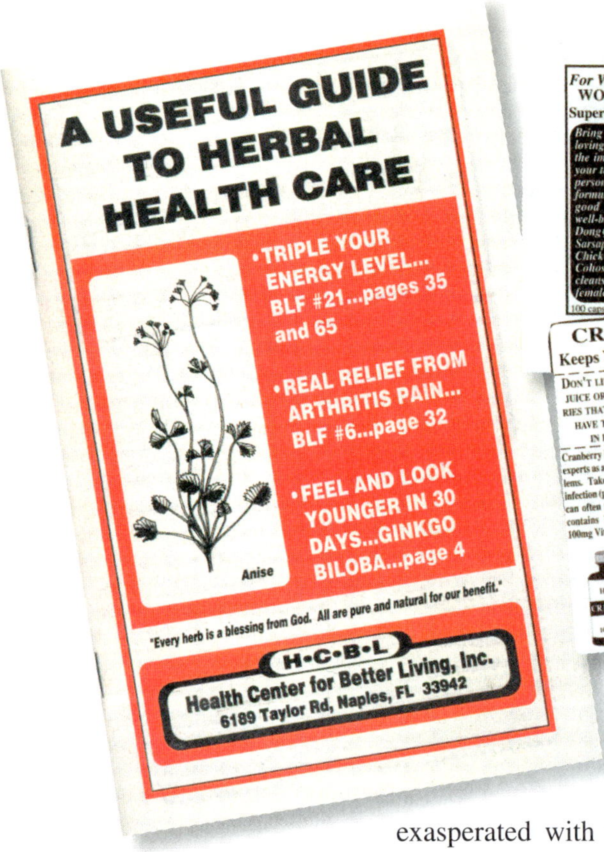


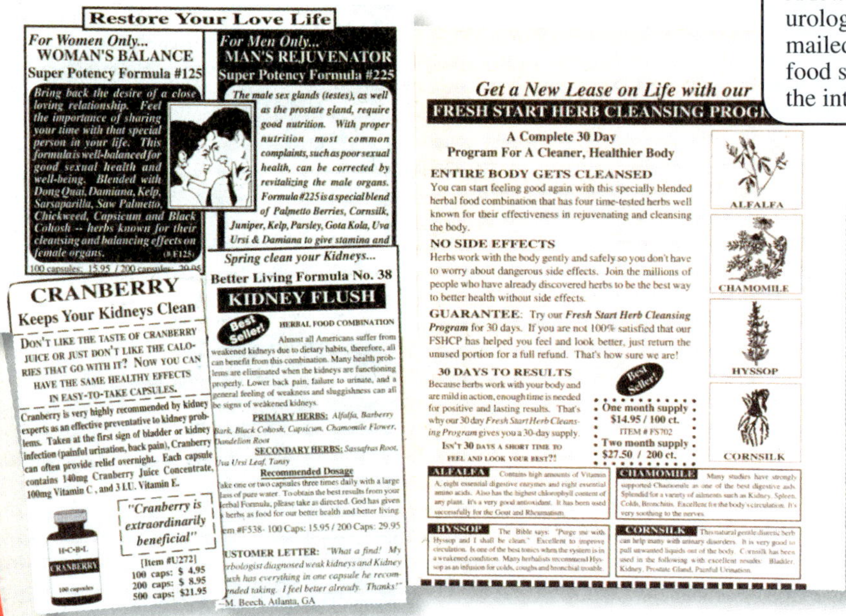


A few examples of the many urological nostrums offered in mailed catalogues, in health food store brochures and on the internet.

strength of consumers—otherwise known as patients. The patients have become exasperated with the shortfalls of conventional medicine. This primarily involves delivery and attitude rather than its body of knowledge. All too often the practitioners and systems can be impersonal, short on time, expensive, and fixated on technological prowess, rather than building therapeutic relationships with patients. Call it "alternative," "complementary," "integrative," or "holistic" medicine. By whatever name you choose, this non-traditional therapeutic practice has become increasingly prominent and provocative as part of the U.S. medical landscape.

No longer willing to let health plans dictate to them or to take their doctor's word as gospel, patients are investing time and money in their own care. They are big spenders, shelling out in 1997 alone more than $27 billion from their own pockets for alternative medicine. This amount, up 45 percent from 1990, is almost equivalent to the estimated $29 billion that patients spent for all non-reimbursed physician services. Taking both of these amounts together means that consumers are willing to spend $56 billion of their own money on health care. That amount is up for grabs among the health care providers who can meet consumers' demands. It is expected that the amount for alternative treatment will increase. Medical schools are also buying in. According to the *Journal of the American Medical Association* of 1998, 75 out of 117 schools now include some form of training in alternative medicine within their core curriculum or as electives. Even flinty-eyed health

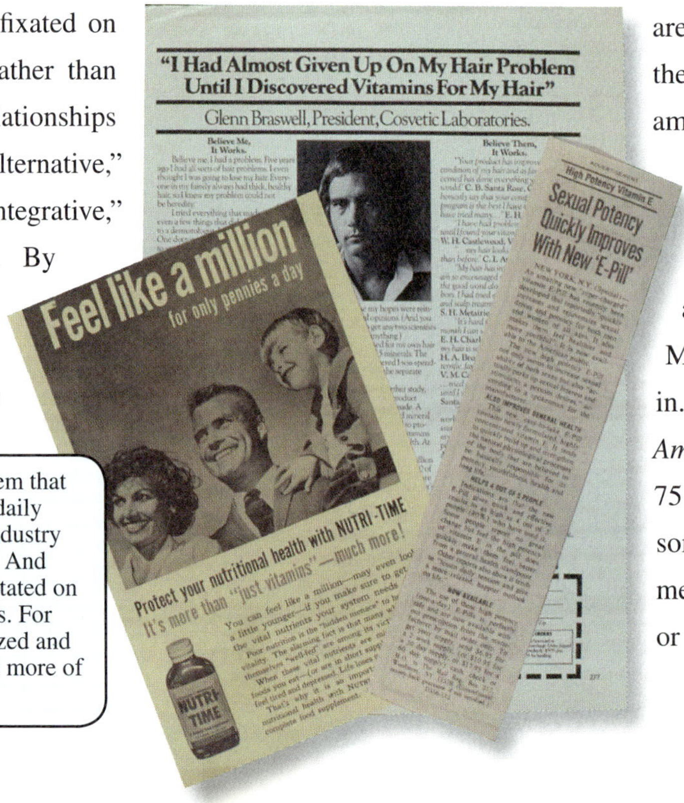


The subtleties of vitamin E highlight the problem that confronts the millions of Americans who take daily vitamin supplements. The $6 billion vitamin industry is loosely regulated by the federal government. And there are often discrepancies between what is stated on the label and what the capsule actually contains. For example, seven vitamin E products were analyzed and were discovered to have from 41% less to 57% more of the stated active ingredient!(8)

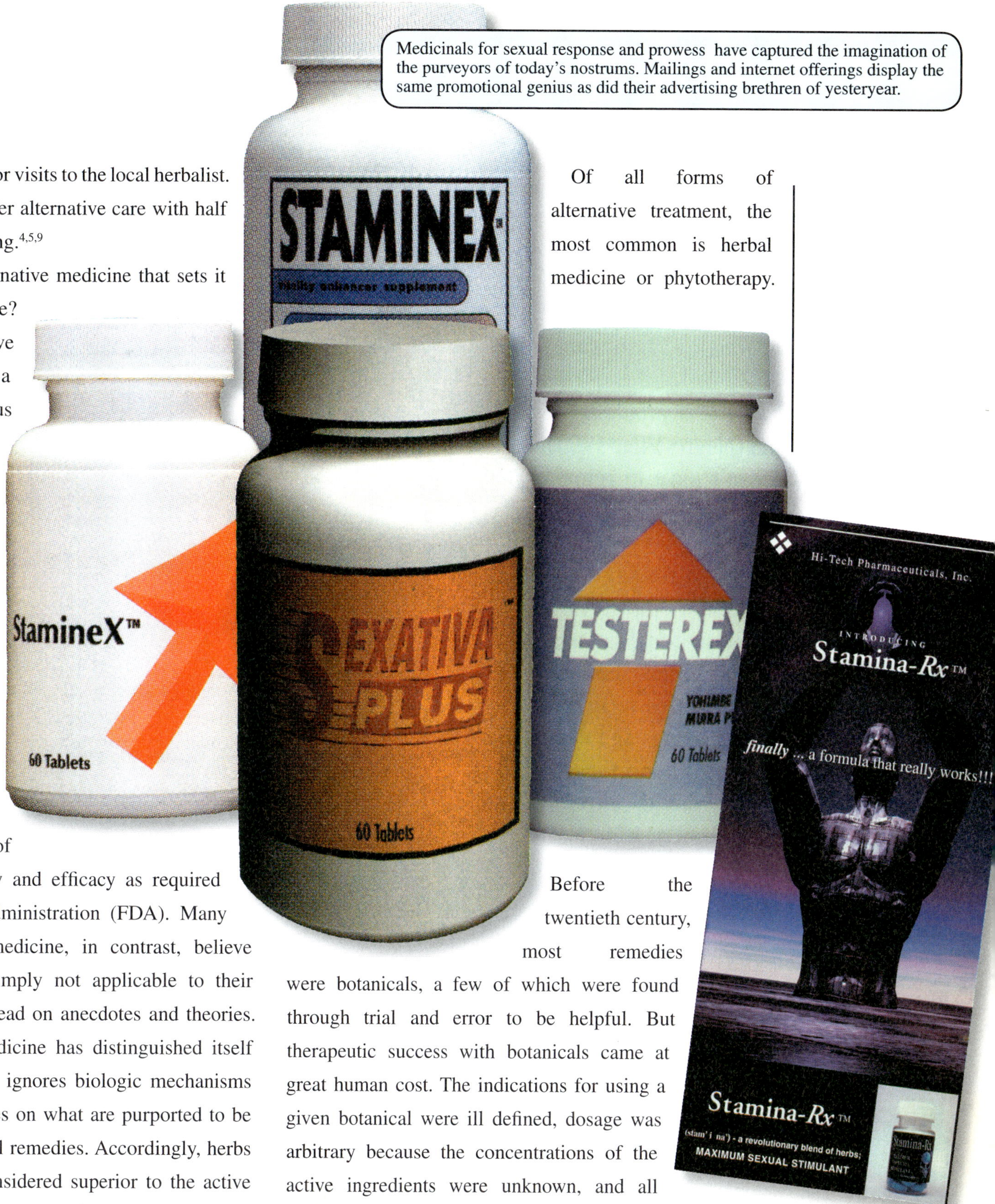


Medicinals for sexual response and prowess have captured the imagination of the purveyors of today's nostrums. Mailings and internet offerings display the same promotional genius as did their advertising brethren of yesteryear.

insurers are starting to pay for visits to the local herbalist. Two out of three HMOs offer alternative care with half their subscribers participating.[4,5,9]

What is there about alternative medicine that sets it apart from ordinary medicine? The term, alternative medicine, refers to a remarkably heterogeneous group of theories and practices—as disparate as acupuncture, homeopathy, therapeutic touch, yoga, herbal medicine, or phytotheraphy. What most sets alternative medicine apart is that it has not been scientifically tested and its advocates largely deny the need for such testing. By testing is meant the marshalling of rigorous evidence of safety and efficacy as required by the Food and Drug Administration (FDA). Many advocates of alternative medicine, in contrast, believe the scientific method is simply not applicable to their remedies and they rely instead on anecdotes and theories. Specifically, alternative medicine has distinguished itself by an ideology that largely ignores biologic mechanisms and modern science. It relies on what are purported to be ancient practices and natural remedies. Accordingly, herbs or mixture of herbs are considered superior to the active components isolated in the laboratory.[2]

Of all forms of alternative treatment, the most common is herbal medicine or phytotherapy.

Before the twentieth century, most remedies were botanicals, a few of which were found through trial and error to be helpful. But therapeutic success with botanicals came at great human cost. The indications for using a given botanical were ill defined, dosage was arbitrary because the concentrations of the active ingredients were unknown, and all manner of contaminants were often present.

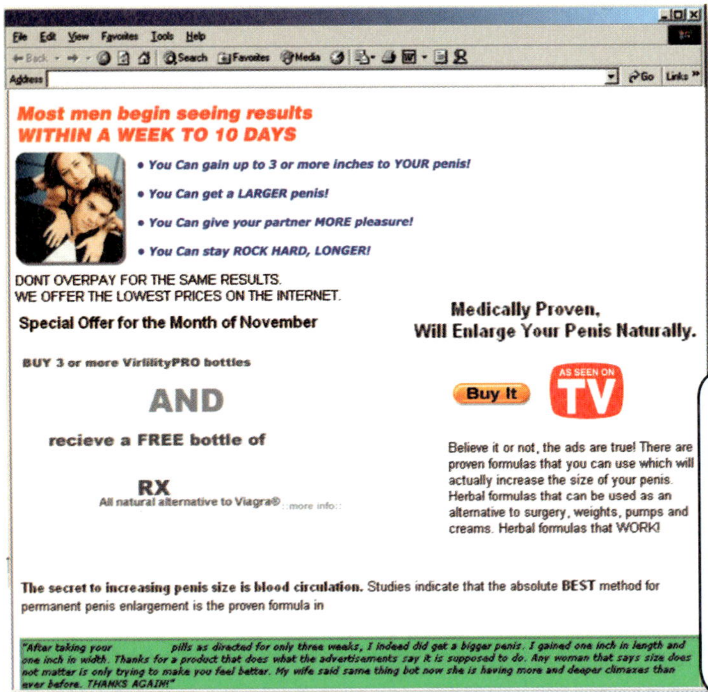


Along with the information explosion on the internet has come an abundance of health related advice. Unfortunately some of the information is deliberately deceitful. Offered are scams and products of dubious value.

Most importantly, many of the remedies simply did not work, and some were harmful and even deadly. The only way to separate the beneficial from the useless or hazardous was through anecdotes relayed mainly by word of mouth.[6,10]

A significant problem today is patient reporting. Of the millions of Americans using alternative medicines only a third of them report it to their doctor. The American Society of Anesthesiology for example reported alarming side effects with anesthesia because of the unknown use of gingko, St. John's wort, or ginseng. It is imperative that patients taking alternative medicinals must also assume the responsibility of reporting such use.[1]

What about the FDA? Shouldn't it be monitoring the safety and efficacy of these remedies? Not any longer, according to the United States Congress. In response to the lobbying efforts of the multi-billion dollar "dietary supplement" industry, Congress in 1994 exempted their products from FDA regulation. Since then, these products have flooded the market, subject only to the scruples of their manufacturers.[3,11] They may contain the substances listed on the label in the amounts claimed, but they may not, and there is no one to prevent their sale if they don't. Herbal remedies may also be sold without any knowledge of their mechanism of action. The only legal requirement in the sale of such products is that they not be marketed to specifically prevent or treat disease. To comply with that stipulation, euphemistic phrases and insinuating labeling are used. Nevertheless, it is clear what is meant. For example saw palmetto is sold to "promote prostate health." Let the buyer beware! The FDA can intervene only after the fact, when it is shown that a product is harmful.[2,7]

Consequently it is time for the scientific community to discontinue its laissez-faire attitude toward alternative medicine. Continuation only reinforces the public's notion that alternative therapies are devoid of potential harm. There cannot be two kinds of medicine—conventional and alternative. There is only medicine that has been adequately tested and medicine that has not, medicine that works and medicine that may or may not work. When a treatment has been tested vigorously, it no longer matters whether it was once considered an herbal medicinal. If it is found to be reasonably safe and effective, it will be accepted. Alternative treatments should be subjected to scientific testing no less rigorous than that required for conventional therapy.[2]

Chapter 20

# A Case In Point: Phytotherapy For Urinary Tract Symptoms

During the patent medicine era human complaints were treated with thousands of different medicinal concoctions from liquid nostrums to pills, plasters, and teas. Despite the probable widespread incidence of lower urinary tract symptoms, there was a significant paucity of its mention in almanac and trade card advertising. There was only a rare patent medicine available for this complaint.

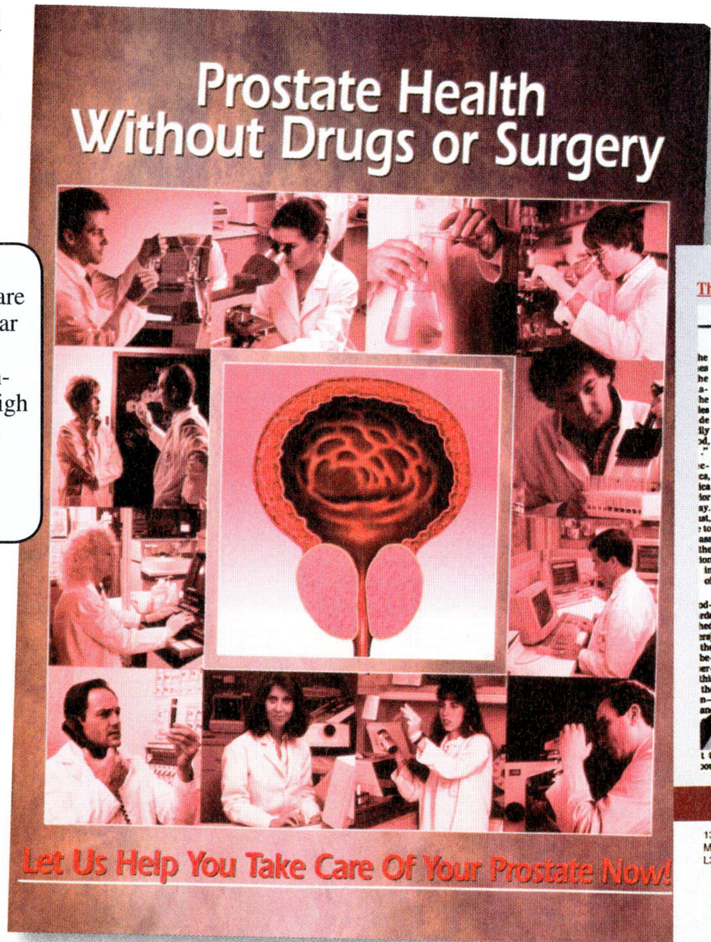


**Prostate Health Brochures**
Today's proprietary nostrums are advertised in a strikingly similar style to that of yesteryear. The brochure reads like an old fashioned almanac. Contained is high praise for the maker's product, disparagement of the medical profession and many dramatic anecdotal testimonials.

However, today, while complementary or alternative medicine continues to offer treatment to a wide variety of medical conditions,[1,2] there is also a significant selection of botanicals for the complaint of lower tract symptoms.[3,4,5] Herbal remedies have become particularly popular for men with lower urinary tract symptoms since the primary goal of treatment in most men with benign prostatic obstruction (BPH) is a subjective relief in voiding complaints.[6,7]

Often there is a decrease in symptom scores and an increase in urinary flow rates in men receiving placebos.[8] This, as well as the unpredictable natural history of BPH,[9] have led some to suggest that "maybe a placebo for BPH is not so terrible."[10] Although there is a general perception that herbal products are at worst a harmless placebo, growing evidence today suggests that this is not always true.

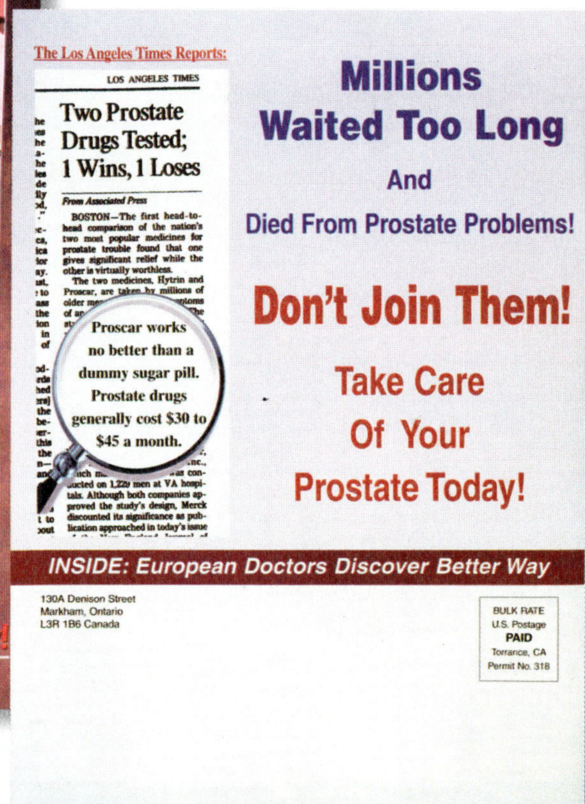


With the increased popularity of alternative medicine has come increased scrutiny regarding its efficacy and safety.[11] Di Paola and others reported that an eight herbal combination mixture, PC-SPES, which is claimed to bolster the immune system of men with prostate cancer, has significant hormonal (estrogenic) activity.[12] It is promoted as a nonestrogenic food supplement. Of

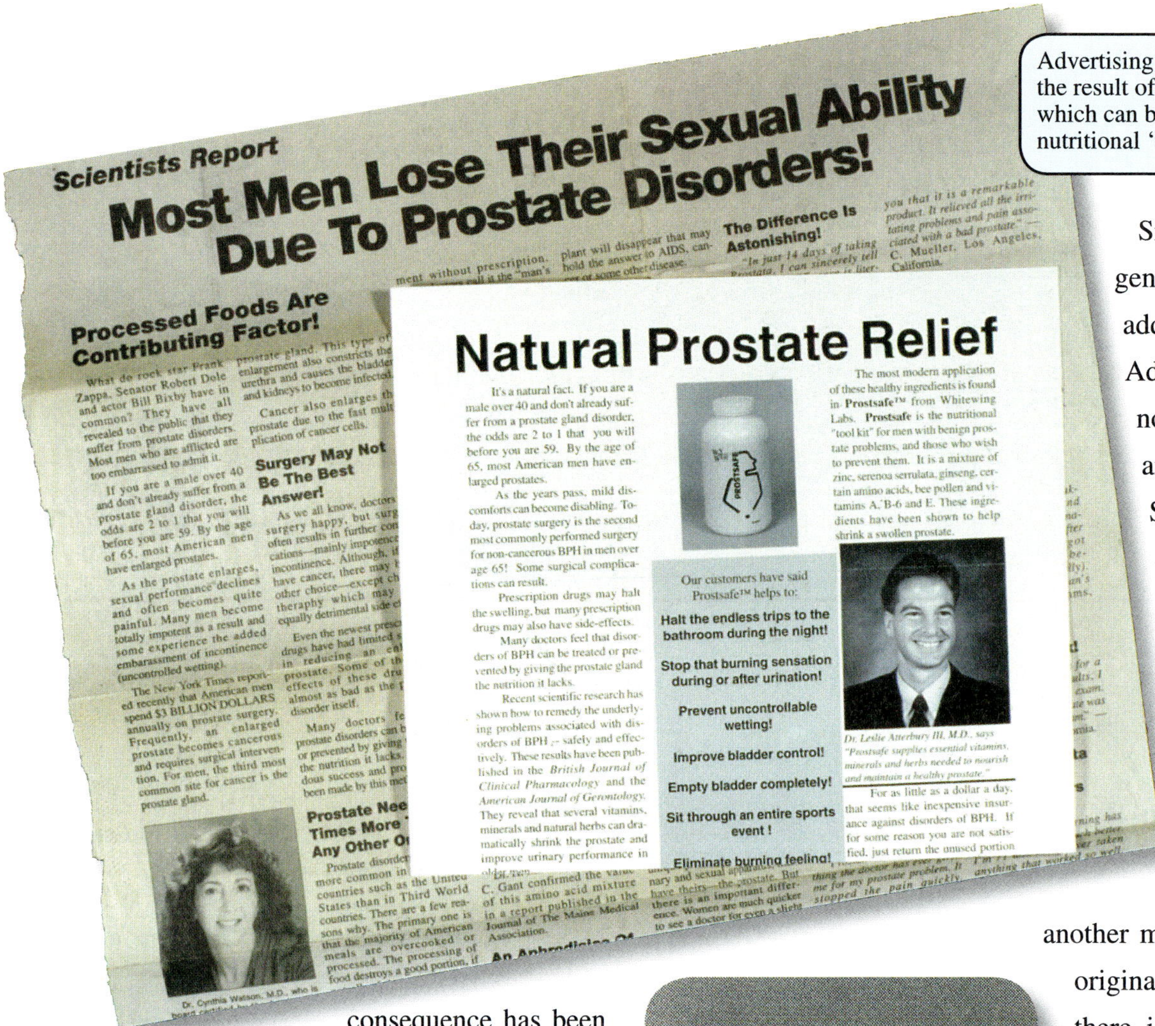

Scientists Report

# Most Men Lose Their Sexual Ability Due To Prostate Disorders!

## Processed Foods Are Contributing Factor!

What do rock star Frank Zappa, Senator Robert Dole and actor Bill Bixby have in common? They have all revealed to the public that they suffer from prostate disorders. Most men who are afflicted are too embarrassed to admit it.

If you are a male over 40 and don't already suffer from a prostate gland disorder, the odds are 2 to 1 that you will before you are 59. By the age of 65, most American men have enlarged prostates.

As the prostate enlarges, sexual performance declines and often becomes quite painful. Many men become totally impotent as a result and some experience the added embarassment of incontinence (uncontrolled wetting).

The New York Times reported recently that American men spend $3 BILLION DOLLARS annually on prostate surgery. Frequently, an enlarged prostate becomes cancerous and requires surgical intervention. For men, the third most common site for cancer is the prostate gland.

## Natural Prostate Relief

It's a natural fact. If you are a male over 40 and don't already suffer from a prostate gland disorder, the odds are 2 to 1 that you will before you are 59. By the age of 65, most American men have enlarged prostates.

As the years pass, mild discomforts can become disabling. Today, prostate surgery is the second most commonly performed surgery for non-cancerous BPH in men over age 65! Some surgical complications can result.

Prescription drugs may halt the swelling, but many prescription drugs may also have side-effects.

Many doctors feel that disorders of BPH can be treated or prevented by giving the prostate gland the nutrition it lacks.

Recent scientific research has shown how to remedy the underlying problems associated with disorders of BPH -- safely and effectively. These results have been published in the *British Journal of Clinical Pharmacology* and the *American Journal of Gerontology*. They reveal that several vitamins, minerals and natural herbs can dramatically shrink the prostate and improve urinary performance in older men.

Our customers have said Prostsafe™ helps to:

**Halt the endless trips to the bathroom during the night!**

**Stop that burning sensation during or after urination!**

**Prevent uncontrollable wetting!**

**Improve bladder control!**

**Empty bladder completely!**

**Sit through an entire sports event !**

**Eliminate burning feeling!**

The most modern application of these healthy ingredients is found in **Prostsafe™** from Whitewing Labs. **Prostsafe** is the nutritional "tool kit" for men with benign prostate problems, and those who wish to prevent them. It is a mixture of zinc, serenoa serrulata, ginseng, certain amino acids, bee pollen and vitamins A, B-6 and E. These ingredients have been shown to help shrink a swollen prostate.

*Dr. Leslie Atterbury III, M.D., says "Prostsafe supplies essential vitamins, minerals and herbs needed to nourish and maintain a healthy prostate."*

For as little as a dollar a day, that seems like inexpensive insurance against disorders of BPH. If for some reason you are not satisfied, just return the unused portion

Advertising that: "prostate disease is the result of improperly processed foods which can be treated with a natural nutritional 'tool kit'".

consequence has been the estrogen related side effects, such as venous thrombosis. The treatment may be inappropriate for patients already receiving other hormonal agents, as it may confound follow up for those with prostate cancer by altering prostate specific antigen (PSA) values. There are also the potentially adverse interactions between nonprescription "dietary supplements" and conventional medicines.[13,14]

Since herbal preparations are generally categorized as food additives by the Food and Drug Administration there is little or no oversight of their production and distribution in the United States. The absence of regulatory control is likely to lead to marked differences in purity and content among botanicals.[11,13] Because of the lack of standardization in plant extract synthesizing, the resulting botanical products of one manufacturer cannot be reliably extrapolated to another manufacturer's product even if they originated from the same plant.[14] Also, there is a natural variability among the plants themselves.

Although the efficacy and safety of botanicals can only be determined reliably through placebo controlled studies, clinically relevant information can be gained from comparative and observational trials. Herbal preparations have been tested in randomized trials both with and without a placebo arm.[15,16,17] The findings of meta-analysis regarding the results achieved

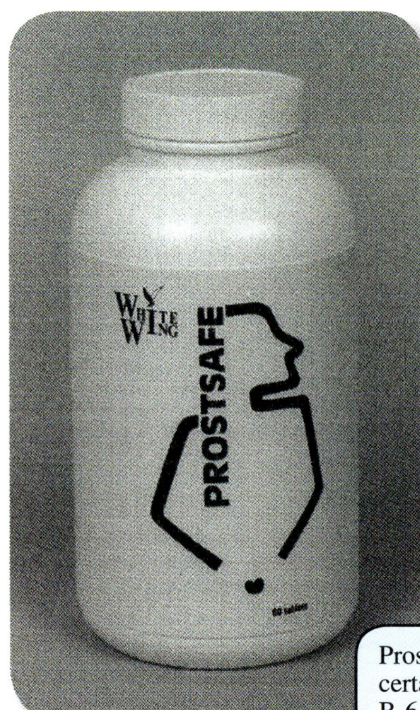


Prostsafe is a mixture of Serenoa serrulata, ginseng, certain amino acids, bee pollen, zinc, vitamins A, B-6 and E.

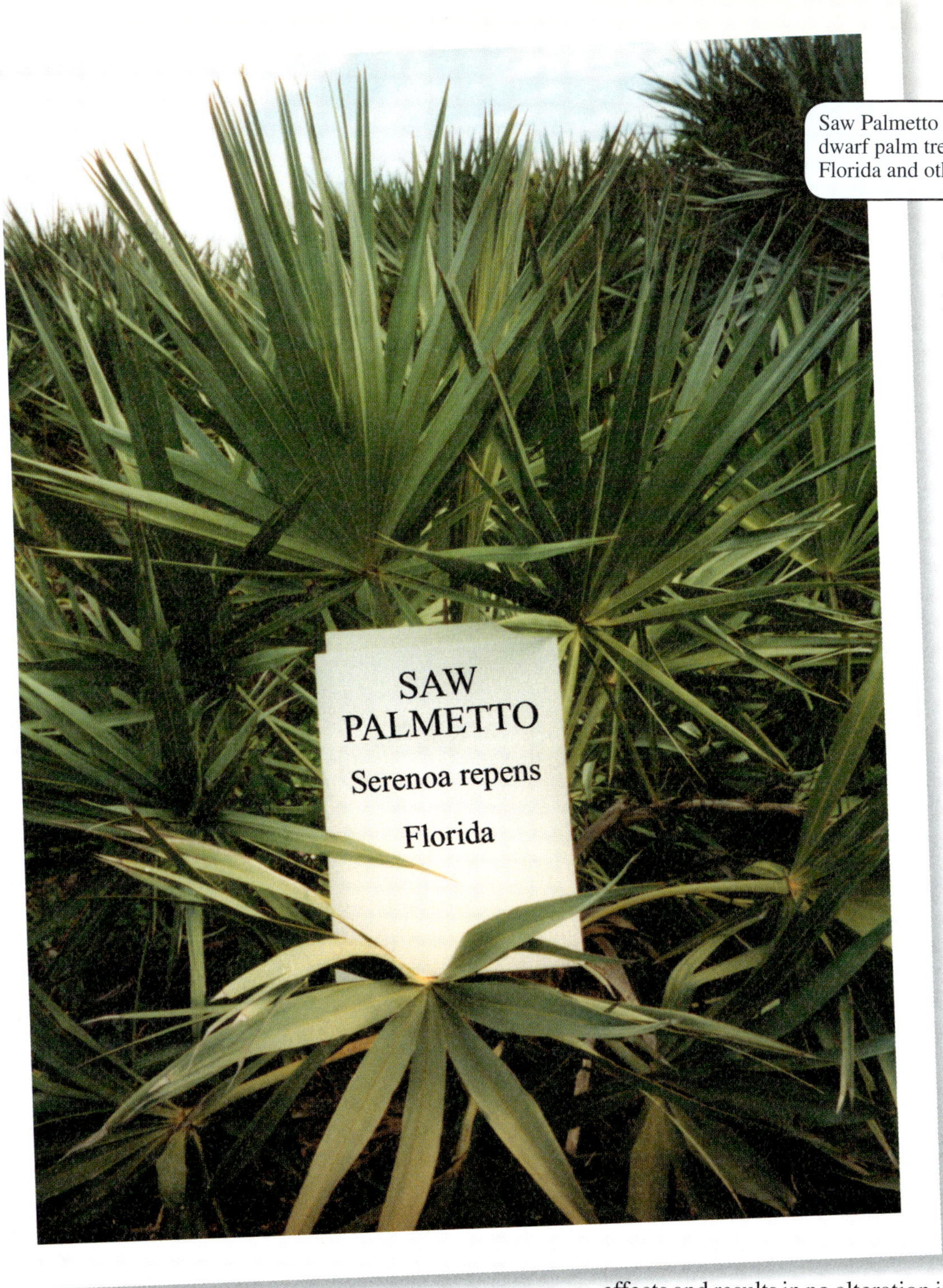


Saw Palmetto extract is derived from the American dwarf palm tree, Serenoa repens, which is found in Florida and other areas of southeastern United States.

suggest the benefits of these agents. However, multiple methodological difficulties make it harder to accept the reliability of these conclusions. Limitations include treatment intervals of only one to three months, small numbers of patients, and failure to use standardized testing, such as symptom scores. Until data from large-scale placebo-controlled studies are presented, questions will continue regarding the efficacy and safety of phytotherapeutic agents in men with lower urinary tract symptoms.[18,19]

Today's patient can choose from a variety of phytotherapeutic agents. Saw palmetto is the most commonly used and most widely studied herbal remedy in the United States and Europe.[19] Saw palmetto extract is derived from the American dwarf palm tree, *Serenoa repens*, which is found in southeastern United States.[18] Saw palmetto has been demonstrated to have no adverse side effects and results in no alteration in serum PSA. Clinical studies suggest mild improvement in symptoms and in flow rates.[18] *Pygeum africanum* extract (Tadenan) comes from the bark of the African plum tree and is used primarily in Europe. Other formulations such as Prostata are available in the United States.[20] The list of additional botanicals includes *Urtica dioica* which is derived as an extract from the roots of the stinging nettle.[3] *Secale cereale* is extracted by microbial digestion of rye pollen and is known as Cernilton.[21] *Hypoxis roopere* extracted from South African star grass is sold as Harzol.[22] These herbal medicinals may be marketed and sold alone or as combination products. Most "prostate health" pills are combinations of plant extracts although there are no data to suggest either increased efficacy or synergy in such products.[6]

Overall, preliminary trials with phytotherapeutic agents for lower urinary tract symptoms suggest a significant benefit. However, these herbal medicinals serve as a case in point. In spite of a variety of botanicals that show promise as safe and effective medications, there is critical need for well-established proof with laboratory testing and clinical trials.

Prostrata is a combination of "proprietary compounds" including an extract mixture of Serenoa, Pygeum africanum, Panax, hydrangeas, zinc, several amino acids, Vitamin B-6 and bee pollen.

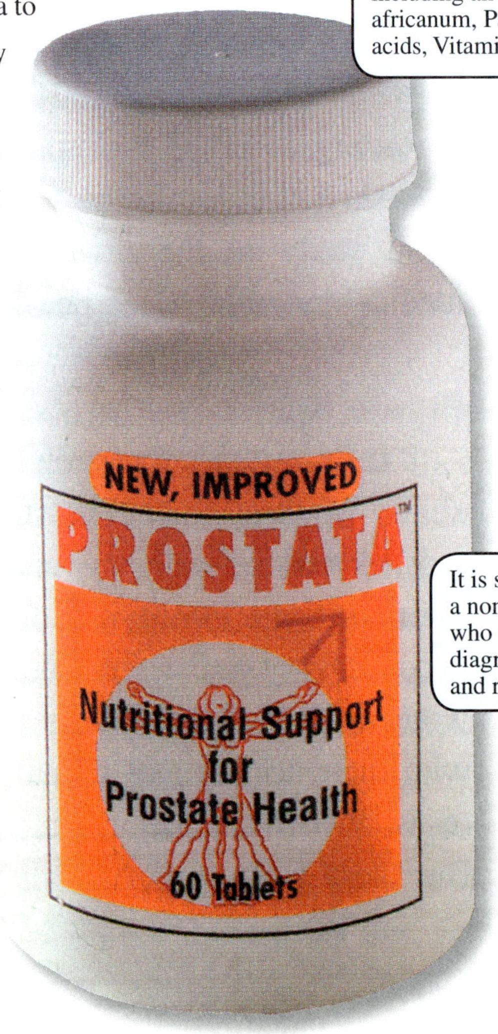


It is significant that the American Botanical Council, a non-profit herbal organization, emphasizes that men who suspect prostate problems should get a proper diagnosis from their doctor before taking saw palmetto and related herbal medicine.

Chapter 21

# Today's FDA: Wounded Giant & Weakened Champion

The Food and Drug Administration touches the lives of virtually every American every day. The FDA regulates over one trillion dollars worth of products, which account for 25 cents of every dollar spent annually by American consumers. It is the FDA's job to see that the food we eat is safe and wholesome, the cosmetics we use won't hurt us, the medicines and medical devices we use are safe and effective, and that radiation-emitting products such as microwave ovens won't do us harm. In addition the FDA ensures that all of these products are labeled truthfully with information that consumers need to use them properly.[1,2]

These emphases on the dual goals of the FDA—ensuring the timely availability of safe and effective new products (pre-market), and ensuring the highest level of safety for marketed products (post-market)—have allowed our nation to continue as the world leader in new product innovation and development, while still giving Americans round–the-clock protection. International leadership in medicine and medical device production with safety assurance has occurred in spite of a seven-fold increase in expenditures in recent years for drug research. Consequently the FDA must address an environment both domestically and internationally that continues to broaden in scope and complexity.[1,5]

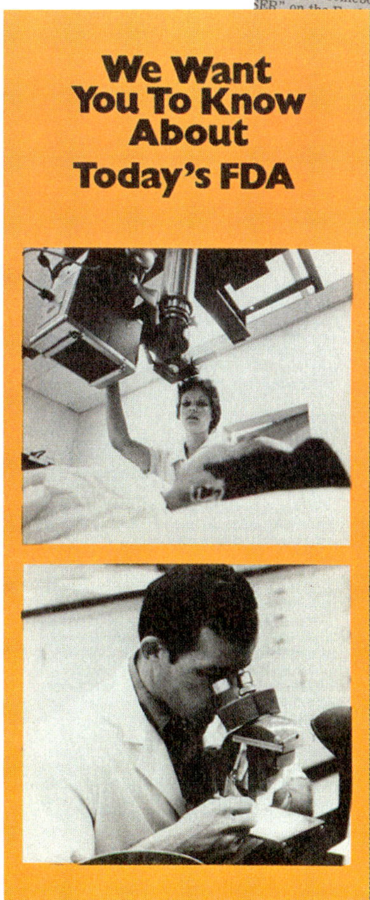


First and foremost, the FDA is a public health agency that enforces the Federal Food, Drug and Cosmetic Act and several related public health laws. To carry out this mandate of consumer protection, the FDA has approximately 9000 employees with 1,100 investigators and inspectors who cover the country's 95,000 FDA-regulated businesses.[1,2,6]

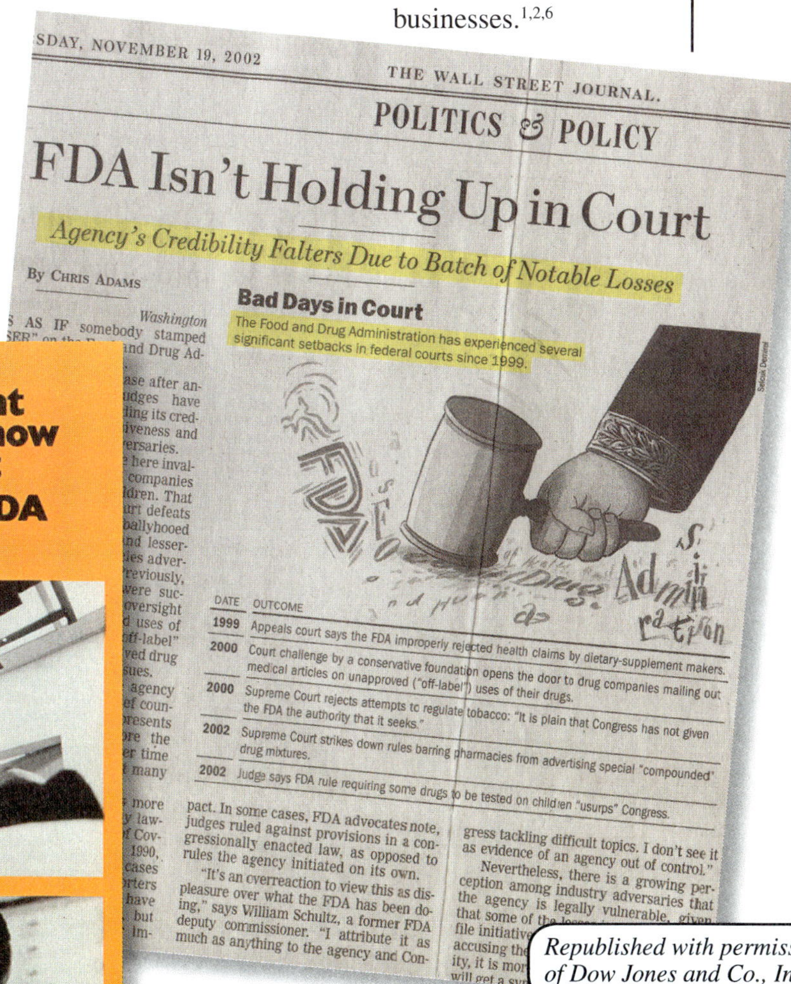
SDAY, NOVEMBER 19, 2002 THE WALL STREET JOURNAL.

POLITICS & POLICY

FDA Isn't Holding Up in Court

*Agency's Credibility Falters Due to Batch of Notable Losses*

By Chris Adams

*Washington*

AS IF somebody stamped ...

**Bad Days in Court**

The Food and Drug Administration has experienced several significant setbacks in federal courts since 1999.

| DATE | OUTCOME |
| --- | --- |
| 1999 | Appeals court says the FDA improperly rejected health claims by dietary-supplement makers. |
| 2000 | Court challenge by a conservative foundation opens the door to drug companies mailing out medical articles on unapproved ("off-label") uses of their drugs. |
| 2000 | Supreme Court rejects attempts to regulate tobacco: "It is plain that Congress has not given the FDA the authority that it seeks." |
| 2002 | Supreme Court strikes down rules barring pharmacies from advertising special "compounded" drug mixtures. |
| 2002 | Judge says FDA rule requiring some drugs to be tested on children "usurps" Congress. |

pact. In some cases, FDA advocates note, judges ruled against provisions in a congressionally enacted law, as opposed to rules the agency initiated on its own.

"It's an overreaction to view this as displeasure over what the FDA has been doing," says William Schultz, a former FDA deputy commissioner. "I attribute it as much as anything to the agency and Congress tackling difficult topics. I don't see it as evidence of an agency out of control."

Nevertheless, there is a growing perception among industry adversaries that the agency is legally vulnerable, given that some of the ...

*Republished with permission of Dow Jones and Co., Inc.(7)*

However, there is a critical gap between the agency's current capacity, and the goals of statutory requirements and public expectations. Unsafe, ineffective, and fraudulent medicinal products present a real danger to public health. The FDA's ability to physically verify the safety of

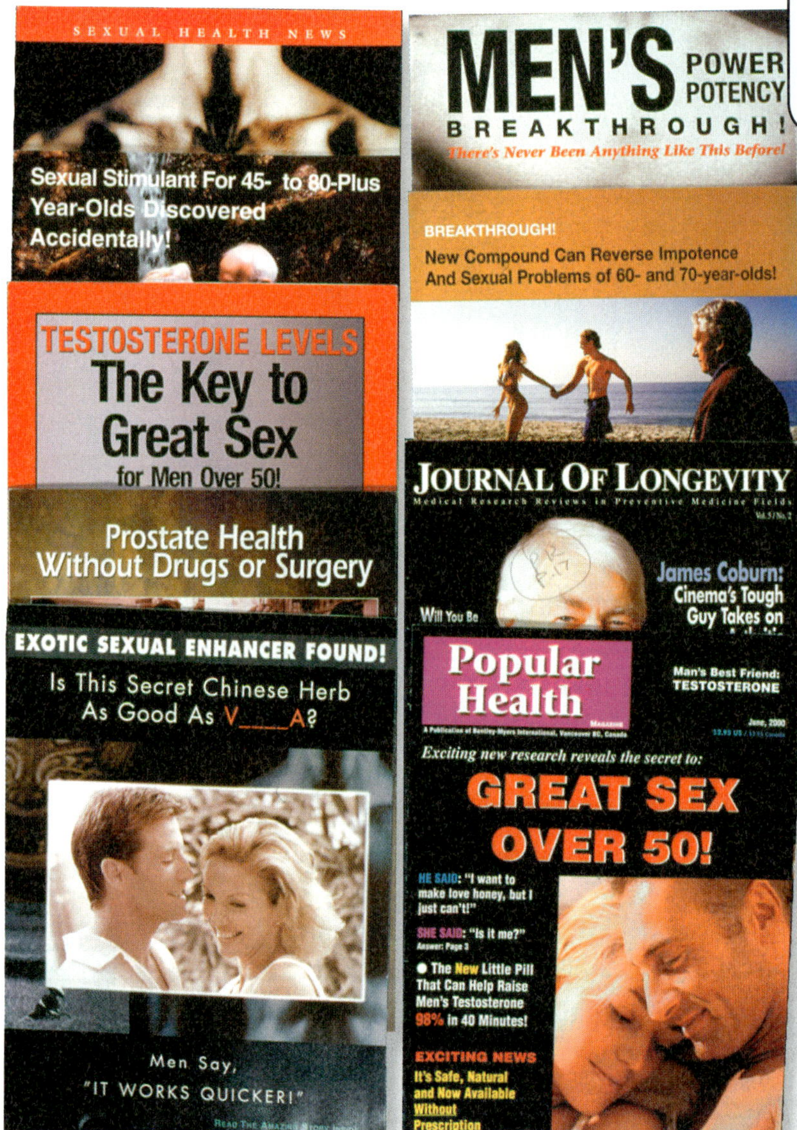


**Mailed Advertising**
Similar to the almanacs of yesteryear, today's sexual brochures extol the virtues of their products with exaggerated claims of success. Also, included are many testimonials of satisfied men and women customers.

domestic and imported products has eroded considerably in all product areas, even as consumer expectations continue to rise. This level of effort is also falling significantly short of the minimum inspection obligations required by the FDA Modernization Act of 1997. Import entries alone increased 14 percent in 1999, and over all, less that one percent of import entries are physically examined. Even in conjunction with its state regulatory partners, the FDA is able to inspect annually less than a third of domestic firms within its purview. The number of FDA inspections for food, drugs, and devices, foreign and domestic, including inspections by State agencies under contract to the FDA has decreased from 28,000 to 22,000 between 1991 and 1999. This decrease of 6,000 inspections, or 21 percent, reflects the impact of the time required to perform the complex science based inspections now necessary to assess safety, and the almost static numbers of investigational personnel.[1,2]

The herbal medicinal and dietary supplement industry is one of the fastest growing industries in the world. Sales have nearly doubled in the past five years and one study estimates that sales will increase by over 90 percent during the next six years. Surveys show that over half of the American population now uses some form of herbal supplement. The Dietary Supplement Health and Education Act of 1994 is the law that spurred the so-called "herbal renaissance." It is important to remember that all herbal medicinals are now outside the aegis of the FDA and not subject to a pre-market safety review by the FDA. Congress basically decided in 1994 that supplements, most of which had been sold as folk remedies or food additives

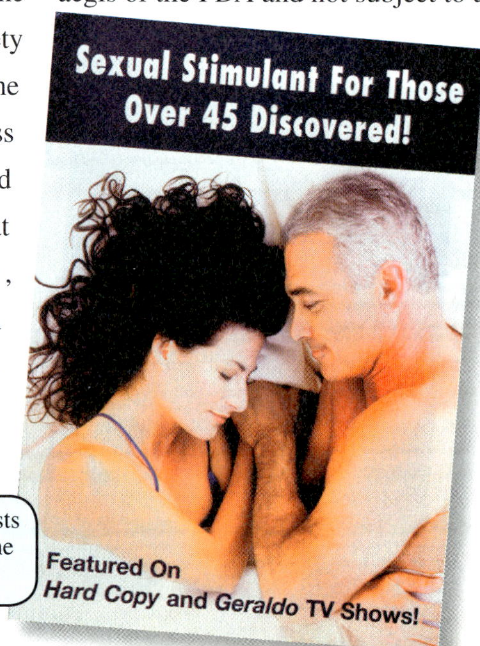


An unregulated industry for nostrums exists today, as it did in the 19th century, with the emphasis on packaging and marketing.

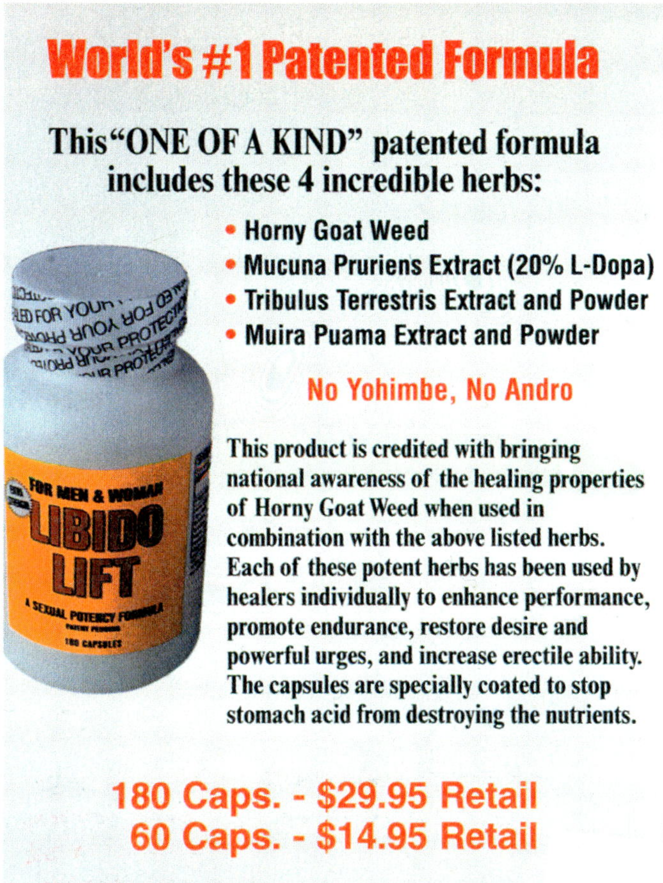


before the law took effect, had been proven safe by years of use. Moreover, herbal medicinal manufacturers are not required to report adverse events associated with the use of their products. Recent experience with serious adverse events—including death associated with the use of such products as ephedra, digitalis, contaminated plantain, and others—underscores the severity of the situation. The FDA's ability to monitor the safety of the industry is truly dependent on the Adverse Event Reporting System. Unfortunately, the system is outdated and does not permit the FDA to adequately monitor and evaluate such events. Because of the large number of new products entering the marketplace and the growing number of Americans using these products, the risk of adverse events is growing exponentially. Also the Internet, while promising enormous benefits to business and consumers, is being used by unscrupulous individuals to unlawfully promote and sell unapproved prescription drugs. State and Federal laws require that certain drugs be dispensed only with a valid prescription.[1,2]

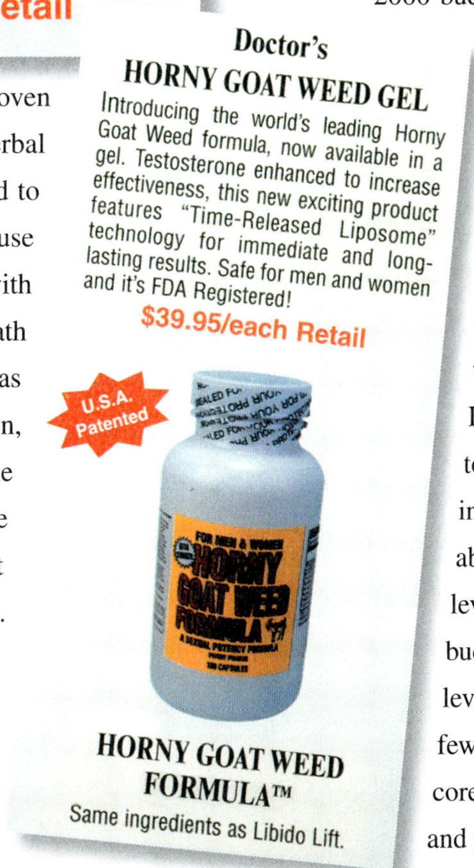


In addition the FDA has incurred a significant decrease in financial funding. On October 28, 1999, Congress passed a government-wide rescission as part of the Omnibus Consolidated Appropriations Act. The department-wide reduction for the year 2000 budget totaled $165.8 million. For the past seven years, the FDA, along with much of the Federal government, has absorbed the annual inflationary increases for pay and non-pay. At first, the impact of absorption was negligible, as the FDA was able to offer efficiencies. However, as new opportunities to streamline disappeared, inflationary increases were absorbed by reducing staffing levels each year. The year 2001 budget reflected a reduced staffing level of 160, which translated into fewer people to perform the FDA's core activities of pre-market review and post-market assurance.[1,2]

You may inquire, "What about

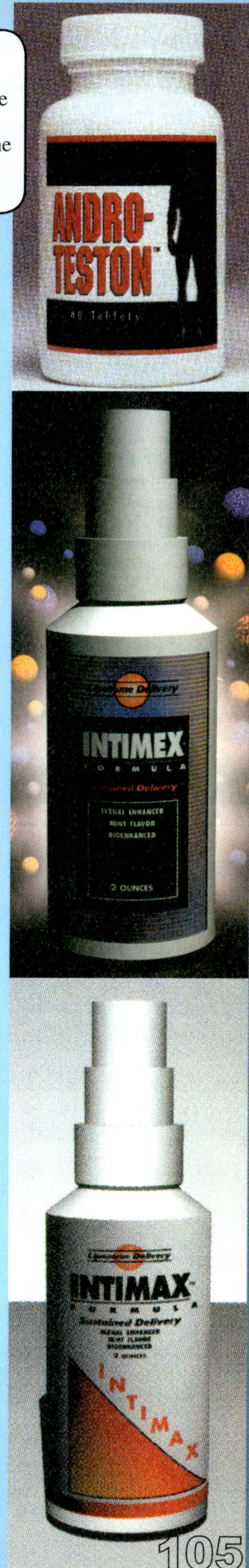


These products contain several herbal preparations that reportedly stimulate testosterone production. Two anabolic steroids are present in addition. Of significance is the absence in their literature of any warning concerning the ill effects to those men that are harboring an unknown prostate cancer. The prevalence of prostate cancer in this age group makes such a qualifying statement necessary.

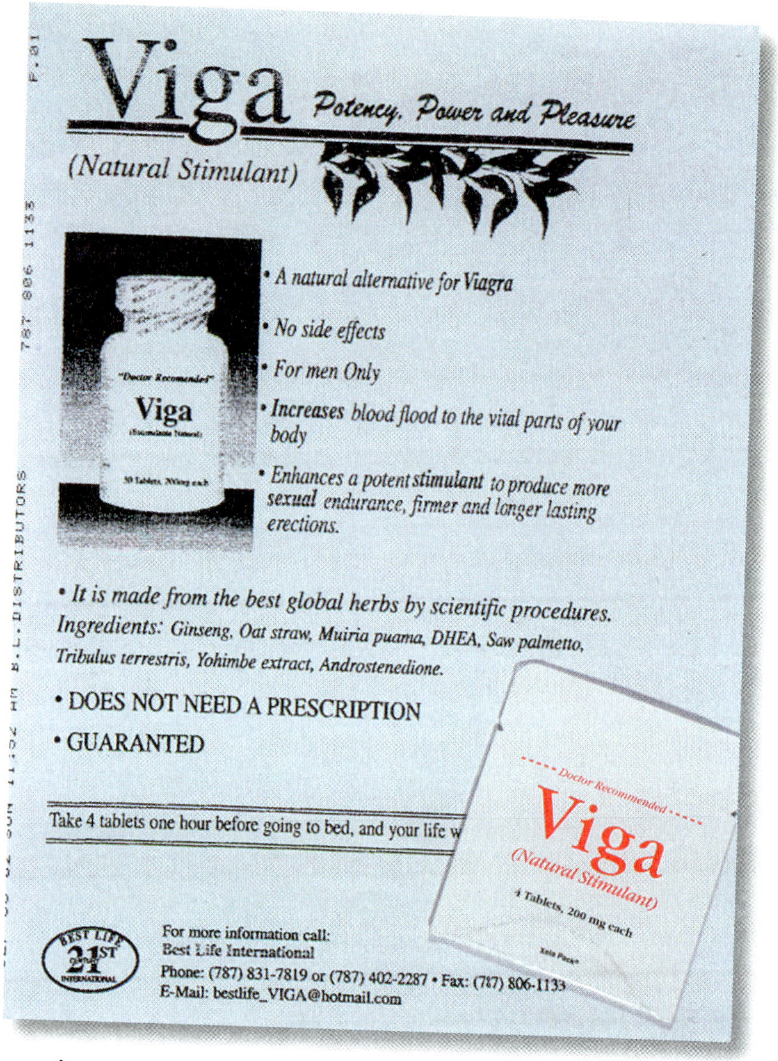


the Federal Trade Commission?" The FDA and the FTC work together under a long-standing agreement governing the division of responsibilities between the two agencies. As applied to herbal medicinals, the FDA has responsibility for claims on product labeling while the FTC has primary responsibility for claims in advertising. Specific terms for a product label or ad may be used as long as they do not suggest disease prevention or treatment such as "stimulate," "maintain," "support," "regulate," or "promote." But, some terms are not to be used at all such as "diagnose," "treat," "prevent," "cure," or "mitigate." The FTC's truth-in-advertising law can be boiled down to two propositions: (1) advertising must be truthful and not misleading; and (2) before disseminating an ad, advertisers must have adequate substantiation for all objective product claims. The test of any medical treatment is whether it can be shown to be safe, effective, and appropriate. That is as true for brain surgery as it is for alternative medicine. Adequate substantiation is critical to ensuring that consumers receive truthful and accurate information. However, the FDA and the FTC differ as to what constitutes adequate substantiation. Basically, the FDA abides by a strict code and protocol for conducting relevant research. There are phase I, II, III studies that include lengthy placebo controlled double-blinded clinical trials. The FTC has no fixed formula for the number or type of studies required or more specific parameters like sample size and study duration. It is possible under FTC law to have a health claim in advertising that has not been authorized for labeling by the FDA. Thus, departmental differences continue to create a tension as to procedural methods that standardize what is appropriate and substantiated.[1,3,4,6]

Consequently the FDA will be unable to address the 21st century consumer protection challenges by working independently. To perform its regulatory role effectively, the FDA will have to join forces with other health regulatory partners. At times it will have to work with the U.S. Customs Services, the Drug Enforcement Administration, the Postal Service, and the Federal Trade Commission. Increasing coordination with other health partners should result in a new and challenging expansion of the FDA's traditional inspection role.[2]

Chapter 22

# Conclusion: "Quackery and Idolatry are All But Immortal"

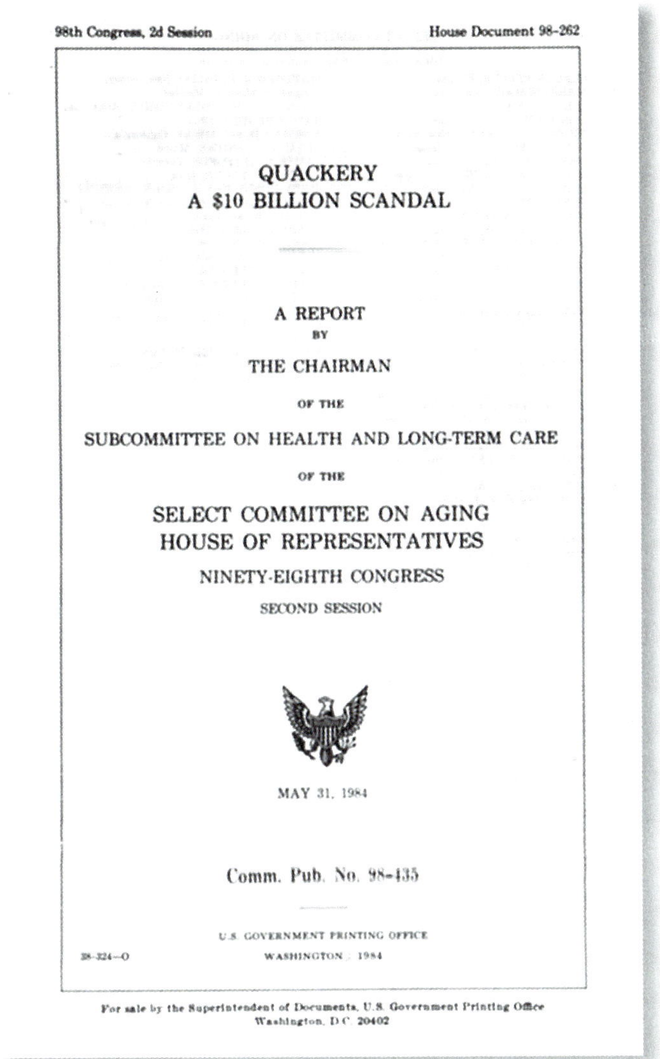

98th Congress, 2d Session — House Document 98-262

QUACKERY
A $10 BILLION SCANDAL

A REPORT
BY
THE CHAIRMAN
OF THE
SUBCOMMITTEE ON HEALTH AND LONG-TERM CARE
OF THE
SELECT COMMITTEE ON AGING
HOUSE OF REPRESENTATIVES
NINETY-EIGHTH CONGRESS
SECOND SESSION

MAY 31, 1984

Comm. Pub. No. 98-435

38-324-O

U.S. GOVERNMENT PRINTING OFFICE
WASHINGTON : 1984

For sale by the Superintendent of Documents, U.S. Government Printing Office
Washington, D.C. 20402

The 98th Congress House Select Committee on Aging reported in depth on health fraud and quackery. A $10 billion per year scandal is described in detail.

Quackery has traveled far from the days of the pitchman and the covered wagon. With the advance of medicine and the development of scientific procedures, the distinction between quackery and medicine becomes apparent. Although the practice of quackery has changed, it has not diminished, but grown in size and sophistication. Quackery may now affect nearly every aspect of our lives. The easy-to-recognize and somewhat comic figure of the pitchman of the past has been supplanted by sophisticated and shrewd hucksters with a keen sense of the vulnerability of potential customers, the limitations of the law, and the profitability of exploiting both. Those who orchestrate and profit from the sale and promotion of these "health" products are precise, polished and persistent.[2,9]

Quackery is a complex and evolving problem. The reliance on unproven health methods is as old as man, spawned in pain and desperation. When symptoms are intense and prolonged, the temptation "to try anything" is almost irresistible. As stated by Oliver Wendell Holmes, "the persons who seek the aid of health professionals are very honest and sincere in their wish to get rid of their complaints . . . there is nothing people will not do, there is nothing they have not done, to recover their health and save their lives."[7,8]

The definition of quackery is inclusive. There is usually the common denominator of conscious deliberate deceit. However, quackery often attracts adherents with near religious zeal who place unquestioning faith in the health nostrum and serve to further the cause unwittingly. As Benjamin Franklin said, "quacks are the greatest liars in the world except their patients." Also, there is a disregard for scientific testing and proof. Quackery reflects pseudo-science at best. In the words of Oliver Wendell Holmes, "probably in many nostrums and in some pseudo-medical treatments of disease or disturbances there is a grain or two of truth, which, however, has been so magnified and lauded for financial gain that nothing but quackery, deceit or insanity is left."[5,6,7,8]

> "Credulity is bred less by a lack of brains than by a dearth of knowledge. We are all credulous when we wander in fields that are strange to us. Knowledge, rather than intelligence, is the best antidote for credulity. The quack, who knows how to word his appeal, can gull the intelligentsia as easily as he can fool the illiterate. Talleyrand boiled down the philosophy of the quack in the statement: 'To succeed in this world, it is much more necessary to possess the penetration to discover who is the ignoramus, than to discover who is the wise man.'"
> *Nostrums and Quackery and Psuedo-Medicine. Vol.III, Introduction p.7, 1936.*

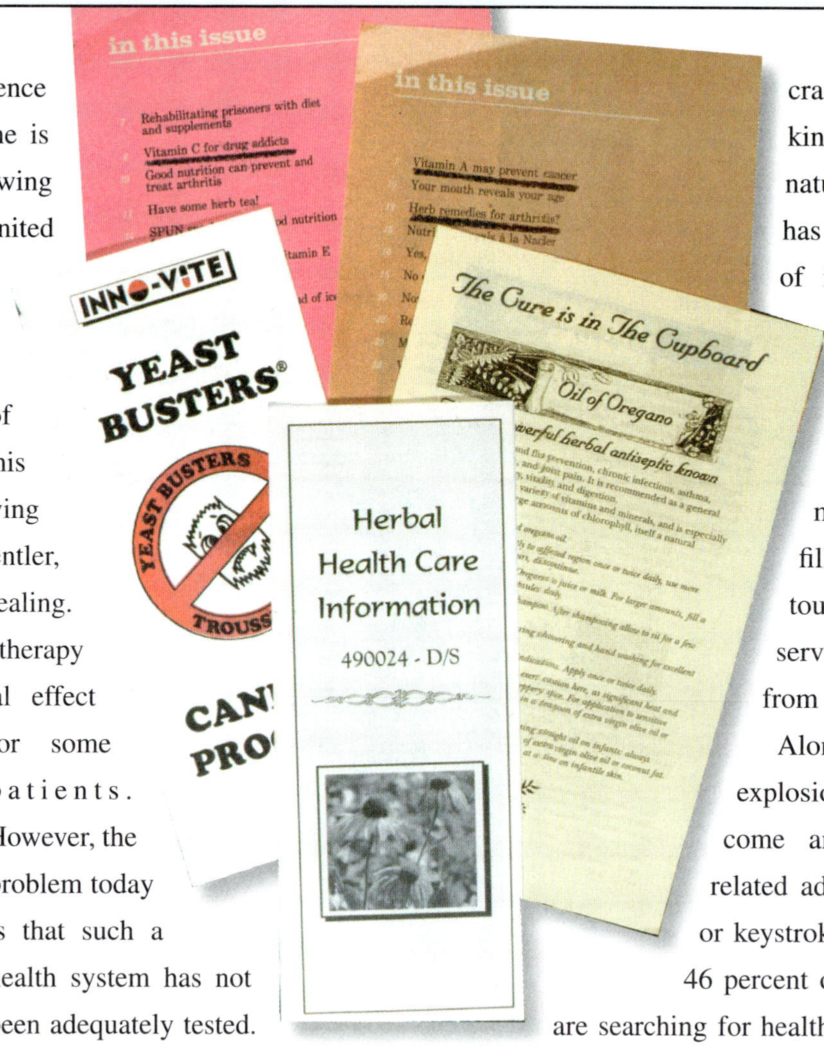


It is of consequence that alternative medicine is one of the fastest growing industries in the United States today. An estimated 50 percent of all Americans has turned to some type of alternative therapy. This shift may reflect a growing public yearning for gentler, less invasive forms of healing. And it is true that such therapy may have a beneficial effect for some patients. However, the problem today is that such a health system has not been adequately tested. Unfortunately the result has been two separate health delivery systems—one system that has been scientifically tested and one that has not—conventional and alternative treatment forms. Alternative medicine is further divided into different therapeutic practices such as visceral manipulation, yoga, craniosacral therapy, applied kinesiology, acupuncture, naturopathy, none of which has had scientific proof of its validity. As a result unconventional potions and practices afford rich opportunities for quackery. Health-food magazines and web sites are filled with advertisements touting miracle cures that serve only to separate the sick from their money.[1,2]

Along with the information explosion on the Internet has come an abundance of health-related advice that lies but a click or keystroke away. By one estimate, 46 percent of those who surf the net are searching for health enlightenment. Much of this information can improve public knowledge, but unfortunately, much of it is fraudulent. In June, 1999, the FTC issued a Consumer Alert warning that, "some unscrupulous marketers are using cyberspace to peddle 'miracle' treatments and cures to vulnerable consumers." Any number of unauthorized prescription medications are available. Recently shut down was a web-site which freely dispensed Viagra. The FTC and the FDA also issued warnings about unapproved HIV home test kits sold on the

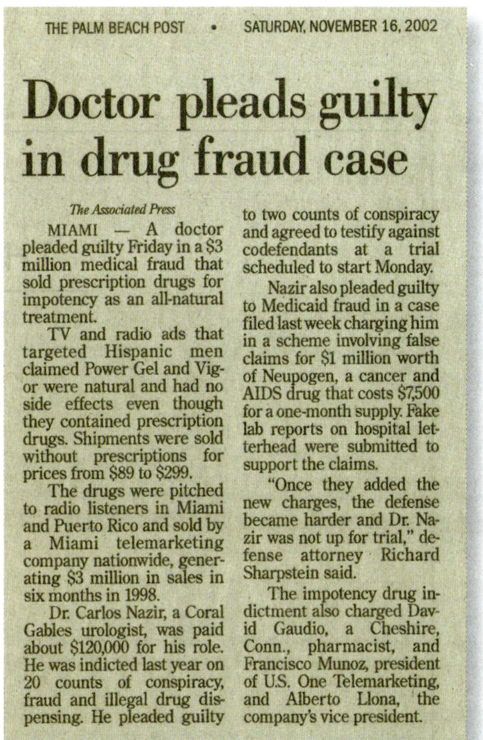

THE PALM BEACH POST • SATURDAY, NOVEMBER 16, 2002

## Doctor pleads guilty in drug fraud case

*The Associated Press*

MIAMI — A doctor pleaded guilty Friday in a $3 million medical fraud that sold prescription drugs for impotency as an all-natural treatment.

TV and radio ads that targeted Hispanic men claimed Power Gel and Vig-or were natural and had no side effects even though they contained prescription drugs. Shipments were sold without prescriptions for prices from $89 to $299.

The drugs were pitched to radio listeners in Miami and Puerto Rico and sold by a Miami telemarketing company nationwide, generating $3 million in sales in six months in 1998.

Dr. Carlos Nazir, a Coral Gables urologist, was paid about $120,000 for his role. He was indicted last year on 20 counts of conspiracy, fraud and illegal drug dispensing. He pleaded guilty to two counts of conspiracy and agreed to testify against codefendants at a trial scheduled to start Monday.

Nazir also pleaded guilty to Medicaid fraud in a case filed last week charging him in a scheme involving false claims for $1 million worth of Neupogen, a cancer and AIDS drug that costs $7,500 for a one-month supply. Fake lab reports on hospital letterhead were submitted to support the claims.

"Once they added the new charges, the defense became harder and Dr. Nazir was not up for trial," defense attorney Richard Sharpstein said.

The impotency drug indictment also charged David Gaudio, a Cheshire, Conn., pharmacist, and Francisco Munoz, president of U.S. One Telemarketing, and Alberto Llona, the company's vice president.

Quackery is alive and well today.

*Reprinted with permission of The Associated Press.*

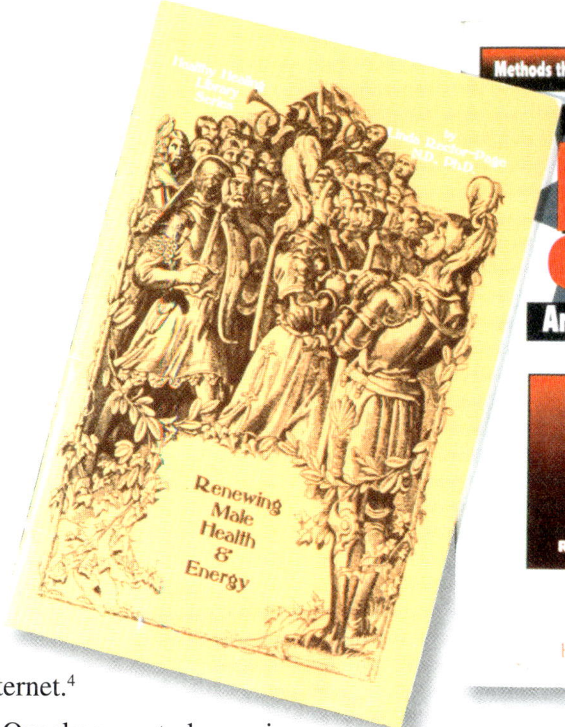


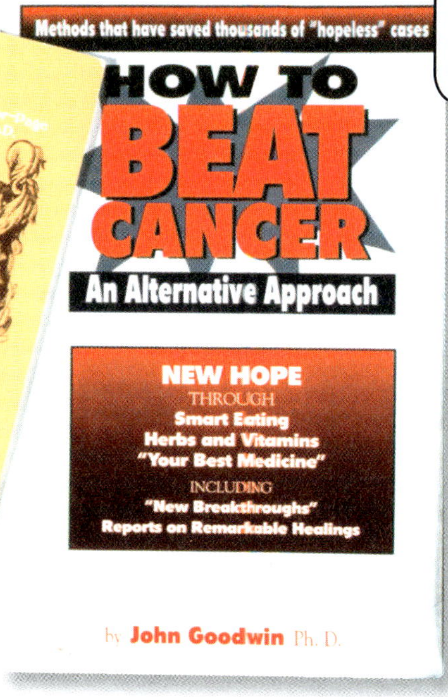


Today there are many books that describe curative methods for treating serious disease. It may be a nostrum or an herbal combination with a diet. Assurances of cure are given for cancer, arthritis, reversal of the aging process and more.

Internet.[4]

Quackery today is big business. Purveyors of quackery provide a panacea for virtually all human ailments. The modern quack's prime target is the senior citizen with his chronic or incurable diseases. Eighty percent of seniors have at least one chronic health condition. The purveyor's approach is the illustrated brochure, the supermarket press, television commercials, "testimonial" ads, and phony foundations providing "scientific" information, and storefront clinics. Voltaire said, "quackery began when the first knave met the first quack." Since quackery is big business, there must be many of both types. It is estimated that medical quacks rob senior citizens and other unsuspecting Americans of more than $20 billion per year. The cost in human terms, measured in disillusionment, pain, and relief forsaken or postponed because of reliance on unproven methods, is more difficult to measure, but nonetheless real. At times the purchaser paid with his life.[2,6]

In the year 2001 purveyors were selling "colloidal silver," a centuries old substance that federal regulators called a total scam. This nostrum allegedly could cure acne, herpes, cancer, leprosy, and the bubonic plague—"more than 650 different disease causing viruses." Ads boasted that it gave the body a "superior second immune system" and Viagra-like power to spice up one's sex life. Ingesting silver, including colloidal

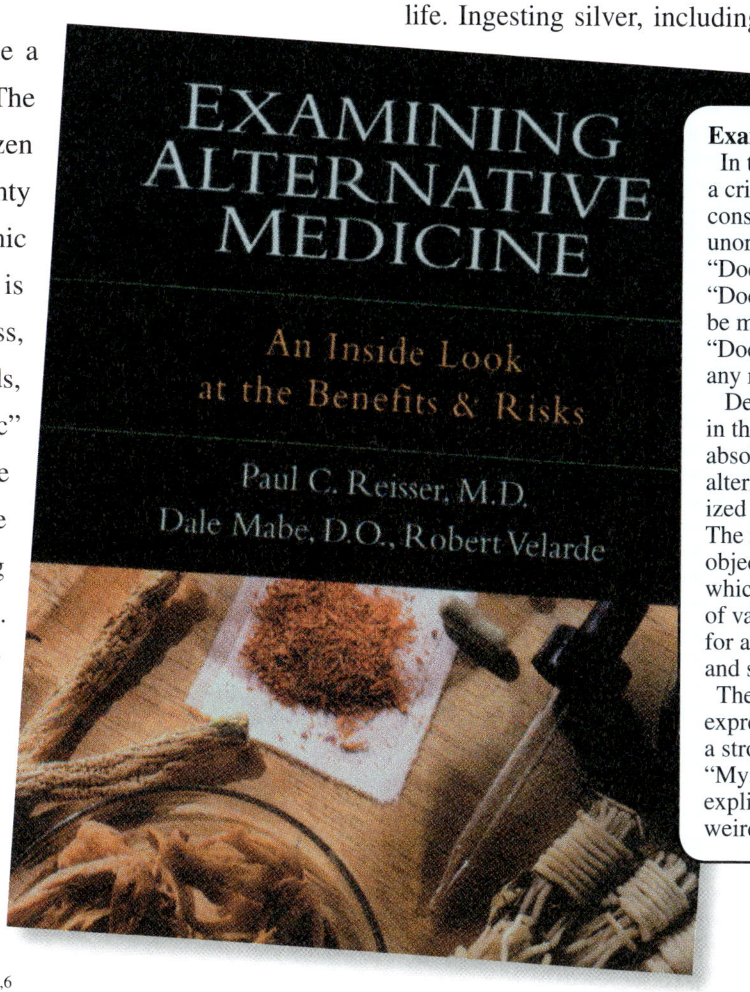


**Examining Alternative Medicine**
In this book the authors ask why a critical thinking people lay such consideration aside when dealing with unorthodox healing methods. Questions, "Does it work?" and more specifically, "Does it make me feel better?" seem to be more important considerations then, "Does it make any sense?" or "Is there any reasonable proof?"

Described are the traditionalists who in theory still hold to the concept of absolute truth while a great majority of alternative practitioners are characterized by the rejection of such a concept. The removal of the idea of discernible objective truth in the physical world, which also downgrades the importance of valid studies and relevant data, allows for an easy entry into spiritual relativism and syncretion.

The authors conclude that most expressions of alternative medicine have a strong "religious" streak to them. "Mysticism, New Age thinking and explicit expressions of Far Eastern weirdness permeate the practice."

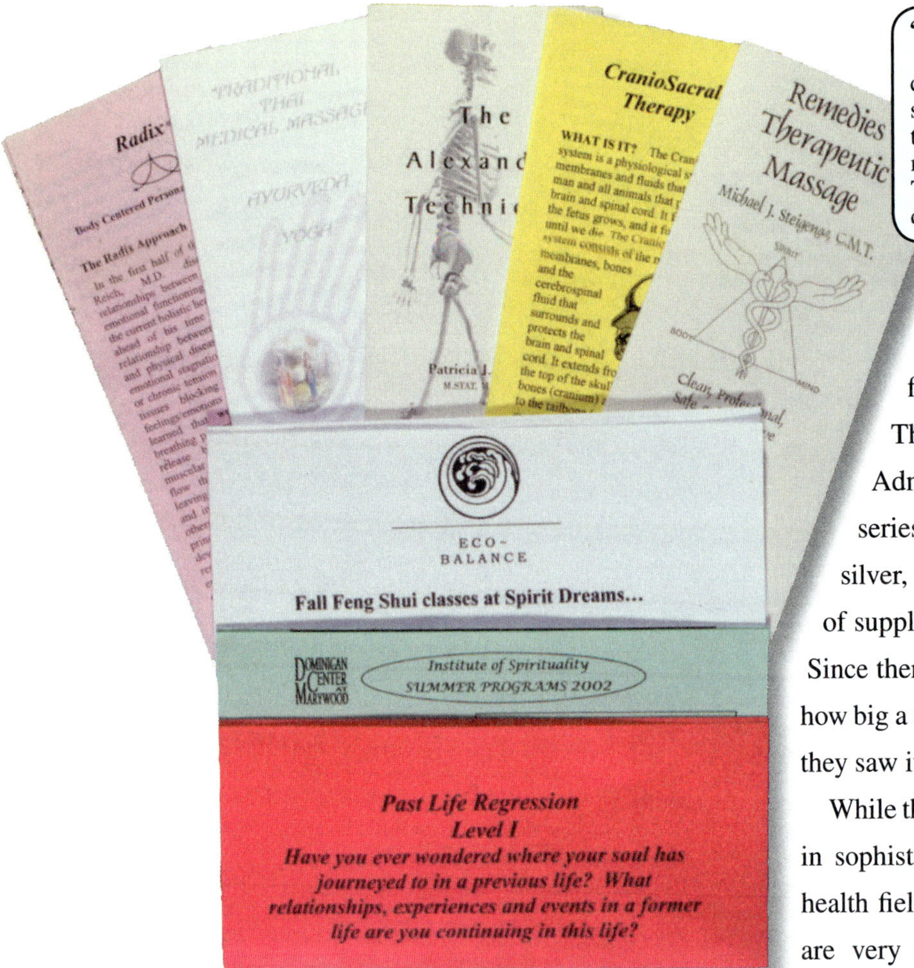


**"Leap of Logic"**

Available today are alternative practices and spiritual healing methods characterized by Mysticism and Far Eastern thought that require a significant "leap of logic". Included are such practices as cranio sacral therapy, sacred touch, Anusara Yoga, Ayurveda Yoga, Thai medical massage, therapeutic massage, the Radix process, Feng Shui, Alexander Technique, Past Life Regression, Interior Alignment, sacred space cleansing, Pranic Crystal Healing, Somato Emotional Release.

silver, does have one documented effect. It can permanently change the color of skin. Tiny bits of silver build up and dye the flesh a shade of blue-gray that darkens with exposure to sunlight. This irreversible condition is called argyria. The Food and Drug Administration and the Federal Trade Commission announced a series of enforcement actions against the Internet retailers of colloidal silver, which the agencies said were engaging in "fraudulent marketing of supplements and other health products." The operators refused to stop. Since there was no easy way to track sales of colloidal silver, no one knew how big a scam it was. All that regulators could do was try to stop it wherever they saw it—and they saw a lot of it online.[3]

While the impact of quackery on our lives has been increasing and growing in sophistication, the misinformed public believes that advertisers in the health field are so rigorously policed and regulated that serious distortions are very unlikely. Unfortunately, policing and regulating efforts have diminished, been redirected or disbanded. The Food and Drug Administration, once a formidable force for controlling quackery, now directs a very limited percentage of its budget to the control of quackery. The Federal Trade Commission's efforts to control misleading advertising are even less significant.[6] Unfortunately the purveyors of quackery live on to build and prosper beneath their mask of respectability despite disillusionment, despair, misery, and death.

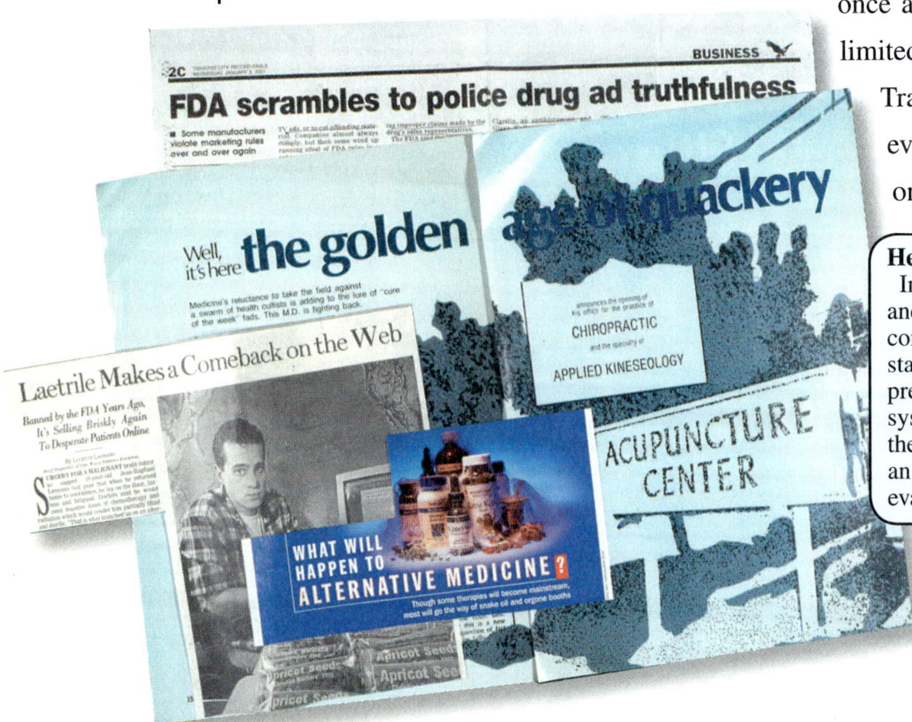


**Headlines**

In conclusion, the regulation of quackery and health fraud would be much better controlled without the current double standard of care. As a consequence, the presence of two separate health delivery systems affords abundant opportunity for the existence of quackery. Unfortunately an aversion to scientific testing and proper evaluating continues.

We would all do well to remember a saying of the Buddha: "Believe nothing, no matter where you read it, or who said it, no matter if I have said it, unless it agrees with your own reason and your own common sense."

# References


**Chapter 1 Patent Medicine - What Is It?**

1. Aikman, Lonnelle. *Nature's Healing Arts, From Folk Medicine to Modern Drugs.* Washington, D.C., The National Geographic Society, 1977.
2. Bingham, A. Walker. *The Snake Oil Syndrome.* Hanover, Mass., The Christopher Publishing House, 1994.
3. Ketchum, Jr., William C. *A Treasury of American Bottles.* Indianapolis/New York, The Bobbs-Merrill Company, Inc., 1975.

**Chapter 2 Nostrum Container – the Glass Bottle**

1. Agee, Bill. *Collecting All Cures.* Waco, Texas, Texian Press, 1973.
2. Harden, Donald B. *Glass of the Caesars.* Milan, Italy, Olivetti, 1987.
3. Kendrick, Grace. *The Mouth-Blown Bottle.* Ann Arbor, Michigan, Edwards Brothers, Inc., 1968.
4. Ketchum, Jr., William C. *A Treasury of American Bottles.* Indianapolis/New York, The Bobbs-Merrill Company, Inc., 1975.
5. McKearin, George S. and Helen. *American Glass.* New York, Crown Publishers, 1941.
6. McKearin, Helen and George. *Two Hundred Years of American Blown Glass* New York, Bonanza Books, 1949-1950.
7. Sauzay, A. *Wonders of Glass and Bottle Making.* Fort Davis, Texas, Frontier Book Co., 1969.
8. Spillman, Jane Shadel. *Glassmaking America's First Industry.* Corning, New York, 1976.

**Chapter 3 From Medicine Men to Men of Medicine**

1. Bingham, A. Walker. *The Snake Oil Syndrome.* Hanover, Mass., The Christopher Publishing House, 1994.
2. Carson, Gerald. *One For a Man, Two For a Horse.* New York, Bramhall House, 1961.
3. Chernow, Ron. *Titan: The Life of John D. Rockefeller, Sr.* New York: Random House, 1998.
4. Hechtlinger, Adelaide. *The Great Patent Medicine Era.* New York, Grosset and Dunlop, Inc., 1970.
5. Holbrook, Stewart H. *The Golden Age of Quackery.* New York: The Macmillan Company, 1959.
6. Karolevitz, Robert F. *Doctors of the Old West.* New York: Bonanza Books, 1967.
7. Odell, John. *Indian Battles and Brands.* John Odell, 1997, Intro.
8. Munsey, Cecil. *He Was a Patent Medicine Vender, A Bigamist and Father of the World's Richest Man.* Bottles and Extras. 11: 3–8, 2000.
9. Young, James Harvey. *The Toadstool Millionaires.* Princeton, New Jersey, Princeton University Press, 1961.
10. Young, James Harvey. *The Medical Messiahs.* Princeton, New Jersey, Princeton University Press, 1967.

**Chapter 4 Rise and Fall**

1. Janssen, Wallace F. *The U.S. Food and Drug Law: How It Came—How It Works.* U.S. Dept. of Health and Human Services Publication No. 79-1054.
2. Auburn, Steve. *A Brown Bitter Flood.* Santa Rosa, Calif., The Federation Letter, 8: 4-12, 1978.
3. Young, James Harvey. *The Toadstool Millionaires.* Princeton, New Jersey, Princeton University Press, 1961, Chapter 13.
4. Natenberg, Maurice. *The Legacy of Dr. Wiley*. Chicago: Regent House, 1957, pp. 47-57.
5. Federal Food and Drugs Act 34, Stat. 768.
6. American Medical Association. *Nostrums and Quackery*. Chicago: American Medical Association Press, 1912.

**Chapter 5 Bitters**

1. Ketchum, Jr., William C. *A Treasury of American Bottles.* Indianapolis/New York, The Bobbs-Merrill Company, Inc., 1975.
2. Munsey, Cecil. *The Illustrated Guide to Collecting Bottles.* New York, Hawthorn Books, Inc., 1970.
3. Ring, Carlyn, Ham, W.C. *Bitters Bottles.* Downieville, CA, 1998
4. Watson, Richard. *Bitters Bottles.* New York, Thomas Nelson and Sons, 1965.
5. Watson, Richard. *Supplement to Bitters Bottles.* Camden, New Jersey, Thomas Nelson and Sons, 1971.
6. Wichmann, Jeff. *Antique Western Bitters Bottles.* Sacramento, CA, 1999.
7. Wilson, Bill and Betty. *Western Bitters.* Santa Rosa, CA, Northwestern Printing Co., 1969.
8. Wilson, Bill and Betty. *19th Century Medicine In Glass.* Eau Gallie, FL, 19th Century Hobby & Publishing Co., 1971.
9. Young, James Harvey. *The Toadstool Millionaires.* Princeton, New Jersey, Princeton University Press, 1961.

**Chapter 6 Cures**

1. Agee, Bill. *Collecting the Cures.* Waco, Texas, Texian Press, 1969.
2. Agee, Bill. *Collecting All Cures.* Waco, Texas, Texian Press, 1973.
3. Bingham, A. Walker. *The Snake Oil Syndrome.* Hanover, Mass., The Christopher Publishing House, 1994.
4. McEwen, Alan. *Collecting "Quack Cures."* West Yorkshire, England, Alan McEwen, 1977.
5. Stecher, Jack. *H.H. Warner–World Renowned Patent Medicine King–A Biographical Sketch.* Antique Bottle & Glass Collector. 18: (2) 34–38, 2001.
6. Wilson, Bill and Betty. *19th Century Medicine in Glass.* Eau Gallie, Florida, 19th Century Hobby and Publishing Co., 1971.
7. Wolf, John. Personal communication.

**Chapter 7 Teas**

1. Aikman, Lonnelle. *Nature's Healing Arts, From Folk Medicine to Modern Drugs.* Washington, D.C., The National Geographic Society, 1977.
2. Bingham, A. Walker. *The Snake Oil Syndrome*. Hanover, Mass., The Christopher Publishing House, 1994.
3. Edwards, Tamala M. *Tea Time Once Again*. Time, 154: 95, 1999.
4. Ketchum, Jr., William C. *A Treasury of American Bottles*. Indianapolis/New York, The Bobbs-Merrill Company, Inc., 1975.

**Chapter 8 Pills**

1. Devner, Kay. *At The Sign Of The Mortar.* Tucson, Arizona, The Tombstone Epitaph, 1970.
2. Richardson, Lillian C. and Charles G. *The Pill Rollers.* Harrisionburg, Virginia, Old Fort Press, 1992.
3. Young, James Harvey. *The Toadstool Millionaires.* Princeton, New Jersey, Princeton University Press, 1961.

**Chapter 9 Venereal Disease**

1. Bingham, A Walker. *The Snake Oil Syndrome.* Hanover, Mass., The Christopher Publishing House, 1994.
2. Cannon, Richard. *Swift's Syphilitic Specific and Billy Bowlegs.* Antique Bottle and Glass Collector. 9: (6) 48-49, 1992.
3. Carson, Gerald. *One For a Man, Two For a Horse.* New York, Bramhall House, 1961.
4. Herman, John R. *Urology—A View Through the Retrospectroscope.* Hagerstown, Maryland, Medical Department, Harper and Row Publishers, Inc., 1973.
5. Lyons, Albert S. and Petrucelli, II, R. Joseph. *Medicine, An Illustrated History.* Harry N. Abrans, Inc., Publishers, New York, 1978.
6. Wilson, Bill and Betty. *19th Century Medicine In Glass.* Eau Gallie, Fl, 19th Century Hobby & Publishing Co., 1971.
7. Young, James Harvey. *The Toadstool Millionaires.* Princeton, New Jersey, Princeton University Press, 1961.
8. Young, James Harvey. *The Medical Messiahs.* Princeton, New Jersey, Princeton University Press, 1967.

**Chapter 10 Virility Aids**

1. Bingham, A. Walker. *The Snake Oil Syndrome*. Hanover, Mass., The Christopher Publishing House, 1994.
2. Carson, Gerald. *One For a Man, Two For a Horse*. New York, Bramhall House, 1961.
3. Hechtlinger, Adelaide. *The Great Patent Medicine Era*. New York, Grosset and Dunlop, Inc., 1970.
4. Herman, John R. *Urology—A View Through the Retrospectroscope*. Hagerstown, Maryland, Medical Department, Harper and Row, Publishers, Inc. 1973.
5. Wilson, Bill and Betty. *19th Century Medicine In Glass.* Eau Gallie, Fl, 19th Century Hobby & Publishing Co., 1971.

**Chapter 11 Lithontriptics – Urinary Stone Dissolvers**

1. Bigelow, Henry J. *Rapid Lithotrity with Evacuation*. Boston, A. Williams Publisher, 1878.
2. Butt, Arthur J. *Treatment of Urinary Lithiasis*. Springfield, Illinois, Charles C. Thomas Publisher, 1960.
3. Cannon, Richard. *Vaughn's U.S.A. Hosp. Dept. and the Window.* Antique Bottle and Glass Collector, 15: (3) 14, 1998.
4. Haeger, Knut. *The Illustrated History of Surgery*. New York, Bell Publishing Co., 1988.
5. Herman, John R. *Urology*—A *View Through the Retrospectroscope*. Hagerstown, Maryland, Medical Department, Harper and Row Publishers, Inc., 1973.
6. Swerdlow, Joel L. *Nature's Medicine—Plants that Heal*. Washington, D.C., National Geographic, 2000.
7. Tolet, Francios. *Traité de la Lithotomie*. 4th Edition, Paris, 1693.

**Chapter 12 Mineral Spring Waters**

1. Devner, Kay. *At the Sign of the Mortar.* Tucson, Arizona, The Tombstone Epitaph, 1970.
2. Fountain, John C. and Colcleaser, Donald. *Dictionary of Soda and Mineral Water Bottles.* Sacramento, California, Ole Empty Bottle House Publishing Co., 1968.
3. Munsey, Cecil. *The Illustrated Guide to Collecting Bottles.* New York, Hawthorn Books, Inc., 1970.
4. Percival, Pamela. *The Thirst Quencher—The Sugar-Free, Calorie-Free Drink Is Sweeping the Nation.* Scripps Howard News Service, August 20, 1998.

**Chapter 13 H.H. Warner – The Rise and Fall**

1. Atwater, Edward C. *Hulbert Harrington Warner and the Perfect Pitch: Sold Hope; Made Millions.* New York History, 56: 1975, pp. 154-190.
2. Carson, Gerald. *One For Man, Two For a Horse*. New York, Bramhall House, 1961.
3. Kaidy, Mitchell. *Rochester's Medicine Man*. New York, Upstate, Mar. 29, 1981, pp. 21-25.
4. Seeliger, Michael W. *H.H. Warner, His Company and His Bottles*. Madison, Wisconsin, 1974.

5. Stecher, Jack. *H.H. Warner—World Renowned Patent Medicine King—A Biographical Sketch.* Antique Bottle and Glass Collector. 18: (2) 34-38, 2000.
6. Young, James Harvey. *The Toadstool Millionaires.* Princeton, Princeton University Press, 1961.

**Chapter 14 Swamproot, the Kidney Cure**

1. Bingham, A. Walker. *The Snake Oil Syndrome.* Hanover, Mass., The Christopher Publishing House, 1994.
2. Cannon, Richard. *Dr. Kilmer and Co.* Antique Bottle and Glass Collector. 3: (3) 50-55, 1986.
3. Carson, Gerald. *One For a Man, Two For a Horse.* New York, Bramhall House, 1961, p. 75.
4. Golley, John E. *The Kilmers of Binghamton, New York.* 14: (2) 6–9, 1997.
5. Hagenbuch, Jim. *Dr. Kilmer—Alive and Keeping People Well.* Antique Bottle and Glass Collector. 4: (2)14–20, 1987.
6. Ketchum, Jr., William C. *A Treasury of American Bottles.* Indianapolis/New York, The Bobbs-Merrill Company, Inc., 1975, p. 86.

**Chapter 15 Dr. Chase and his Recipe Book**

1. Hechtlinger, Adelaide. *The Great Patent Medicine Era.* New York, Grosset and Dunlop, Inc., 1970.
2. *Dr. A. W. Chase's Calendar–Almanac.* Buffalo, New York, Dr. A.W. Chase Medicine Co., 1909.
3. Massie, Larry. *Michigan Back When.* Press News Service, 1982.

**Chapter 16 Trade Cards**

1. Barry, Kit. *The Advertising Trade Card.* Monson, Mass., Blatchley's Printers, 1981.
2. Cheadle, Dave. *Victorian Trade Cards.* Paducah, Kentucky, Collector Books, 1996, pp. 5–13.
3. Jay, Robert. *The Trade Card in Nineteenth-Century America.* Columbia, Mo., University Press, 1987.
4. Rickards, Maurice. *Collecting Printed Ephemera.* New York, Abbeville Press, 1988.
5. Mascieri, Russell. *Trade Cards and Ephemera.* Marlton, New Jersey, Victorian Images, 1998.
6. Young, James Harvey. *The Toadstool Millionaires.* Princeton, New Jersey, Princeton University Press, 1961.

**Chapter 17 Almanacs**

1. Bingham, A. Walker. *The Snake Oil Syndrome.* Hanover, Mass., The Christopher Publishing House, 1994, pp. 125–128.
2. Hechtlinger, Adelaide. *The Great Patent Medicine Era.* New York, Grosset and Dunlop, Inc., 1970.
3. Ketcham, Steve. *Almanacs Are Timely Reminders of Days Gone By.* Bottles and Extras, 11: 12–14, 2000.
4. Sagendorph, Robb. *America and Her Almanacs.* Boston, Little Brown and Co., 1970.
5. Young, James Harvey. *The Toadstool Millionaires.* Princeton, New Jersey, Princeton University Press, 1961, p. 125–143.

**Chapter 18 Medicine Shows**

1. Bingham, A. Walker. *The Snake Oil Syndrome.* Hanover, Mass., The Christopher Publishing House, 1994.
2. Calhoun, Mary. *Medicine Show: Conning People And Making Them Like It.* New York, Hagerstown, San Francisco, London, Harper & Row Publishers, 1976.
3. Carson, Gerald. *One For a Man, Two For a Horse.* New York, Bramhill House, 1961.
4. Holbrook, Stewart H. *The Golden Age Of Quackery.* New York: The Macmillan Company, 1959.
5. Young, James Harvey. *The Toadstool Millionaires.* Princeton, New Jersey, Princeton University Press, 1961.

**Chinese Medicine**

1. Beinfield, H. and Korngold, E. *Between Heaven and Earth: A Guide to Chinese Medicine.* New York, Ballantine Books, 1992.
2. Haeger, K. *The Illustrated History of Surgery.* New York, Bell Publishing Co., 1988.
3. Hoizey, D. and Hoizey, M.J. *A History of Chinese Medicine.* Edinburgh, Edinburgh Univ. Press, 1993.
4. Pheric-Walton, L. and Murray, V. *Toxicity of Chinese Herbal Remedies.* Lancet 340: 673, 1992.
5. Swerdlow, J.L. *Nature's Medicine: Plants that Heal.* Washington, D.C., National Geographic, 2000.

**Chapter 19 What About Alternative Medicine?**

1. Ang-Lee, M.K., Moss, J., Yaun, C.-S. *Herbal Medicines and Perioperative Care.* JAMA, 286: 208, 2001.
2. Angell, M. and Kassirer, J. P. *Alternative Medicine—The Risks of Untested and Unregulated Remedies.* N Engl J Med, 339: 839, 1998.
3. Dietary Supplement Health and Education Act of 1994. (Public Law 103-417).
4. Eisenberg, D.M., Kessler, R.C., Foster, C. et al. *Unconventional Medicine in the United States—prevalence, costs and*

*patterns of use.* N Engl J Med, 328: 246, 1993.
5. Eisenberg, D.M., Davis, R.B., Ettner, S.L. et al. *Trends in Alternative Medicine Use in the United States, 1990-1997.* JAMA, 280: 1569, 1998.
6. Fontanarosa, P.B. *Alternative Medicine—An Objective Assessment.* Chicago, JAMA, Frankos Pub., 2000.
7. Love, L.A. *The Med Watch Program.* Clin Toxicol, 36: 263, 1998.
8. Peifer, A.H., Fleshner, N.E., Klotz, L. *Analytical accuracy and reliability of commonly used nutritional supplements in prostate disease.* J Urol, 168: 150-154, 2002.
9. Spiegel, D., Stroud, P., Fyke, A. *Complementary Medicine.* West J Med, 168: 241, 1998.
10. Swerdlow, J.L. *Nature's Medicine—Plants that Heal.* Washington, D.C., National Geographic, 2000.
11. Wittes, B. *FDA exemption sought for self-help medicines.* The Recorder. October 7, 1994: 2.

**Chapter 20 A Case In Point: Phytotherapy For Lower Urinary Tract Symptoms**

1. Eisenberg, D. M., Kessler, R.C., Foster, C. et al. *Unconventional medicine in the United States. Prevalence, costs, and patterns of use.* N Engl J Med, 328: 246, 1993.
2. Marwick, C. *Growing use of medicinal botanicals forces assessment by drug regulators.* JAMA, 273: 607, 1995.
3. Ernst, E. *Harmless herbs? A review of the recent literature.* AM J Med, 104: 170, 1998.
4. Wilt, T.J., Ishani, A. Stark, G. et al. *Saw palmetto extracts for treatment of benign prostatic hyperplasia: a systematic review.* JAMA, 280: 1604, 1998.
5. Int Med World Report 13: 8, 1998.
6. Lowe, F.C. and Fagelman, E. *Phytotherapy in the treatment of benign prostatic hyperplasia: an update.* Urology, 53: 671-677, 1999.
7. Buck, A.C. *Phytotherapy for the prostate.* Br J Urol, 78: 325, 1996.
8. Nickel, J.C. *Placebo therapy of benign prostatic hyperplasia: a 25-month study. Canadian Prospect Study Group.* Br J Urol, 81: 383, 1998.
9. Barry, M.J., Fowler, F.J., Jr., Bin, L. et al. *The natural history of patients with benign prostatic hypersplasia as diagnosed by North American Urologists.* J Urol, 157: 10, 1997.
10. Lowe, F.C. *Editorial Comment.* Urology, 51: 1007, 1998.
11. Angell, M. and Kassirer, J.P. *Alternative medicine—the risks of untested and unregulated remedies.* N Engl J Med, 339: 839, 1998.
12. Di Paola, R.S. Zhang, H., Lambert, G.H. et al. *Clinical and biologic activity of an estrogenic herbal combination (PC-SPES) in prostate cancer.* N Engl J Med, 339: 785, 1998.
13. Cui, J., Garle, M. Eneroth, P. et al. *What do commercial ginseng preparations contain?* Lancet, 344: 134, 1994.
14. Driekorn, K, Borkowski A. Broeckman, J. et al. *Other medical therapies:* Proceedings of the Fourth International Consultation on Benign Prostatic Hyperplesia, July 1997. Plymouth, UK, Health Publications, 1998, 635-659.
15. Chopin, D., Perier, A. and Raymond, J.P. *Improvements in benign prostatic hyperplasia (BPH) symptoms are not related to prostatic volume in the Permixon/finasteride comparative study.* Presented at the 4th International Consultation on BPH, Paris, France, 1997.
16. Broechman, J. *The extract of Serenon repens in the treatment of benign prostatic hyperplasia: a multicenter open study.* Curr Ther Res, 55: 776, 1994.
17. Descotes, J.L., Rambeaud, J.J., Deschaseaux, P. et al. *Placebo controlled evaluation of the efficacy and tolerability of Permixon in benign prostatic hyperplasia after exclusion of placebo responders.* Clin Drug Invest, 9: 291, 1995.
18. Gerber, G.S. *Saw palmetto for the treatment of men with lower urinary tract symptoms.* J. Urol, 163: 1408-1412, 2000.
19. Marks, L.S., Partin, A.W., Epstein, J.L., et al. *Effects of a saw palmetto herbal blend in men with symptomatic benign prostatic hyperplasia.* J Urol, 163:1451-1456, 2000.
20. Breza. J., Dzurny, O., Borowka, A. et al. *Efficacy and acceptability of Tadenan (Pygeum africanum extract) in the treatment of benign prostatic hyperplasia (BPH): a multicultural trial in Central Europe.* Curr Med Res Opin, 14: 127-139, 1998.
21. Dutkiewicz, S. *Usefulness of Cernilton in the treatment of benign prostatic hyperplasia.* Int Urol Nephrol, 28: 49-53, 1996.
22. Klippel, K.F., Hilti, D.M., and Schipp, B., for the German BPH—Phytotherapy Study Group. *A multicentric, placebo-controlled, double-blind clinical trial of beta-sitosteral (phytosterol) for the treatment of benign prostatic hypersplasia.* Br J Urol, 80: 427-432, 1997.

**Chapter 21 Today's FDA: Wounded Giant & Weakened Champion**

1. FDA. *Overview of the Food and Drug Administration.* Pub. No. BG 99-2, Jan. 11, 1999.
2. FDA. *Food and Drug Administration FY 2001 Congressional Budget Request.* Executive Summary, 2001.
3. FTC. *Enforcement Policy Statement of Food Advertising.* May, 1994.
4. FTC. Bureau of Consumer Protection. *Dietary Supplements: An Advertising Guide for Industry.* Nov., 2000.
5. Hutt, P.B. *A Historical Introduction.* 45 Food Drug Cosm. L.J. 17, 1990.
6. Hutt, P.B. *Essentials of Functional Foods.* Gaithersburg, M.D., Aspen Publishers, Inc., 2000.
7. Republished with permission of Dow Jones and Co., Inc., from *F.D.A. Isn't Holding Up In Court,* by Chris Adams, 2002: Permission conveyed through Copyright Clearance Center.

**Chapter 22 Conclusion "Quackery and Idolatry Are All But Immortal"**

1. Angell, M. and Kassirer, J.P. *Alternative Medicine—The Risks of Untested and Unregulated Remedies.* N Engl J Med, 339: 839, 1998.
2. Barrett, S. *The Health Robbers.* Philadelphia, PA., Geo. Stickley Co. Publishers, 1980.
3. Carroll, J. *Regulators Crack Down on Web's New Miracle Cure: Colloidal Silver.* Wall Street Journal, 238: June 14, 2001.
4. Forster, J. *Snake Oil On the Internet.* Medical Economics, 76 (18) September 20, 1999.
5. Hudson, R.P. *Immortal Quackery.* Medical Heritage, 1: 14, 1985.
6. Select Committee On Aging—House of Representatives. *Quackery—A $10 Billion Scandal.* Comm. Pub. No. 98-435, May, 1984.
7. Young, J.H. *The Toadstool Millionaires.* Princeton, New Jersey. Princeton University Press, 1961.
8. Young, J.H. *The Medical Messiahs.* Princeton, New Jersey, Princeton University Press, 1967.
9. Youngson, R.M. *Medical Curiosities and Mistakes.* Bath, UK, Parragon Book Publishing, 1999.

# Index

Numbers in ***bold italics*** refer to color images.

Numbers in ***bold italics*** refer to color images.

Numbers in ***bold italics*** refer to color images.

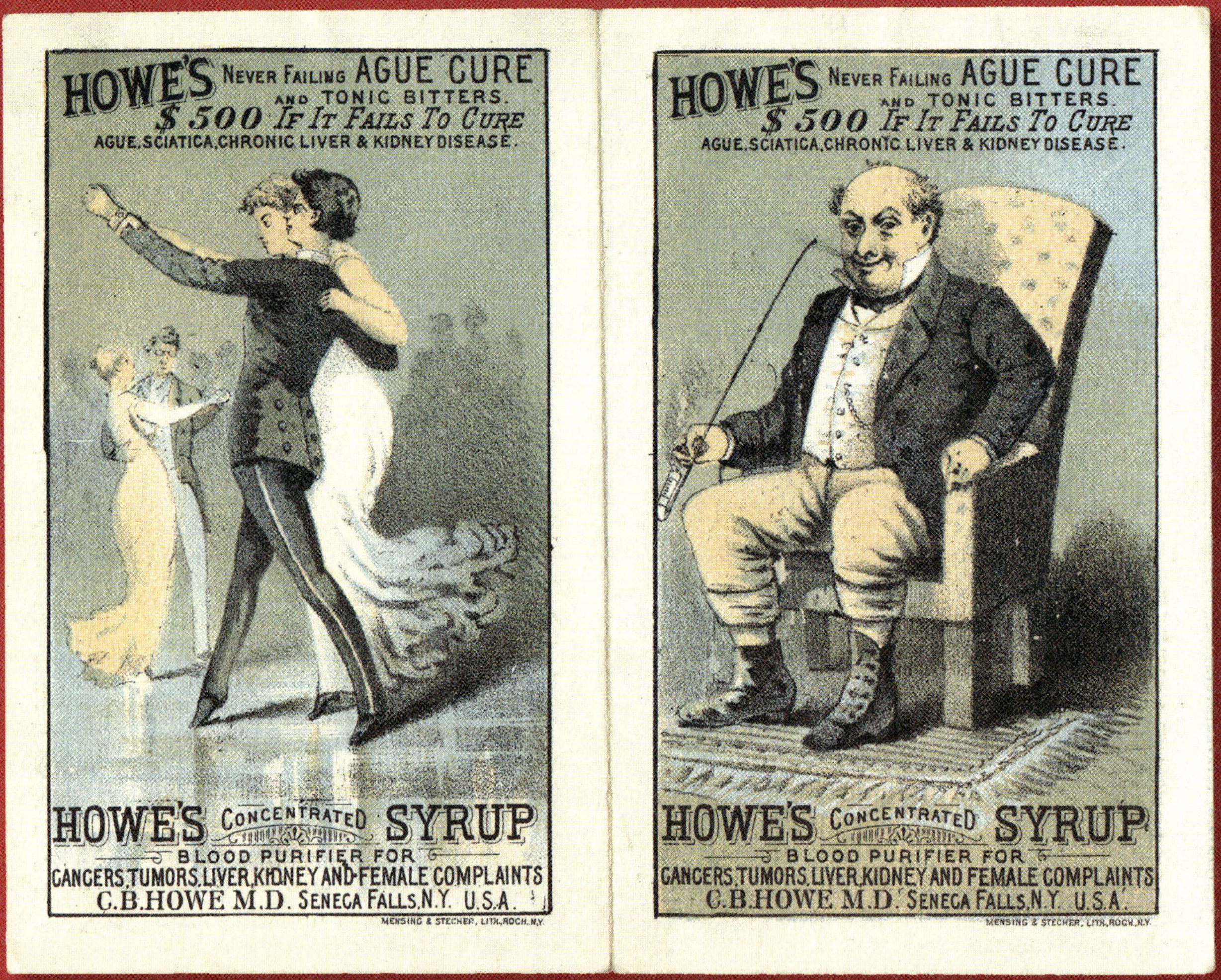
HOWE'S NEVER FAILING AGUE CURE AND TONIC BITTERS.
$500 IF IT FAILS TO CURE
AGUE, SCIATICA, CHRONIC LIVER & KIDNEY DISEASE.
HOWE'S CONCENTRATED SYRUP
BLOOD PURIFIER FOR
CANCERS, TUMORS, LIVER, KIDNEY AND FEMALE COMPLAINTS
C.B. HOWE M.D. SENECA FALLS, N.Y. U.S.A.
MENSING & STECHER, LITH. ROCH. N.Y.
HOWE'S NEVER FAILING AGUE CURE AND TONIC BITTERS.
$500 IF IT FAILS TO CURE
AGUE, SCIATICA, CHRONIC LIVER & KIDNEY DISEASE.
HOWE'S CONCENTRATED SYRUP
BLOOD PURIFIER FOR
CANCERS, TUMORS, LIVER, KIDNEY AND FEMALE COMPLAINTS
C.B. HOWE M.D. SENECA FALLS, N.Y. U.S.A.
MENSING & STECHER, LITH. ROCH. N.Y.